Neurotransmitter-Related Molecular Modeling Studies

Neurotransmitter-Related Molecular Modeling Studies

Editors

Alicja Nowaczyk
Grzegorz Grześk

MDPI • Basel • Beijing • Wuhan • Barcelona • Belgrade • Manchester • Tokyo • Cluj • Tianjin

Editors
Alicja Nowaczyk
Nicolaus Copernicus
University
Poland

Grzegorz Grześk
Nicolaus Copernicus
University
Poland

Editorial Office
MDPI
St. Alban-Anlage 66
4052 Basel, Switzerland

This is a reprint of articles from the Special Issue published online in the open access journal *Molecules* (ISSN 1420-3049) (available at: https://www.mdpi.com/journal/molecules/special_issues/Neurotransmitter_Molecular_Modeling).

For citation purposes, cite each article independently as indicated on the article page online and as indicated below:

LastName, A.A.; LastName, B.B.; LastName, C.C. Article Title. *Journal Name* **Year**, *Volume Number*, Page Range.

ISBN 978-3-0365-4277-5 (Hbk)
ISBN 978-3-0365-4278-2 (PDF)

Cover image courtesy of Łukasz Fijałkowski

Contents

About the Editors vii

Preface to "Neurotransmitter-Related Molecular Modeling Studies" ix

Magdalena Kowalska, Łukasz Fijałkowski, Monika Kubacka, Kinga Sałat, Grzegorz Grześk, Jacek Nowaczyk and Alicja Nowaczyk
Antiepileptic Drug Tiagabine Does Not Directly Target Key Cardiac Ion Channels Kv11.1, Nav1.5 and Cav1.2
Reprinted from: *Molecules* **2021**, *26*, 3522, doi:10.3390/molecules26123522 1

Aathira Sujathan Nair, Jong-Min Oh, Vishal Payyalot Koyiparambath, Sunil Kumar, Sachithra Thazhathuveedu Sudevan, Opeyemi Soremekun, Mahmoud E. Soliman, Ahmed Khames, Mohamed A. Abdelgawad, Leena K. Pappachen, Bijo Mathew and Hoon Kim
Development of Halogenated Pyrazolines as Selective Monoamine Oxidase-B Inhibitors: Deciphering via Molecular Dynamics Approach
Reprinted from: *Molecules* **2021**, *26*, 3264, doi:10.3390/molecules26113264 19

Robert Krysiak, Marcin Basiak and Bogusław Okopień
Cardiometabolic Risk Factors in Rosuvastatin-Treated Men with Mixed Dyslipidemia and Early-Onset Androgenic Alopecia
Reprinted from: *Molecules* **2021**, *26*, 2844, doi:10.3390/molecules26102844 37

Kinga Sałat and Anna Furgała-Wojas
Serotonergic Neurotransmission System Modulator, Vortioxetine, and Dopaminergic D_2/D_3 Receptor Agonist, Ropinirole, Attenuate Fibromyalgia-Like Symptoms in Mice
Reprinted from: *Molecules* **2021**, *26*, 2398, doi:10.3390/molecules26082398 47

Tomasz Guzel and Dagmara Mirowska-Guzel
The Role of Serotonin Neurotransmission in Gastrointestinal Tract and Pharmacotherapy
Reprinted from: *Molecules* **2022**, *27*, 1680, doi:10.3390/molecules27051680 65

Magdalena Hurkacz, Lukasz Dobrek and Anna Wiela-Hojeńska
Antibiotics and the Nervous System—Which Face of Antibiotic Therapy Is Real, Dr. Jekyll (Neurotoxicity) or Mr. Hyde (Neuroprotection)?
Reprinted from: *Molecules* **2021**, *26*, 7456, doi:10.3390/molecules26247456 81

Agnieszka Pawlos, Marlena Broncel, Ewelina Woźniak and Paulina Gorzelak-Pabiś
Neuroprotective Effect of SGLT2 Inhibitors
Reprinted from: *Molecules* **2021**, *26*, 7213, doi:10.3390/molecules26237213 105

Grzegorz Grześk and Alicja Nowaczyk
Current Modulation of Guanylate Cyclase Pathway Activity—Mechanism and Clinical Implications
Reprinted from: *Molecules* **2021**, *26*, 3418, doi:10.3390/molecules26113418 121

Michał Kosowski, Joanna Smolarczyk-Kosowska, Marcin Hachuła, Mateusz Maligłówka, Marcin Basiak, Grzegorz Machnik, Robert Pudlo and Bogusław Okopień
The Effects of Statins on Neurotransmission and Their Neuroprotective Role in Neurological and Psychiatric Disorders
Reprinted from: *Molecules* **2021**, *26*, 2838, doi:10.3390/molecules26102838 137

Anna Pierzchlińska, Magdalena Kwaśniak-Butowska, Jarosław Sławek, Marek Droździk and Monika Białecka
Arterial Blood Pressure Variability and Other Vascular Factors Contribution to the Cognitive Decline in Parkinson's Disease
Reprinted from: *Molecules* **2021**, *26*, 1523, doi:10.3390/molecules26061523 . . . . **157**

About the Editors

Alicja Nowaczyk

Alicja Nowaczy is an associate professor at Ludwik Rydygier Collegium Medicum in Bydgoszcz, Nicolaus Copernicus University in Toruń. As an academic teacher and science popularizer, she holds a postdoctoral degree in pharmaceutical sciences and a doctorate in chemical sciences. She is a member of the Pharmaceutical, Biomedical and Natural Products Analysis Team of the Analytical Chemistry Committee of the Polish Academy of Sciences, the Polish Pharmaceutical Society, and the Polish Chemical Society.

Her research focuses on medical and pharmaceutical sciences in the areas of pharmacometrics and molecular modeling. Her interests concern the predictive modeling of the detailed mechanisms of action and pharmacological efficacy of biologically active compounds in the areas of neuropharmacology, cardiovascular, and safety pharmacology as well as chemical reaction pathways. The following awards prove the importance and validity of her research: the Team Award of the Minister of Health of the Republic of Poland and a number of other awards, including the award of the Rector of the Nicolaus Copernicus University and the award of the Rector of the Medical University of Gdańsk. The research she conducts is interdisciplinary and is assumed to be carried out within larger research groups. Prof. Assoc. Nowaczyk actively cooperates with specialists from Poland, Germany, Denmark, and Spain.

Grzegorz Grześk

Grzegorz Grześk is a full professor at Ludwik Rydygier Collegium Medicum in Bydgoszcz, Nicolaus Copernicus University in Toruń. As a physician and university teacher, he combines theoretical and clinical sciences. He is a specialist in internal medicine, cardiology, and clinical pharmacology. He is the head of the Cardiology Clinic of the Jan Biziel University Hospital No. 2 and the provincial consultant in the two clinical areas of cardiology and clinical pharmacology.

He is also an experienced researcher, especially in the field of experimental pharmacology, including studies in animal models. His interests are particularly focused on issues related to cardiology and the function of blood vessels and vascular endothelium, including the role of the mediators and modulators of reactions affecting the molecular level. It is the primary investigator in numerous clinical and experimental studies. He is a board member of the Polish Society of Clinical Pharmacology as well as a member of the European Society of Cardiology and the Society of Polish Internists. The research he conducts combines molecular and clinical approaches with clinical pharmacology methods in a unique way.

Preface to "Neurotransmitter-Related Molecular Modeling Studies"

The year 2021 is the 100th anniversary of the confirmation of the neurotransmission phenomenon that was originally observed by Otto Loewi. For this reason, we have compiled some of what we consider to be the most interesting research reports and reviews in this field. The aim was to introduce the effects of experimental research into practical and clinical applications.

Neurotransmitters are chemicals that enable communication, i.e., the flow of nerve impulses between nerve cells or between nerve cells and muscles and glands. There are approximately 10^{11} nerve cells in a human brain, each of which can be connected to many other cells. In general, excitatory and inhibitory mediators have been distinguished, both of which are endogenous and exogenous compounds that control the function of the whole organism. Chemically, neurotransmitters belong to many different structural groups, such as amino acids (such as glycine), peptides (such as substance P, somatostatin), monoamines (such as noradrenaline or dopamine), purine derivatives (such as adenosine), gases (such as nitrogen, NO, carbon monoxide CO), and acetylcholine. From a medical point of view, disturbances in the concentration of neurotransmitters in the body mainly result in the occurrence of mood disorders and mental diseases. Thus, a sanguine personality type (sociable optimist) is a personality type that is mainly determined by dopamine. Serotonin mainly determines the temperament of a choleric person (vigorous chief), and acetylcholine implies the personality of a melancholic person (gifted analyst). On the other hand, the influence of the γ-ammino butyric acid determines the phlegmatic personality type (patient caregiver). For this reason, the deficit or excess of a specific neurotransmitter results in disturbances to the balanced mood of a person. Mental disorders such as depression, schizophrenia, and Parkinson's disease contribute to the occurrence of dementia (including Alzheimer's disease), among other disorders. However, the epidemiological problems are much wider. Neural conduction disorders can lead to many cardiovascular diseases and the development of vascular diseases of the brain as well as in many other organs. For example, the digestive system is the second largest cluster of neurons in our body—it has been estimated that it consists of at least 10^8 neuron cells. Enteric neurons are able to produce numerous neurotransmitters such as dopamine and serotonin. The neurons of the enteric nervous system are in regular contact with the microbes in the gut. In all respects, this communication system is very active. Many of the gut microbes produce the substances necessary for the proper functioning of the developing brain.

Year by year, pharmacological interventions try to influence regulatory processes. Such treatments improve survival, reduce the frequency of readmission, and improve patients' quality of life. We are deeply convinced that while 20 years ago, molecular research and its influence on therapeutic processes were the domain of the so-called researchers who only dealt with basic research, at present, knowledge, albeit basic, about the molecular basis of the effects of therapy allows for the better planning and personalization of therapy, which leads to greater effectiveness and a reduction in the number of side effects.

It is with great pleasure that we present readers with a book whose subject matter is very interesting for experienced and young researchers in the field of medical and health sciences: pharmacology and pharmacy and in the field of natural sciences: chemistry. We believe that the presented research results not only deserve the reader's attention but that they can also be helpful for further research development in the described area.

Alicja Nowaczyk and Grzegorz Grześk
Editors

molecules

Article

Antiepileptic Drug Tiagabine Does Not Directly Target Key Cardiac Ion Channels Kv11.1, Nav1.5 and Cav1.2

Magdalena Kowalska [1], Łukasz Fijałkowski [1], Monika Kubacka [2], Kinga Sałat [2], Grzegorz Grześk [3], Jacek Nowaczyk [4] and Alicja Nowaczyk [1,*]

1 Department of Organic Chemistry, Faculty of Pharmacy, Ludwik Rydygier Collegium Medicum in Bydgoszcz, Nicolaus Copernicus University in Toruń, 87-100 Toruń, Poland; magda.kowalska@doktorant.umk.pl (M.K.); l.fijalkowski@cm.umk.pl (Ł.F.)
2 Department of Pharmacodynamics, Chair of Pharmacodynamics, Jagiellonian University Medical College, 9 Medyczna St., 30-688 Krakow, Poland; monika.kubacka@uj.edu.pl (M.K.); kinga.salat@uj.edu.pl (K.S.)
3 Department of Cardiology and Clinical Pharmacology, Faculty of Health Sciences, Collegium Medicum in Bydgoszcz, Nicolaus Copernicus University, 75 Ujejskiego St., 85-168 Bydgoszcz, Poland; g.grzesk@cm.umk.pl
4 Physical Chemistry and Chemistry of Polymers, Faculty of Chemistry, Nicolaus Copernicus University, 7 Gagarina St., 87-100 Toruń, Poland; jacek.nowaczyk@umk.pl
* Correspondence: alicja@cm.umk.pl

Abstract: Tiagabine is an antiepileptic drug used for the treatment of partial seizures in humans. Recently, this drug has been found useful in several non-epileptic conditions, including anxiety, chronic pain and sleep disorders. Since tachycardia—an impairment of cardiac rhythm due to cardiac ion channel dysfunction—is one of the most commonly reported non-neurological adverse effects of this drug, in the present paper we have undertaken pharmacological and numerical studies to assess a potential cardiovascular risk associated with the use of tiagabine. A chemical interaction of tiagabine with a model of human voltage-gated ion channels (VGICs) is described using the molecular docking method. The obtained in silico results imply that the adverse effects reported so far in the clinical cardiological of tiagabine could not be directly attributed to its interactions with VGICs. This is also confirmed by the results from the isolated organ studies (i.e., calcium entry blocking properties test) and in vivo (electrocardiogram study) assays of the present research. It was found that tachycardia and other tiagabine-induced cardiac complications are not due to a direct effect of this drug on ventricular depolarization and repolarization.

Keywords: tiagabine; cardiac voltage-gated ion channels; molecular modeling; ECG study

Citation: Kowalska, M.; Fijałkowski, Ł.; Kubacka, M.; Sałat, K.; Grześk, G.; Nowaczyk, J.; Nowaczyk, A. Antiepileptic Drug Tiagabine Does Not Directly Target Key Cardiac Ion Channels Kv11.1, Nav1.5 and Cav1.2. *Molecules* **2021**, *26*, 3522. https://doi.org/10.3390/molecules26123522

Academic Editor: Diego Muñoz-Torrero

Received: 22 April 2021
Accepted: 8 June 2021
Published: 9 June 2021

1. Introduction

Epidemiological studies have consistently shown that people with epilepsy have a higher prevalence of structural cardiac disease than those without it [1]. The functioning of neurons, muscles and cardiac myocytes is based on action potentials (APs) generated by transmutational ion currents mediated mainly by sodium, calcium and potassium [2,3]. According to the guidelines of the Comprehensive in vitro Proarrhythmia Assay (CiPA), a set of six ion channels has been selected for which currents are important for both the repolarization and depolarization of the cardiac action potential (AP) [4]. There is some evidence, based on the effect of clinical drugs on cardiac APs, indicating the classification of cardiac ion channels into two classes [5–7]. The first class contains the most important cardiac ion channels, such as $K_V11.1$, $Na_V1.5$ and $Ca_V1.2$. The second class comprises $K_V4.3$, K_VLQT1/mink and Kir2.1 and is less critical for the assessment of all drugs under CiPA [7–9].

A common feature of both neurological disorders (e.g., epilepsy and chronic pain) and cardiac dysrhythmias is cell (neuronal cell and cardiac myocyte, respectively) hyperexcitability [2]. Therefore, drugs affecting cell excitability threshold within the nervous tissue can also interact with cardiac cell APs and vice versa [10–12]. It has to be emphasized that this drug-induced effect might sometimes be harmful as it may lead to the occurrence of additional alterations in neuronal or cardiac cell reactivity, thus being a cause for additional drug-induced (iatrogenic) complications. From the safety pharmacology point of view, it is of key importance to recognize these potential risk factors as early as possible. The cardiac VGICs assay is an indispensable step and a high-quality assay must accompany any investigational new drug application. The in silico studies of drug binding to K_V11.1, Na_V1.5 and Ca_V1.2 may be valuable assays for drugs and drug candidates at present [13].

Currently, several antiepileptic drugs were reported to have cardiotoxic and metabolic adverse effects [1,14]. Tiagabine (TGB) is an anticonvulsant drug used to treat partial seizures in humans. Recent results of clinical trials and animal studies indicate that it might be also effective in patients suffering from pain, insomnia or mood disorders and these activities are attributed to its inhibitory effect on GABA uptake [15,16]. TGB is a 96% protein-bound molecule [17]. The drug is a potent inhibitor of [3H]GABA uptake into synaptosomal membranes (IC_{50} = 67 nM) or neurons (IC_{50} = 446 nM) and glial cells (IC_{50} = 182 nM) in primary cell cultures. The in vivo tests have shown that TGB neuronal inhibiting is 2.5-fold more potent than glial GABA uptake [18–20]. The enhancement of GABA neurotransmission due to GABA transporter subtype 1 (GAT-1) inhibition might also explain most of adverse effects of TGB, including drowsiness, confusion and dizziness [18,21]. However, some other TGB-induced complications do not to be directly related to its influence on GABA concentration in the brain and other tissues.

Several recent reports have demonstrated that tachycardia is observed in about 1.0% of patients treated with TGB [18,22] but the mechanisms underlying this cardiotoxic effect are not known. In the literature there is a limited amount of data regarding the influence of TGB on cardiovascular functions and metabolism [23].

Since tachycardia is most frequently caused by impaired ion channel functions [24–27], in the in silico part of the present study a detailed analysis of the interactions between the human K_V11.1, Na_V1.5, Ca_V1.2 and TGB was performed. In order to compare the strength of TGB's binding to individual ion channels terfenadine (TEF) [28], batrachotoxin (BTX) [29,30] and nifedipine (NFD) [31] were selected as compounds strongly affecting these molecular targets.

In the course of present study, in vivo tests in rats were performed. The in vivo assay comprised the assessment of TGB's proarrhythmic potential and its effects on ECG components were studied; i.e., we conducted in vivo evaluation of TGB to assess its influence on PQ, QRS, QT and QTc intervals. Its effect on heart rate was also investigated. The relevant changes in PQ, QRS, QT and QTc intervals were interpreted as the effect of the test drug predominantly on Na_v, K_v and Ca_v channels. In contrast, the changes in heart rate were treated as a measure of the effect of the test compound, particularly, on the Nav1.5 channel or autonomic system function. Calcium blocking properties of TGB were tested in the isolated rat aorta contracted with depolarizing KCl solution.

2. Results

2.1. *Pharmacological Part*

2.1.1. The Effect on Normal Electrocardiogram

In vivo ECG study showed that TGB marked no significant effect on PQ, QRS, QT and QTc intervals. TGB also did not influence the heart rate significantly. It decreased the heart rhythm maximally at 30 min (by 6.9%) but this result did not reach statistical significance (Table 1). What is most important to note is that TGB at a dose as high as 100 mg/kg *i.p* did not prolong QT interval, which suggests that it did not prolong cardiac repolarization and probably did not block I_{KR} currents. Similar observations have also been made in the published studies [32,33]. We also did not observe the prolongation of PQ interval and QRS widening, which reflects the slowed conduction and disturbances in ventricular depolarization, usually due to the I_{Na} block. This is in line with the results obtained and presented here from molecular docking studies, where we found that TGB did not bind to cardiac voltage-gated ion channels K_V11.1 (hERG) and Na_V1.5.

Table 1. Effects of TGB (100 mg/kg *i.p.*) on the heart rate and ECG intervals in anesthetized rat (thiopental 75 mg/kg *i.p.*).

Parameters	Time of Observation (min)							
	0	5	10	20	30	40	50	60
Beats/min	288.0 ± 5.4	275.6 ± 7.6	274.2 ± 7.7	269.5 ± 6.6	268.1 ± 3.0	276.7 ± 4.7	283.7 ± 7.0	289.5 ± 11.3
PQ (ms)	52.6 ± 2.0	56.2 ± 2.0	56.8 ± 2.1	56.6 ± 18	57.2 ± 1.3	55.2 ± 2.2	57.2 ± 1.2	56.8 ± 1.3
QRS (ms)	19.2 ± 0.5	18.4 ± 1.1	19.8 ± 0.9	19.4 ± 0.6	19.4 ± 0.9	19.8 ± 0.5	19.6 ± 0.4	19.0 ± 0.9
QT (ms)	61.0 ± 1.0	60.6 ± 0.4	62.6 ± 1.9	62.8 ± 1.8	60.8 ± 0.8	63.6 ± 1.8	61.2 ± 0.8	61.6 ± 0.9
QTc (ms)	113.8 ± 3.0	115.6 ± 1.5	119.9 ±5.6	121.1 ±3.8	117.4 ± 2.0	121.0 ± 3.8	115.0 ± 2.0	114.8± 3.0

The data are the means of five experiments ± S.E.M. Statistical analysis: one-way analysis of variance (ANOVA) with repeated measurements and followed by Dunnett's post hoc test.

2.1.2. Voltage-Dependent Calcium Channels

During the course of our study, we investigated the calcium entry blocking properties of TGB in vasculature by employing the isolated rat aorta contracted with depolarizing KCl solution. In this experiment, the KCl-induced contraction was caused by an increase in extracellular potassium that leaded to membrane depolarization, which increases calcium influx from extracellular sources involving voltage-dependent calcium channels [34] (Ca_V1.2). The reference compounds we used were verapamil [35] and NFD [36]. TGB was not able to relax KCl-precontracted aortic rings at the range of concentration 1–30 μM (Figure 1). At a higher concentration, TGB was not tested as it precipitated in Krebs–Henseleit solution. NFD, verapamil and voltage-dependent calcium channel blockers relaxed KCl (60 mmol/L)-precontracted aortic rings in a dose-dependent manner (Figure 1) by 95–97%, with the IC_{50} values of 4.7 ± 0.2 nM and 32.9 ± 7.4 nM, respectively [35,36]. On the basis of these results, we may state that TGB does not possess voltage-dependent calcium channel blocking properties at the tested range of concentrations.

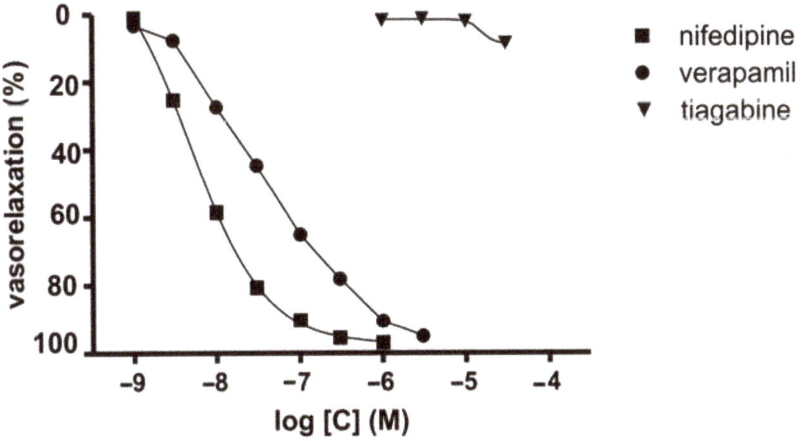

Figure 1. Inhibitory potencies of TGB and reference drugs (NFD and verapamil) on sustained contraction of aortic rings induced by KCl (60 mM).

2.2. *Molecular Docking Studies*

2.2.1. Terfenadine

TEF is (RS)-1-(4-tert-butylphenyl)-4-{4-[hydroxy(diphenyl)methyl]piperidin-1-yl}-butan-1-ol and, from a chemical point of view, belongs to piperidine derivatives (Figure 2).

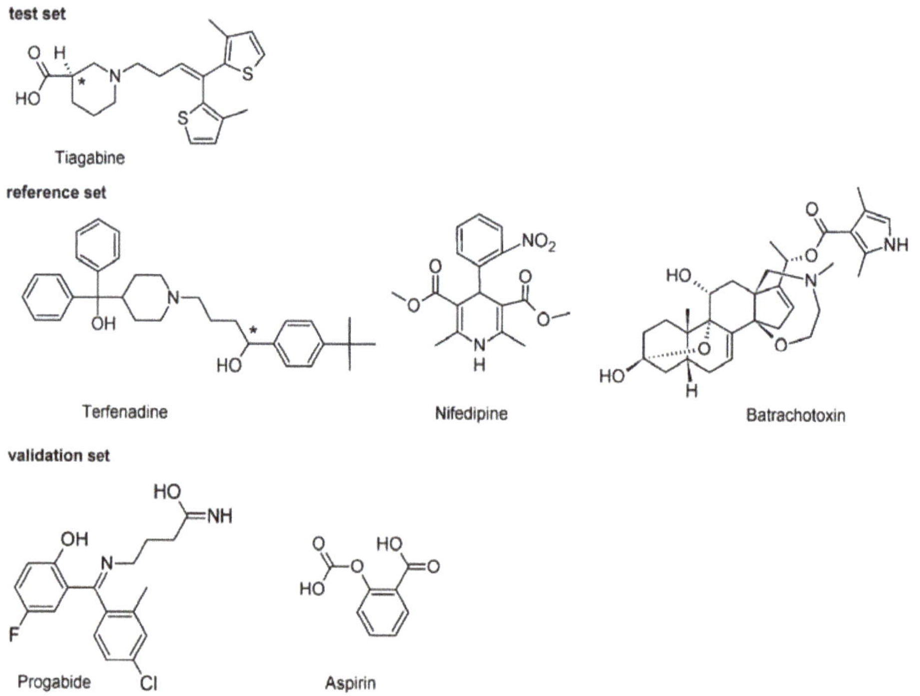

Figure 2. Chemical structure of the investigated compounds. Carbons at a tetrahedral stereogenic center are distinguished by *.

The obtained results from molecular docking confirmed the strongest blocking effects of TEF on the $hK_v11.1$ channel. R-TEF-$hK_v11.1$ is the most stable complex in the studied set. Comparison of the data (such as E_B and pK_i, Table 2) obtained for R-TEF and S-TEF complexes leads to the conclusion that there are significant stereoselective differences in the potential interaction for all studied channels. Docking experimentation predicted more effective potential interactions of all studied channels and S-TEF than its counterpart R-TEF (Table 2). Nevertheless, all calculated h-bonds formed are weak interactions. Moreover, obtained data suggests that R/S-TEF displays non inhibitory effects for $hCa_v1.2$. According to data in Table 2, pKi < 3.5, while by convention $pK_i \leq 4$ indicates the lack of a biological effect. Based on the CiPA studies, including the examination of the effect of 30 clinical drugs on the 7-ion channel [7], it can be concluded that the risk level of torsade de pointes (TdP) is correlated with the blocking effects of $hK_v11.1$, $hNa_v1.5$ and $hCa_v1.2$. Crumb et al. [7,37] in their research proposed a classification of drugs into three categories of TdP entry risk (high, medium and low). According to their studies, drugs belonging to the high and medium risk stand out with block hERG to a much greater extent than any other tested currents. The drugs belonging to the low risk category is distinct with the non-specific blocking of $hK_v11.1$, $hNa_v1.5$ and $hCa_v1.2$ channels (Figure S1). These results clearly indicate the need for testing drug candidates on the ion channel panel. In our study it was found, on the molecular level, that the high risk of TdP is a result of TEF's strong blocking effects on hERG. R-TEF-$hK_v11.1$ complex has one normal h-bond in which the hydroxyl group of the (4-tert-butylphenyl)methanol moieties of R-TEF donates energetically weak (−3.62 kcal/mol), short (2.12 Å) and almost linear interactions (158°) to Tyr652 (Figure S2). Regarding the interaction of R-TEF and S-TEF with the $hNa_v1.5$ channel, it should be noted that both enantiomers of TEF practically strongly interact with this protein ($pK_i > 5$, Table 2), which also indicates their arrhythmogenic effects through the $hNa_v1.5$. This observation is also confirmed by previously presented pharmacological studies [38].

Table 2. The summary of $hNa_v1.5$, $hCa_v1.2$ and $hK_v11.1$ (hERG) channel docking experiment results.

Complex		E_B	pK_i	Amino Acid Residues	H_B		Angle	L_{HB}	E_{HB}
Protein	Ligand	kcal/mol			donor	acc	θ	Å	kcal/mol
$hNa_v1.5$	R-TGB	−5.01	3.74	ASN927	#$CONH_2$	%COO	153.33	2.17	−3.38
	S-TGB	−5.21	3.82	ASN927	#$CONH_2$	%COO	171.54	2.23	−4.05
	NFD	−7.00	5.13	LEU409	%NOH	#CONH	146.945	1.987	−0.07
	R-TEF	−6,83	5.01		none				
	S-TEF	−7.45	5.46	LEU409	%OH	#CONH	163.079	2.014	−1.00
				GLU417	%OH	#COO	129.495	2.178	−0.04
	BTX	−9.01	6.68	SER1458	%NH	#CONH	156.904	2.179	−3.43
$hCa_v1.2$	R-TGB	−5.05	3.70	THR1056	%NH	#OH	168.494	1.868	−7.33
				SER1132	#OH	%COO	176.604	2.116	−5.54
	S-TGB	−4.77	3.50	THR1056	%NH	#OH	150.676	2.155	−4.06
				SER1132	#OH	%COO	137.882	2.092	−0.01
	NFD	−10.71	7.85	THR1462	%NOH	#CONH	124.62	1.68	−3.13
				TYR1508	#PhOH	%NOH	141.07	1.92	−3.84
	R-TEF	−4.16	3.05	THR1133	%OH	#CONH	137.428	2.021	−0.35
	S-TEF	−4.75	3.48	ALA1174	%OH	#CONH	128.006	1.901	−0.35
	BTX	−7.17	5.25	GLN1060	%OH	#CONH2	157.582	1.691	−0.37
				SER1132	#OH	%OH	141.666	2.221	−3.23
				MET1178	%NH-pyrrole	#CONH	156.864	2.028	−4.51
$hK_v11.1$	R-TGB	−5.4	3.32	none					
	S-TGB	−5.2	3.14	TYR652	%NH	#CONH	136.087	1.97	−2.86
				SER660	#OH	%COO	128.896	2.145	−0.04
	NFD	−4.42	3.24	ASN658	#$CONH_2$	%NO	174.448	1.849	−7.63
	R-TEF	−8.4	6.27	TYR652	%OH	#PhOH	158.395	2.121	−3.63
	S-TEF	−8.4	6,56	none					
	BTX	−6.75	4.95	PHE551	%OH	#CONH	171.728	1.933	−0.28
				THR623			140.298	1.933	−2.24

Abbreviations in Table. Components of the investigated complexes: protein-hNav1.5, hCav1.2 and $hK_v11.1$ (hERG); and ligands, R/S-TGB (R/S-tiagabine), NFD (nifedipine), R/S-TEF (R/S-terfenadine), BTX (batrachotoxin). Other abbreviations: H_B—hydrogen bond. acc—hydrogen bond acceptor. Hydrogen bond components: from the ligand % and from the protein #. E_B—complex energy binding. θ—hydrogen bond angle. L_{HB}—hydrogen bond length. E_{HB}—hydrogen bond energy. pK_i was calculated from the AutoDock4 and estimated inhibition constant K_i, which is reported in the AutoDock4 output.

2.2.2. Nifedipine

NFD is a 3,5-dimethyl 2.6-dimethyl-4-(2-nitrophenyl)-1.4-dihydropyridine-3,5-dicarboxylate (Figure 2). It is classified as a dihydropyridine subclass compound. It is a highly apolar photosensitive compound. The NFD docking experiment revealed that this molecule can interact with an active site of all the studied proteins (Table 2). It can be set to the following descending order of binding energies $E_{B(NFD\text{-}hKv11.1)} \approx -4.42$, $E_{B(NFD\text{-}hNav1.5)} \approx -7.00$ and $E_{B(NFD\text{-}hCav1.2)} \approx -10.71$ kcal/mol, respectively. The binding energies obtained in the docking experiment show that NFD forms a more stable complex in the case of the $hCa_v1.2$ channel. The in silico data obtained for blocking of

$hCa_v1.2$ channel (pK_i = 7.85) are in line with data in the literature (pIC_{50} = 7.48) [35] and (pK_i = 7.66) [39]. Based on the predicted binding affinity, the highest affinity was observed with the $hCa_v1.2$ and NFD in all cases of studied channels. Additionally, the blocking effect of NFD with $hNa_v1.5$ was also proven (Table 2). It has to be highlighted that in NFD-$hNa_v1.5$ and NFD-$hK_v11.1$ complexes, NFD interacts via one normal h-bond. In contrast, the complex NFD-$hCa_v1.2$ shows two h-bonds, both of which are short (≈1.68 Å) and strong (≈−3.8 kcal/mol) (Table 2.). The assessment of the data obtained for the hydrogen bonds clearly leads to the conclusion that they all have incomparable energies and bond lengths. Interestingly, NFD forms the strongest h-bond with $hK_v11.1$ and the weakest one with $hNa_v1.5$ channel (Table 2. Figure S2). The h-bond with $hCa_v1.2$ is characterized by an indirect force of influence. However, taking into account the data from Table 2, there is no correlation between the binding affinities of NFD and h-bond energy. The obtained distribution of estimated pK_i measure shows that in case of the $hK_v11.1$ channel, NFD has no inhibitory effect for this channel (pK_i < 4. Table 2). These data prove that NFD has potency only in inhibiting the $hCa_v1.2$ and $hNa_v1.5$ channel, which is in agreement with the pharmacological data previously presented in pharmacological literature [40].

2.2.3. Batrachotoxin

BTX as a steroidal alkaloid belongs to class A channel opening toxins [41]. Its molecule contains an oxazepane ring with tertiary amine and an aromatic pyrrole ring connected to the rigid polycyclic steroidal core via the ester group (Figure 2). Its 3D structure adopts a horseshoe conformation [42,43]. The outer surface of the horseshoe is hydrophobic, while the inner one is rather hydrophilic and forms the oxygen triad (at C3, C9 and C11) [44,45]. The outer surface of the horseshoe is hydrophobic, while the inner one is rather hydrophilic and forms oxygen triad (at C3, C9 and C11) [44]. It was suggested in the literature that this oxygen triad forms a hydrophilic arc, which can be regarded as a chelating site attracting some cations [46]. In the preliminary analysis of the docking, it was observed that BTX interacts with the active site of all studied proteins (Figure S2). The achieved data demonstrated that $Na_v1.5$ forms one h-bond, while $hCa_v1.2$ and $hK_v11.1$ form two h-bonds. The energies obtained in the present in silico experiment show that $hCa_v1.2$ and $hK_v11.1$ form more and form stronger hydrogen bonds than the remaining one ($hNa_v1.5$). The predicted binding affinity can be arranged in the following increasing order: $hK_v11.1 < hCa_v1.2 < hNa_v1.5$ (Table 2). Obtained results revealed that BTX-$hNa_v1.5$ is an energetically more stable complex with a binding energy of −9.01 kcal/mol. The stability of the complex with the $hCa_v1.2$ and $hK_v11.1$ is slightly lower than that with $hNa_v1.5$ (i.e., $E_{B\ BTX\text{-}hCav1.2}$ = −7.17 and $E_{B\ BTX\text{-}hKv11.1}$ = −6.75 kcal/mol, respectively). The calculated BTX affinity value of pKi = 6.68 is consistent with the relevant inhibitory potential data known from the specialized literature (pIC_{50} = 6.71) [47]. The BTX-$hNa_v1.5$ complex is formed via a single key interaction with residues of $hNa_v1.5$. The hydroxyl group at position C-11 of the steroid skeleton donates one h-bond to the sulfur atom of Ser1458. This interaction is non-linear (157°) and with weak energy, i.e., −3.43 kcal/mol and a small bond length equal to 2.18 Å. This is in line with the literature data according to which the atom included in oxygen triad is responsible for the toxic interaction of BTX with its molecular target [44]. We can treat these data as a strong argument proving that BTX acts on the cytoplasmic side of the channel just as other Class A neurotoxic compounds do, as it is shown in Figure S2.

For $hCa_v1.2$ and $hK_v11.1$ channels, BTX has pK_i ≈ 5.2, which suggests comparable blocking effects. The BTX-$hCa_v1.2$ complex is a more energetically stable form than the BTX-$hNa_v1.5$ complex (Table 2). This complex has one normal h-bond. In the bifurcated h-bond, the major component is Ser1132 and the minor component is Gln1060; the associated energies are weak (E_{HB} = −0.37 kcal/mol and −3.23 kcal/mol, respectively). The distances of the hydrogen bonds lay in the range from 1.69 to 2.22 Å and, due to this, the three-centered hydrogen bond is highly not symmetric. In the case of BTX-$hCa_v1.2$ complex, it is formed via one normal h-bond interaction (Table 2).

2.2.4. Tiagabine

As it can be seen from the data collected in Table 2, TGB complexes between $hNa_v1.5$, $hCa_v1.2$ and $hK_v11.1$ have a calculated $pK_i \leq 4$, which is commonly used as a threshold and this drug can thus be considered as an inactive ligand for those proteins. These data refer to both R/S enantiomers of TGB (Figure 3). Docking TGB into the $hNa_v1.5$ channel showed the highest pK_i value in Table 2, however, the value is still below the activity threshold level of $pK_i > 4$. The lowest pK_i was observed for $hK_v11.1$. We can treat these data as a partial explanation of the reported adverse TGB interactions in the cardiovascular system. It also seems that a small percentage of the observed cardiac disorders can be attributed to the fact that TGB does not interact with hKv11.1, for which inhibition is responsible for QT_c prolongation. In all analyzed cases, R-TGB shows slightly higher binding affinities than S-TGB. This observation is in line with many previous pharmacological studies indicating the greater biological activity of R enantiomers compared to the S ones [10–12]. It is also worth emphasizing that all h-bonds formed between $hCa_v1.2$ channels and R/S-TGB possess very favorable key interaction energy values ($E_{HB} \approx -7.32$ for $hCa_v1.2$-R-TGB and -5.54 kcal/mol for $hCa_v1.2$-S-TGB, Table 2) and geometrically nonlinear systems.

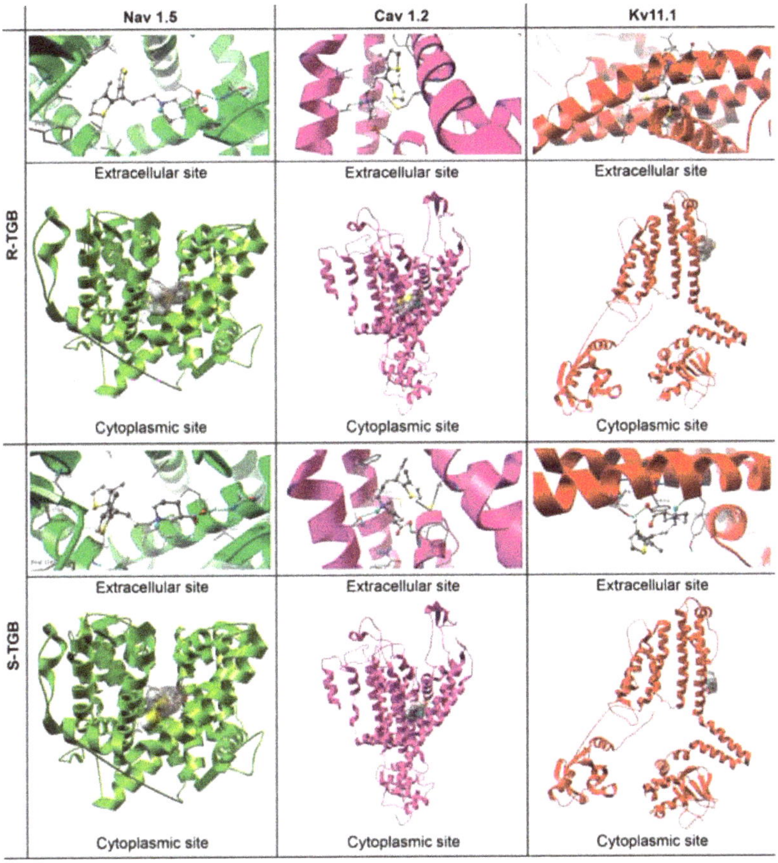

Figure 3. Pocket locations and binding modes of (R/S)-Tiagabine (R/S-TGB) and the investigated channels: hNav1.5, hCav1.2 and hKv11.1. Ligands (ball and stick model) and calculated hydrogen bonds (dashed green lines).

To sum up, the docking experiment revealed that R/S-TGB has lower intermolecular forces with all studied ion channels ($E_B \approx -5.30$ kcal/mol, Table 2). The combination of the above-mentioned docking data with pharmacological as well as literature data regarding the risk for tachycardia due to TGB administration suggests that this adverse effect observed in humans is not likely to result from TGB interaction with molecular anti-targets (i.e., ion channels tested in this study) used for the cardiac risk assessment. The data obtained in this study allowed the supplementation of information on the impact of TGB on other than GAT-1 molecular targets. As is currently known, TGB has no significant affinity to other uptake systems, such as those for dopamine, noradrenaline, acetylcholine, adenosine, serotonin, histamine, opiate, glycine, glutamate or GABA [48,49]. It only has a weak affinity towards benzodiazepine receptors and does not affect K^+ and Ca^{2+}, while it slightly affects Na^+ and cardiovascular channel function [19].

2.3. Validation Experiment

The validation was carried out by the docking of molecules with no affinity to $hNa_v1.5$, $hCa_v1.2$ and $hK_v11.1$ channels, such as progabide (PRG) [50,51] and acetylsalicylic acid (ASA) [52]. This choice of PRG and ASA was made based on their chemical and biological similarity to TGB (ATC code: N03AG06 [53]). PRG (ATC code: N03AG05 [53]) is a first-generation antiepileptic drug without analgesic properties [12,54]. ASA (ATC code: N02BA01 [52]) is a classical and peripherally-acting nonsteroidal anti-inflammatory drug that is inactive at GAT and recommended for the prevention of several cardiovascular diseases due to its antiplatelet activity [52].

The results of the validation experiments, such as the complex binding energies, the specific hydrogen bond components and detailed data of the hydrogen bond features (energies, lengths and angles) are gathered in Table 3. The binding modes between $hNa_v1.5$, $hCa_v1.2$ and $hK_v11.1$; and the control compound are illustrated in Figure S3 in the supplementary file. As it can be observed from the data, all control complexes have a calculated $pK_i < 4$, which is commonly used as the threshold and therefore the test compounds can be considered to be inactive ligands for those proteins. In addition, all control complexes have higher binding energy values and lower hydrogen bond energy than the TGB-hVGICs complex.

Table 3. The summary of validation experiment results.

Complex		E_B	pKi	Amino Acid Residues	H_B		Angle	L_{HB}	E_{HB}
Protein	Ligand				donor	acc	θ	Å	kcal/mol
$hNa_v1.5$	PRG	−3.90	2.86	ASP945	%CONH1	#COO	157.949	1.998	−5.425
				ASN1474	%CONH2	#CO	155.21	2.00	−5.04
				ASN1474	#NH2	%CO	141.795	1.987	−2.731
	ASA	−3.29	2.41	LYS1477	#NH1	%CO	159.455	1.905	−2.071
				LYS1477	#NH2	%COO	157.938	1.737	−0.015
$hCa_v1.2$	PRG	−3.29	2.41	THR1056	%OH	#OH	163.88	1.99	−4.82
				SER1132	#OH	%CONH	156.74	1.94	−3.02
	ASA	−2.41	1.77	THR1056	#OH	%COO	159.14	1.84	−2.30
				SER1132	#OH	%CO	176.21	1.945	−6.00
$hK_v11.1$	PRG	−3.4	2.50	TYR652	%CONH2	#PhOH	139.884	1.902	−2.015
				TYR652	%NH	#PhOH	139.121	2.182	−1.695
				SER660	%OH	#OH	170.052	2.129	−0.893
	ASA	−3.26	2.39	ASN658	#CONH2	%COO	167.92	1.78	−7.29

Abbreviations in Table. Components of the investigated complexes: protein-hNav1.5, hCav1.2 and hKv11.1 (hERG); and ligands, ASA—acetylsalicylic acid, PRG—Progabide. Other abbreviations: H_B—hydrogen bond. acc—hydrogen bond acceptor. Hydrogen bond components: from the ligand % and from the protein #. E_B—complex energy binding. θ—hydrogen bond angle. L_{HB}—hydrogen bond length. E_{HB}—hydrogen bond energy. pKi was calculated from the AutoDock4 and estimated inhibition constant K_i, which is reported in the AutoDock4 output [55].

3. Discussion

Taking into consideration the new action profile of drugs already on the market, pharmacological safety is a particularly important issue. The main reason for this is the fact that for drugs with an extended therapeutic range (i.e., repurposed medications), the number of patients for whom a given drug is recommended will increase significantly. TGB discussed in this study belongs to this group of drugs. TGB is an anticonvulsant medication. It is also used in the treatment of anxiety-related disorders, as are a few other anticonvulsants [21]. In the case of this drug, the above mentioned point is particularly important because TGB was originally prescribed to a relatively small group of patients due to its narrow range of indicators (adjunctive treatment of partial seizures in adults and children 12 years of age and older) [56]. However, when we consider its analgesic and anxiolytic effects in our considerations, we include therapeutic indications for a significantly larger group of patients. Reports presented in the scientific literature indicate an approximate 70% increase in the number of patients on TGB therapy [57]. This is all the more important as the safety and efficacy of TGB have not been systematically evaluated for indications other than epilepsy.

Modern technology provides us with many different possibilities, the use of which should create the conditions to learn about safety pharmacology. Undoubtedly, in silico research is one of many possibilities for seeking answers in this regard. It seems to us that the research presented above makes some important contributions to this issue. The study tried to answer the question about the cardiovascular safety assessment of TGB. This is all the more important in the light of the recent expert discussions focused on extending the pharmacological profile of TBG. Many modern studies indicate that, in addition to the therapeutic use of TGB in epilepsy, we should strongly consider its utilization for non-epileptic indications. On the other hand, it is known that drugs that show this type of biological activity might have a strong effect on a heart. This, in turn, undoubtedly forces us to increase the effort focused on assessing cardiac safety. Considering the assessment of the effect of the compound on so-called anti-targets adopted from CiPA in the cardiac risk assessment, the TGB interaction was investigated with the following channels: $hK_V11.1$, $hNa_V1.5$ and $hCa_V1.2$. Drugs strongly affecting individual channels (such as TEF, BTX and NFD) were selected as reference compounds for this study. TEF is a prodrug metabolized by intestinal CYP3A4 to fexofenadine, the active form being a selective histamine H1-receptor antagonist with antihistaminic and non-sedative effects. As it is well known, antihistamines may increase the rate of heart beat [58,59]. TEF causes prolonged repolarization, as is reflected in the broadening of the electrocardiographic QT interval, with the potential for serious ventricular arrhythmia and death [60–62]. Due to this, in the U.S. TEF was superseded by its active metabolite fexofenadine in the 1990s [59]. Numerous studies have proven that the ability of TEF to extend the QT interval depends on its binding to the Kv11.1 (Figure S1) protein encoded by hERG [63,64]. Nevertheless, TEF does not readily cross the blood–brain barrier and due to this its CNS, depression is minimal. NFD is a calcium channel blocker, a specific antagonist of Cav1.2 channels [65]. It is used to treat hypertension and chronic stable angina. NFD binds directly to inactive calcium channels and stabilizes their inactive conformation. By inhibiting the influx of calcium in smooth muscle cells, NFD prevents calcium-dependent myocyte contraction and vasoconstriction [31,40]. BTX was chosen as a reference compound in our docking experiment study due to its extremely potent cardiotoxic and neurotoxic characteristics [29,42,46,47,66]. In animals, BTX inactivates sodium channels in nerve cells and muscle cells, thereby interfering with the electrical signals sent throughout the body and causing fibrillation, arrhythmias, cardiac failure and death [29]. It is worth emphasizing that the obtained data from molecular modeling confirmed the high selectivity of the reference compounds for the appropriate ion channels (Table 2). The response obtained from molecular studies also indicates that the mechanisms underlying tachycardia in patients treated with TGB appear to be unrelated to its effect on the $hNa_V1.5$, $hCa_V1.2$ and $hK_V11.1$ heart ion channels. Moreover, it is known that one of the most common mechanisms of drug-induced ventricular tachycardia is the blocking of hERG channels [67,68]. For this reason, additional evidence supporting the conclusions of the in silico study appears to provide epidemiological data (pharmacological reports) in which tachycardia is noted in approximately 1.0% of patients treated with TGB. In light of these facts, if TGB-induced tachycardia contacts the $hK_v11.1$, $hNa_v1.5$ and $hCa_v1.2$. blocking mechanism, one would expect a higher rate of these side effects. In addition to the above-mentioned in vivo tests, as a part of safety pharmacology experiments, the TGB effects on PQ, QRS and QT intervals and the effects of TGB on heart rate were assessed. Many years of research have demonstrated that proarrhythmic effect, QT prolongation and hERG blocking cannot be treated as the only determinants of the occurrence of TdP. For instance, verapamil and ranolazines are examples of drugs that are strong inhibitors of the hERG channel and are simultaneously devoid of the risk of inducing arrhythmias and, vice versa, devoid of serious disorders of cardiomyocyte electrophysiology caused by drugs that are weak hERG inhibitors (e.g., sotalol and alfuzosin) [24,69]. Thus, this proves the insufficient specificity of the tests based only on the assessment of the hERG channel blocking potential. The risk of drug-induced TdP is rather balanced by multiple internal cardiac ionic currents that define ventricular repolarization. Therefore, studies that utilize the whole tissue seem to be a good option for the reflection of pharmacodynamics and potential adverse effects of a drug in a living organism. The in vivo results obtained from studies in rats showed that TGB did not prolong the QT interval or alter the QRS complex which suggests that it did not affect ventricular depolarization and repolarization. Taking into account that as in many other animal models of human diseases and also in this particular rat model, there might be basic translational problems. Some fundamental differences in the cardiac electrophysiology and myocyte calcium/potassium handling between rodents and humans have been suggested [70], but, nonetheless, the ECG in rats is still a widely applied experimental method in basic cardiovascular research. The technique of ECG recordings is simple; however, the interpretation of electrocardiographic parameters might be challenging. This is because the analysis may be biased by experimental settings, such as the type of anesthesia and the strain or age of animals. Furthermore, differences and similarities between rat and human ECG are frequently discussed in the context of translational cardiovascular research. Despite this, rat electrocardiography is an important investigational tool in experimental cardiology, even if the interpretation of electrocardiographic parameters is problematic [71]. In addition to this, a number of studies have shown that cardiotoxic drugs prolong QT interval in rodents and ECG recordings in rats have been used as a screening tool to assess the cardiotoxicity of various drugs. However, it needs to be stressed that the translation of the results of those studies to human application also possesses limitations. This is because rats' hearts do not express hERG, whereas the cardiotoxicity of drugs is strongly associated with the blockade of hERG-related potassium channels. However, rat hearts express a variant of Ether-à-go-go-Related Gene (rat ERG, also known as Kcnh2) [72,73], which may also play a key role in the assessment of drug-induced cardiotoxicity. Taken together, we are aware that extrapolating the results from our rat model to humans should be performed extremely cautiously and this, of course, should be regarded as the main limitation of our study. Therefore, one can assume that its direct interaction with heart sodium and potassium channels can be neglected. TGB also marks no significant effect on the PQ interval, which suggests that it does not influence the atrio-ventricular conduction time. Consequently, we can postulate that TGB has low pro-arrhythmic potential, at least, after a single administration. Given that tachycardia may result due to a number of different mechanisms and not all of them directly affect ion channels, it is also necessary to evaluate the effects of TGB on several neurotransmitters/neuromodulators and the activity of the autonomic nervous system. However, these effects were not investigated in the present research. Further studies are necessary to assess the effect of TGB on the cardiovascular system, especially after chronic administration. On the basis of our research, we can state that TGB did not bind to voltage-gated ion channels and did not affect them directly. Furthermore, the observed accidents of tachycardia are probably not due to the direct effect of TGB on voltage-gated ion channels.

4. Methods

4.1. Pharmacological Studies General Information

The experiments were carried out using male Wistar rats (Krf:(WI) (WU), 200–250 g). The animals were housed in constant temperature facilities exposed to 12:12 h light/dark cycles and were maintained on a standard pellet diet with tap water given ad libitum. All procedures were conducted according to guidelines of ICLAS (International Council on Laboratory Animal Science) and approved by the Second Local Ethics Committee in Krakow, Poland (resolution No. 106/2016, 14 June 2016).

4.1.1. Voltage-Dependent Calcium Channels—Functional Assays

In order to investigate the calcium entry blocking properties of TGB, it was tested on isolated rat aorta precontracted with KCl. Rats were anaesthetized with thiopental sodium (75 mg/kg, i.p., Rotexmedica, Germany) and the thoracic aorta was dissected, cleaned, denuded of endothelium, cut and mounted as described earlier [35]. Briefly, aorta rings were incubated in 30 mL chambers filled with a Krebs–Henseleit solution (NaCl 118 mM, KCl4.7 mM, $CaCl_2$ 2.25 mM, $MgSO_4$ 1.64 mM, KH_2PO_4 1.18 mM, $NaHCO_3$ 24.88 mM, glucose 10 mM, $C_3H_3O_3Na$ 2.2 mM and EDTA 0.05 mM) at 37 °C and pH 7.4 with constant oxygenation (O_2/CO_2, 19:1) and connected to an isometric FDT10-A force displacement transducer (BIOPAC Systems, Inc., COMMAT Ltd., Ankara, Turkey). The aortic rings were stretched and maintained at an optimal tension of 2 g and permitted to equilibrate for 2 h. The aortic rings were contracted to submaximal tension with KCl (60 mmol/L). Once the plateau was attained, concentration-relaxation curves were obtained by the addition of cumulative doses of tiagabine to the precontracted preparations.

Concentration-response curves were analyzed using GraphPad Prism 5.0 software (GraphPad Software Inc., San Diego, CA, USA). Relaxations are expressed as a percentage of inhibition of the maximal tension obtained with the contractile agent (Emax = 100%). Data are the means ± SEM of at least 4 separate experiments.

4.1.2. The Effect on Normal Electrocardiogram

In vivo electrocardiographic investigations were carried out using an ASPEL ASCARD B5 apparatus (Aspel, Poland), standard lead II and paper speed of 50 mm/s. The ECG was recorded just prior to and also at 1, 5, 10, 20, 30, 40, 50 and 60 min following the i.p. administration of TGB at a dose of 100 mg/kg. The QT_c was calculated according to the formula of Bazzett: $QT_c = QT/\sqrt{RR}$ [74]

4.2. In Silico Studies

The calculation procedures applied in the study are typical for the processing of docking studies.

4.2.1. Ligand Preparation

For the 3D molecular structure calculations, the Gaussian 09 (version D.01. for Unix/Linux) package was used [75]. The initial acceptable 3D structures of 6 studied compounds (Figure 2) were downloaded (as mol2 file) from ZINC [76]. Later, the GaussView [75,77] was applied for preparation of Gaussian input files. All the molecules were geometry-optimized in water as described by the PCM (polarizable continuum model). DFT/B3LYP level of theory 6311 + G(d, p) basis set was used. After geometrical optimization, (the root-mean-square gradient value smaller than 10^{-6} a.u.) compounds were saved as mol2 files using the GaussView. Subsequently, torsionals and the number of active torsions for ligands were defined and the Gasteiger charges were assigned to each compound via AutoDockTools (ADT) [78]. Finally, ligands prepared for docking were saved as pdbqt files.

4.2.2. Voltage-Gated Ion Channels Preparation

- $hNa_v1.5$ preparation:

The lack of crystal structure of $hNa_V1.5$ pore domain causes the need for preparing homology 3D models for this protein. For our research, the sequence for the $hNa_v1.5$ protein was gained from the Swiss Model Repository (SMR). SMR is a database which currently holds over 400,000 high quality 3D protein structure models generated by the automated SWISS-MODEL homology modeling pipeline [79]. The pdb file was downloaded from SWISS-MODEL SERVER (accession number Q14524) [80]. For this alignment, X-ray structure of human $Na_v1.2$-β2-KIIIA ternary complex (PDB entry 6J8E) was employed. Sequence identity between template and the monomer of sodium channel protein type 5 subunit α is 66.70%. Subsequently, the pdb file was opened in ADT [78]. ADT read coordinates, added charges, merged non-polar hydrogens and assigned appropriate atom types. Before formatting a molecule for AutoDock, we removed 9Z9 ((3β,14β,17β,25R)-3-[4-methoxy-3-(methoxymethyl)-butoxyl]-spirost-5-en), which is irrelevant molecule in this experiment. Finally, the prepared protein was saved as a pdbqt file. In the computational part of the study, we pondered the interaction between the investigated ligands and the intracellular pore gate formed from the proper residues of chain A.

- $hCa_v1.2$ preparation

The dearth of a 3D structure of $hCa_v1.2$ proper region also causes need for preparing homology models of this protein. The sequence for the $hCa_v1.2$ was gained from the SMR as well (accession number Q13936). For this alignment, X-ray structures of nifedipine complex with rabbit $Ca_v1.1$ (PDB entry 6JP5) were employed. The sequence identity between template and isoform 4 of CAC1C_HUMAN Voltage-dependent L-type calcium channel subunit alpha-1C is 70.31% and, according to the best of our knowledge, this is one of the highest identities currently available. Subsequently, similar to the hNav1.5 protein, the pdb file was opened in ADT [58]. The next steps were also analogous. Before the docking experiment, we removed C8U (methyl (4~{S})-2,6-dimethyl-5-nitro-4-[2-(trifluoromethyl)phenyl]-1,4-dihydropyridine-3-carboxylate)), which is a pointless ligand in this case. The pore forming and dihydropiridyne binding residues (from ARG1109 to LYS1198) were considered as the ligand binding site [81].

- $hK_v11.1$ preparation:

The sequence for the potassium voltage-gated channel subfamily H member 2 protein was downloaded from the Research Collaboratory for Structural Bioinformatics (RCSB) Protein Data Bank (PDB entry 5va2) as the crystal structure [82]. As in previous proteins, the pdb file was opened in ADT, read coordinates, added charges, merged non-polar hydrogens and assigned the appropriate atom types. As usual, we also removed crystallographic waters from 5va2. The binding pocket of the studied molecule were composed of the pore forming segment H5 and transmembrane helical fragment-Segment S6 [83].

4.2.3. Molecular Docking

Molecular docking was performed using the AutoDockTools 4.2 suite of the program [55]. A grid box with a dimension of $60 \times 60 \times 60$ Å^3 and grid spacing of 0.375 Å, which is large enough for a free rotation of a ligands, was built in the middle of the binding pockets of the studied Voltage Gated Ion Channels (VGICs) channels, which are composed using the appropriate residues (Table 4).

Torsionals in the residuals of the binding pocket were not rotatable. The rigid docking was carried out using the Lamarckian genetic algorithm 4. The optimized docking parameters were set as default values, with the exception of the number of genetic algorithms run which was 100. Torsionals in the ligands were rotatable-6 active torsions in each ligand (except for terfenadine, where it was 11). A cluster analysis was performed using RMS tolerance of 2 Å. In each case, the best docking result was considered as the complex with the lowest binding energy. Interactions between ligands and the related channel models were analyzed using the AutoDockTools program (ADT. Version 1.5.4) [78].

Table 4. The composition of the binding pocket of the analyzed channel models: hNav1.5, hCav1.2 and hKv11.1.

Protein	Intramembrane Pore-Forming Region Sequences
hNav1.5	358–382 (Phe, Ala, Trp, Ala, Phe, Leu, Ala, Leu, Phe, Arg, Leu, Met, Thr, Gly, Leu, Ans, Asp, Cys, Trp, Glu, Arg, Leu, Tyr, Gly, Leu, Ans, Gly, Leu, Ans, Thr, Leu) 884–904 (Phe, Phe, His, Ala, Phe, Leu, Ile, Ile, Phe, Arg, Ile, Leu, Cys, Gly, Glu, Trp, Ile, Glu, Thr, Met, Trp) 1406–1427 (Gly, Ala, Gly, Tyr, Leu, Ala, Leu, Leu, Gly, Leu, Ans, Val, Ala, Thr, Phe, Lys, Gly, Trp, Met, Asp, Ile, Met, Tyr, Ala) 1697–1719 (Phe, Ala, Ans, Ser, Met, Leu, Cys, Leu, Phe, Gly, Leu, Ans, Ile, Thr, Thr, Ser, Ala, Gly, Trp, Asp, Gly, Leu, Leu, Ser, Pro) [84,85]
hCav1.2	351–372 (Phe, Ala, Met, Leu, Thr, Val, Phe, Gly, Leu, Ans, Cys, Ile, Thr, Met, Glu, Glu, Trp, Thr, Asp, Val, Leu, Tyr, Trp, Val) 694–715 (Gly, Leu, Ans, Ser, Leu, Leu, Thr, Val, Phe, Gly, Leu, Ans, Ile, Leu, Thr, Gly, Glu, Asp, Trp, Ans, Ser, Val, Met, Tyr, Asp, Gly) 1122–1142 (Leu, Ala, Ala, Met, Met, Ala, Leu, Phe, Thr, Val, Ser, Thr, Phe, Glu, Gly, Trp, Pro, Glu, Leu, Leu, Tyr) 1453–1471 (Ala, Val, Leu, Leu, Leu, Phe, Arg, Cys, Ala, Thr, Gly, Glu, Ala, Trp, Gly, Leu, Ans, Asp, Ile, Met, Leu) [86,87]
hKv11.1	612–632 (Val, Thr, Ala, Leu, Tyr, Phe, Tphe, Ser, Ser, Leu, Thr, Ser, Val, Gly, Phe, Gly, Ans, Vsp) [88,89]

Supplementary Materials: The following are available online, Figure S1: Model transport proteins selected for the study: hNav1.5, hCav1.2, Kv11.1. Figure S2: Figure S3: Binding modes between hNav1.5, hCav1.2 and Kv11.1 and the four tested compounds () and two validated compounds

Author Contributions: A.N. and M.K. (Magdalena Kowalska) conceived and directed the project. K.S., Ł.F., M.K. (Magdalena Kowalska) and A.N. designed the study. K.S., Ł.F., M.K. (Magdalena Kowalska), M.K collected the data and carried out the experiments. K.S., Ł.F., M.K. (Magdalena Kowalska), M.K. and A.N. analyzed the data. A.N., M.K. (Magdalena Kowalska), Ł.F., M.K., G.G., J.N. and K.S. interpreted the results and wrote the manuscript. All authors have read and agreed to the published version of the manuscript.

Funding: This study was supported by a research grant from the National Science Centre UMO-2015/17/B/NZ7/02937.

Institutional Review Board Statement: The study was conducted according to the guidelines of the Declaration of Helsinki, and approved by the Institutional Review Board the Second Local Ethics Committee in Krakow, Poland (resolution No. 106/2016, 14 June 2016).

Informed Consent Statement: Not applicable.

Data Availability Statement: Not applicable.

Conflicts of Interest: None of the authors declare any conflicts of interest with respect to this study.

Sample Availability: Samples of the compounds are not available from the authors.

Abbreviations

AP	Cardiac action potential
(R/S)-TGB	(R/S)-Tiagabine
(R/S)-TEF	((R/S)-Terfenadine
NFD	Nifedipine
BTX	Batrachotoxin
#	Hydrogen bond components: from the protein
%	Hydrogen bond components: from the ligand
Acc	Hydrogen bond acceptor
EB	Complex energy binding
EHB	Hydrogen bond energy
θ	Hydrogen bond angle
VGICs	Voltage-Gated Ion Channels
VGKCs	Voltage-Gated Potassium. Channels
VGNaCs	Voltage-Gated Sodium Channels
VGCaCs	Voltage-Gated Calcium Channels
KV11.1 (hERG)	Cardiac Voltage-Gated Potassium Channels
NaV1.5	Cardiac Voltage-Gated Sodium Channels
CaV1.2	Cardiac Voltage-Gated Calcium Channels

References

1. Shmuely, S.; Van der Lende, M.; Lamberts, R.J.; Sander, J.W.; Thijs, R.D. The heart of epilepsy: Current views and future concepts. *Seizure* **2017**, *44*, 176–183. [CrossRef]
2. Shah, R.R. Cardiac Effects of Antiepileptic Drugs. In *Atlas of Epilepsies*; Springer: London, UK, 2010; pp. 1479–1486.
3. Alberts, B.; Johnson, A.; Lewis, J.; Raff, M.; Roberts, K.; Walter, P. *Molecular Biology of the Cell*, 4th ed.; Garland Science: New York, NY, USA, 2015.
4. Fermini, B.; Hancox, J.C.; Abi-Gerges, N.; Bridgland-Taylor, M.; Chaudhary, K.W.; Colatsky, T.; Correll, K.; Crumb, W.; Damiano, B.; Erdemli, G. A new perspective in the field of cardiac safety testing through the comprehensive in vitro proarrhythmia assay paradigm. *J. Biomol. Screen.* **2016**, *21*, 1–11. [CrossRef]
5. Cheung, S.; Parkinson, J.; Wählby-Hamrén, U.; Dota, C.; Kragh, Å.; Bergenholm, L.; Vik, T.; Collins, T.; Arfvidsson, C.; Pollard, C. A tutorial on model informed approaches to cardiovascular safety with focus on cardiac repolarisation. *J. Pharmacokinet. Pharmacodyn.* **2018**, *45*, 365–381. [CrossRef]
6. Obejero-Paz, C.A.; Bruening-Wright, A.; Kramer, J.; Hawryluk, P.; Tatalovic, M.; Dittrich, H.C.; Brown, A.M. Quantitative profiling of the effects of vanoxerine on human cardiac ion channels and its application to cardiac risk. *Sci. Rep.* **2015**, *5*, 1–15. [CrossRef]
7. Crumb, W.J., Jr.; Vicente, J.; Johannesen, L.; Strauss, D.G. An evaluation of 30 clinical drugs against the comprehensive in vitro proarrhythmia assay (CiPA) proposed ion channel panel. *J. Pharmacol. Toxicol. Methods* **2016**, *81*, 251–262. [CrossRef]
8. Li, Z.; Dutta, S.; Sheng, J.; Tran, P.N.; Wu, W.; Chang, K.; Mdluli, T.; Strauss, D.G.; Colatsky, T. Improving the in silico assessment of proarrhythmia risk by combining hERG (human ether-à-go-go-related gene) channel–drug binding kinetics and multichannel pharmacology. *Circ. Arrhythmia Electrophysiol.* **2017**, *10*, e004628. [CrossRef] [PubMed]
9. Kramer, J.; Obejero-Paz, C.A.; Myatt, G.; Kuryshev, Y.A.; Bruening-Wright, A.; Verducci, J.S.; Brown, A.M. MICE models: Superior to the HERG model in predicting Torsade de Pointes. *Sci. Rep.* **2013**, *3*, 2100. [CrossRef]
10. Nowaczyk, A.; Fijałkowski, Ł.; Zaręba, P.; Sałat, K. Selective neuronal and astrocytic inhibition of human GABA transporter isoform 1 (hGAT1) inhibitors in the mechanism of epilepsy and pain-molecular docking and pharmacodynamics studies, part I. *JMGM* **2018**, *85*, 171–181.
11. Nowaczyk, A.; Fijałkowski, Ł.; Kowalska, M.; Podkowa, A.; Sałat, K. Studies on the activity of selected highly lipophilic compounds toward hGAT1 inhibition: Part II. *ACS Chem. Neurosci.* **2019**, *10*, 337–347. [CrossRef] [PubMed]
12. Fijałkowski, Ł.; Sałat, K.; Podkowa, A.; Zaręba, P.; Nowaczyk, A. Potential role of selected antiepileptics used in neuropathic pain as human GABA transporter isoform 1 (GAT1) inhibitors—Molecular docking and pharmacodynamic studies. *Eur. J. Pharm. Sci.* **2017**, *96*, 362–372. [CrossRef]
13. Kirsch, G.E.; Kramer, J.; Bruening-Wright, A.; Obejero-Paz, C.; Brown, A.M. *The Comprehensive In Vitro Proarrhythmia Assay (CiPA) Guide: A New Approach to Cardiac Risk Assessment*; Charles River Laboratories International: Wilmington, MA, USA, 2016.
14. Raj, S.R.; Stein, C.M.; Saavedra, P.J.; Roden, D.M. Cardiovascular effects of noncardiovascular drugs. *Circulation* **2009**, *120*, 1123–1132. [CrossRef]
15. Schwartz, T.L.; Nihalani, N. Tiagabine in anxiety disorders. *Expert Opin. Pharmacother.* **2006**, *7*, 1977–1987. [CrossRef]
16. Sałat, K.; Podkowa, A.; Kowalczyk, P.; Kulig, K.; Dziubina, A.; Filipek, B.; Librowski, T. Anticonvulsant active inhibitor of GABA transporter subtype 1, tiagabine, with activity in mouse models of anxiety, pain and depression. *Pharmacol. Rep.* **2015**, *67*, 465–472. [CrossRef] [PubMed]
17. Brodie, M.J. Tiagabine pharmacology in profile. *Epilepsia* **1995**, *36*, S7–S9. [CrossRef] [PubMed]
18. Spiller, H.; Wiles, D.; Russell, J.; Casavant, M. Review of toxicity and trends in the use of tiagabine as reported to US poison centers from 2000 to 2012. *Hum. Exp. Toxicol.* **2016**, *35*, 109–113. [CrossRef] [PubMed]
19. Schachter, S.C. Tiagabine. In *Antiepileptic Drugs Pharmacology and Therapeutics*; Springer: New York, NY, USA, 1999; pp. 447–463.
20. Braestrup, C.; Nielsen, E.B.; Sonnewald, U.; Knutsen, L.J.; Andersen, K.E.; Jansen, J.A.; Frederiksen, K.; Andersen, P.H.; Mortensen, A.; Suzdak, P.D. (R)-N-[4, 4-bis (3-methyl-2-thienyl) but-3-en-1-yl] nipecotic acid binds with high affinity to the brain γ-aminobutyric acid uptake carrier. *J. Neurochem.* **1990**, *54*, 639–647. [CrossRef] [PubMed]
21. Khouzam, H.R. A Review of Anticonvulsants use in Psychiatric Conditions. *EC Neurol.* **2019**, *11*, 579–591.
22. Spiller, H.A.; Winter, M.L.; Ryan, M.; Krenzelok, E.P.; Anderson, D.L.; Thompson, M.; Kumar, S. Retrospective evaluation of tiagabine overdose. *Clin. Toxicol.* **2005**, *43*, 855–859. [CrossRef]
23. Jankovic, S.M.; Dostic, M. Choice of antiepileptic drugs for the elderly: Possible drug interactions and adverse effects. *Expert Opin. Drug Metab. Toxicol.* **2012**, *8*, 81–91. [CrossRef] [PubMed]
24. Kowalska, M.; Nowaczyk, J.; Nowaczyk, A. KV11.1, NaV1.5 and CaV1.2 transporter proteins as antitarget for drug cardiotoxicity. *Int. J. Mol. Sci.* **2020**, *21*, 8099. [CrossRef]
25. Passman, R.; Kadish, A. Polymorphic ventricular tachycardia, long QT syndrome and torsades de pointes. *Med. Clin. N. Am.* **2001**, *85*, 321–341. [CrossRef]
26. Rosso, R.; Hochstadt, A.; Viskin, D.; Chorin, E.; Schwartz, A.L.; Tovia-Brodie, O.; Laish-Farkash, A.; Havakuk, O.; Gepstein, L.; Banai, S. Polymorphic ventricular tachycardia, ischaemic ventricular fibrillation, and torsade de pointes: Importance of the QT and the coupling interval in the differential diagnosis. *Eur. Heart J.* **2021**. [CrossRef] [PubMed]
27. Rahm, A.-K.; Lugenbiel, P.; Schweizer, P.A.; Katus, H.A.; Thomas, D. Role of ion channels in heart failure and channelopathies. *Biophys. Rev.* **2018**, *10*, 1097–1106. [CrossRef]
28. Triggle, D.; Janis, R. Calcium channel ligands. *Annu. Rev. Pharmacol. Toxicol.* **1987**, *27*, 347–369. [CrossRef]

29. Albuquerque, E.; Daly, J.; Witkop, B. Batrachotoxin: Chemistry and pharmacology. *Science* **1971**, *172*, 995–1002. [CrossRef] [PubMed]
30. Gilchrist, J.; Olivera, B.M.; Bosmans, F. Animal toxins influence voltage-gated sodium channel function. *Volt. Gated Sodium Channels* **2014**, *221*, 203–229.
31. Sorkin, E.; Clissold, S.; Brogden, R. Nifedipine. *Drugs* **1985**, *30*, 182–274. [CrossRef]
32. Pensel, M.C.; Nass, R.D.; Taubøll, E.; Aurlien, D.; Surges, R. Prevention of sudden unexpected death in epilepsy: Current status and future perspectives. *Expert Rev. Neurother.* **2020**, *20*, 497–508. [CrossRef]
33. Goodnick, P.J.; Parra, F.; Jerry, J. Psychotropic drugs and the ECG: Focus on the QTc interval. *Expert Opin. Pharmacother.* **2002**, *3*, 479–498. [CrossRef]
34. Godfraind, T.; Miller, R.; Wibo, M. Calcium antagonism and calcium entry blockade. *Pharmacol. Rev.* **1986**, *38*, 321–416.
35. Kubacka, M.; Szkaradek, N.; Mogilski, S.; Pańczyk, K.; Siwek, A.; Gryboś, A.; Filipek, B.; Żmudzki, P.; Marona, H.; Waszkielewicz, A.M. Design, synthesis and cardiovascular evaluation of some aminoisopropanoloxy derivatives of xanthone. *Bioorganic Med. Chem.* **2018**, *26*, 3773–3784. [CrossRef]
36. Kubacka, M.; Mogilski, S.; Filipek, B.; Marona, H. The hypotensive activity and alpha1-adrenoceptor antagonistic properties of some aroxyalkyl derivatives of 2-methoxyphenylpiperazine. *Eur. J. Pharmacol.* **2013**, *698*, 335–344. [CrossRef] [PubMed]
37. Strauss, D.G.; Gintant, G.; Li, Z.; Wu, W.; Blinova, K.; Vicente, J.; Turner, J.R.; Sager, P.T. Comprehensive in vitro proarrhythmia assay (CiPA) update from a cardiac safety research consortium/health and environmental sciences institute/FDA Meeting. *Ther. Innov. Regul. Sci.* **2019**, *53*, 519–525. [CrossRef] [PubMed]
38. Orvos, P.; Kohajda, Z.; Szlovák, J.; Gazdag, P.; Árpádffy-Lovas, T.; Tóth, D.; Geramipour, A.; Tálosi, L.; Jost, N.; Varró, A. Evaluation of Possible Proarrhythmic Potency: Comparison of the Effect of Dofetilide, Cisapride, Sotalol, Terfenadine, and Verapamil on hERG and Native I Kr Currents and on Cardiac Action Potential. *Toxicol. Sci.* **2019**, *168*, 365–380. [CrossRef] [PubMed]
39. Balasubramanian, B.; Imredy, J.P.; Kim, D.; Penniman, J.; Lagrutta, A.; Salata, J.J. Optimization of Cav1. 2 screening with an automated planar patch clamp platform. *J. Pharmacol. Toxicol. Methods* **2009**, *59*, 62–72. [CrossRef] [PubMed]
40. Khan, K.M.; Schaefer, T.J. Nifedipine. In *StatPearls [Internet]*; StatPearls Publishing: Treasure Island, FL, USA, 2019. Available online: https://www.ncbi.nlm.nih.gov/books/NBK537052/ (accessed on 22 April 2019).
41. Kosower, E.M. A hypothesis for the mechanism of sodium channel opening by batrachotoxin and related toxins. *FEBS Lett.* **1983**, *163*, 161–164. [CrossRef]
42. Du, Y.; Garden, D.P.; Wang, L.; Zhorov, B.S.; Dong, K. Identification of New Batrachotoxin-sensing Residues in Segment IIIS6 of the Sodium Channel. *J. Biol. Chem.* **2011**, *286*, 13151–13160. [CrossRef]
43. Tokuyama, T.; Daly, J.; Witkop, B.; Karle, I.L.; Karle, J. The structure of batrachotoxinin A, a novel steroidal alkaloid from the Columbian arrow poison frog, Phyllobates aurotaenia. *J. Am. Chem. Soc.* **1968**, *90*, 1917–1918. [CrossRef]
44. Khodorov, B.I.; Yelin, E.A.; Zaborovskaya, L.D.; Maksudov, M.Z.; Tikhomirova, O.B.; Leonov, V.N. Comparative analysis of the effects of synthetic derivatives of batrachotoxin on sodium currents in frog node of Ranvier. *Cell. Mol. Neurobiol.* **1992**, *12*, 59–81. [CrossRef]
45. Tikhonov, D.B.; Zhorov, B.S. Sodium channel activators: Model of binding inside the pore and a possible mechanism of action. *FEBS Lett.* **2005**, *579*, 4207–4212. [CrossRef]
46. Wang, S.-Y.; Tikhonov, D.B.; Mitchell, J.; Zhorov, B.; Wang, G.K. Irreversible block of cardiac mutant Na+ channels by batrachotoxin. *Channels* **2007**, *1*, 179–188. [CrossRef]
47. Toma, T.; Logan, M.M.; Menard, F.; Devlin, A.S.; Du Bois, J. Inhibition of sodium ion channel function with truncated forms of batrachotoxin. *ACS Chem. Neurosci.* **2016**, *7*, 1463–1468. [CrossRef] [PubMed]
48. Vossler, D.G.; Morris, G.L.; Harden, C.L.; Montouris, G.; Faught, E.; Kanner, A.M.; Fix, A.; French, J.A. The Postmarketing Antiepileptic Drug Survey (PADS) group study investigators. Tiagabine in clinical practice: Effects on seizure control and behavior. *Epilepsy Behav.* **2013**, *28*, 211–216. [CrossRef] [PubMed]
49. Masuda, N.; Peng, Q.; Li, Q.; Jiang, M.; Liang, Y.; Wang, X.; Zhao, M.; Wang, W.; Ross, C.A.; Duan, W. Tiagabine is neuroprotective in the N171-82Q and R6/2 mouse models of Huntington's disease. *Neurobiol. Dis.* **2008**, *30*, 293–302. [CrossRef]
50. Davydov, O. Antiepileptic Drugs Beyond Epilepsy (use of anticonvulsants in the treatment of pain syndromes). *Neurosci. Behav. Physiol.* **2014**, *44*, 772–778. [CrossRef]
51. Pack, A.M. Epilepsy Overview and Revised Classification of Seizures and Epilepsies. *Contin. Lifelong Learn. Neurol.* **2016**, *25*, 306–321. [CrossRef] [PubMed]
52. Desborough, M.J.; Keeling, D.M. The aspirin story–from willow to wonder drug. *Br. J. Haematol.* **2017**, *177*, 674–683. [CrossRef]
53. ATC Anatomical Therapeutic Chemical Classification System. Available online: http://www.atccode.com/ (accessed on 22 April 2019).
54. Asif, M. A review on antiepileptic drug and their uses, mechanism of actions, adverse effects and drug interaction. *Curr. Sci. Perspect.* **2016**, *2*, 19–38.
55. Morris, G.M.; Huey, R.; Lindstrom, W.; Sanner, M.F.; Belew, R.K.; Goodsell, D.S.; Olson, A.J. AutoDock4 and AutoDockTools4: Automated docking with selective receptor flexibility. *J. Comput. Chem* **2009**, *30*, 2785–2791. [CrossRef]
56. Meldrum, B.S.; Chapman, A.G. Basic Mechanisms of Gabitril (Tiagabine) and Future Potential Developments. *Epilepsia* **1999**, *40* (Suppl. 9), S2–S6. [CrossRef]

57. Flowers, C.M.; Racoosin, J.A.; Kortepeter, C. Seizure activity and off-label use of tiagabine. *N. Engl. J. Med.* **2006**, *354*, 773–774. [CrossRef]
58. Yarborough, M.; Johnson, J.G. Histamine Modulators. In *Essentials of Pharmacology for Anesthesia, Pain Medicine, and Critical Care*; Springer: New York, NY, USA, 2015; pp. 365–379.
59. Li, M.; Ramos, L.G. Drug-induced QT prolongation and torsades de pointes. *Pharm. Ther.* **2017**, *42*, 473–477.
60. Woosley, R.L.; Chen, Y.; Freiman, J.P.; Gillis, R.A. Mechanism of the cardiotoxic actions of terfenadine. *JAMA* **1993**, *269*, 1532–1536. [CrossRef]
61. Sorkin, E.; Heel, R. Terfenadine A review of its pharmacodynamic properties and terapeutic efficiecy. *Drugs* **1985**, *29*, 34–56. [CrossRef]
62. Ajayi, F.O.; Sun, H.; Perry, J. Adverse drug reactions: A review of relevant factors. *J. Clin. Pharmacol.* **2000**, *40*, 1093–1101.
63. Koch, E.; Plassmann, S. Critical Aspects of Integrated Nonclinical Drug Development: Concepts, Strategies, and Potential Pitfalls. In *A Comprehensive Guide to Toxicology in Nonclinical Drug Development*; Elsevier: Amsterdam, The Netherlands, 2017; pp. 7–38.
64. Roy, M.-L.; Dumaine, R.; Brown, A.M. HERG, a primary human ventricular target of the nonsedating antihistamine terfenadine. *Circulation* **1996**, *94*, 817–823. [CrossRef] [PubMed]
65. Pratt, P.F.; Bonnet, S.; Ludwig, L.M.; Bonnet, P.; Rusch, N.J. Upregulation of L-type Ca^{2+} channels in mesenteric and skeletal arteries of SHR. *Hypertension* **2002**, *40*, 214–219. [CrossRef]
66. Worley, J.; French, R.J.; Krueger, B.K. Trimethyloxonium modification of single batrachotoxin-activated sodium channels in planar bilayers. Changes in unit conductance and in block by saxitoxin and calcium. *J. Gen. Physiol.* **1986**, *87*, 327–349. [CrossRef]
67. Yap, Y.G.; Camm, A.J. Drug induced QT prolongation and torsades de pointes. *Heart* **2003**, *89*, 1363–1372. [CrossRef]
68. Huang, H.; Pugsley, M.K.; Fermini, B.; Curtis, M.J.; Koerner, J.; Accardi, M.; Authier, S. Cardiac voltage-gated ion channels in safety pharmacology: Review of the landscape leading to the CiPA initiative. *J. Pharmacol. Toxicol. Methods* **2017**, *87*, 11–23. [CrossRef]
69. Mirams, G.R.; Cui, Y.; Sher, A.; Fink, M.; Cooper, J.; Heath, B.M.; McMahon, N.C.; Gavaghan, D.J.; Noble, D. Simulation of multiple ion channel block provides improved early prediction of compounds' clinical torsadogenic risk. *Cardiovasc. Res.* **2011**, *91*, 53–61. [CrossRef] [PubMed]
70. Zhang, X.; Ai, X.; Nakayama, H.; Chen, B.; Harris, D.M.; Tang, M.; Xie, Y.; Szeto, C.; Li, Y.; Li, Y. Persistent increases in Ca^{2+} influx through Cav1. 2 shortens action potential and causes Ca^{2+} overload-induced afterdepolarizations and arrhythmias. *Basic Res. Cardiol.* **2016**, *111*, 1–16. [CrossRef] [PubMed]
71. Konopelski, P.; Ufnal, M. Electrocardiography in rats: A comparison to human. *Physiol. Res.* **2016**, *65*, 717–725. [CrossRef]
72. Chun, K.; Koenen, M.; Katus, H.A.; Zehelein, J. Expression of the IKr components KCNH2 (rERG) and KCNE2 (rMiRP1) during late rat heart development. *Exp. Mol. Med.* **2004**, *36*, 367–371. [CrossRef]
73. Matus, M.; Kucerova, D.; Kruzliak, P.; Adameova, A.; Doka, G.; Turcekova, K.; Kmecova, J.; Kyselovic, J.; Krenek, P.; Kirchhefer, U. Upregulation of SERCA2a following short-term ACE inhibition (by enalaprilat) alters contractile performance and arrhythmogenicity of healthy myocardium in rat. *Mol. Cell. Biochem.* **2015**, *403*, 199–208. [CrossRef]
74. De Clerck, F.; Van de Water, A.; D'Aubioul, J.; Lu, H.R.; Van Rossem, K.; Hermans, A.; Van Ammel, K. In vivo measurement of QT prolongation, dispersion and arrhythmogenesis: Application to the preclinical cardiovascular safety pharmacology of a new chemical entity. *Fundam. Clin. Pharmacol.* **2002**, *16*, 125–140. [CrossRef]
75. Frisch, M.J.; Trucks, G.W.; Schlegel, H.B.; Scuseria, G.E.; Robb, M.A.; Cheeseman, J.R.; Zakrzewski, V.G.; Montgomery, J.A.; Stratmann, R.E.; Burant, S.; et al. *Gaussian 09*; Revision D.01; Gaussian, Inc.: Wallingford, CT, USA, 2009.
76. Irwin, J.J.; Sterling, T.; Mysinger, M.M.; Bolstad, E.S.; Coleman, R.G. ZINC: A free tool to discover chemistry for biology. *J. Chem. Inf. Model.* **2012**, *52*, 1757–1768. [CrossRef] [PubMed]
77. Dennington, R.; Keith, T.; Millam, J. *GaussView, Version 5*; Semichem Inc.: Shawnee Mission, KS, USA, 2009.
78. Morris, G.M.; Goodsell, D.S.; Halliday, R.S.; Huey, R.; Hart, W.E.; Belew, R.K.; Olson, A.J. Automated docking using a Lamarckian genetic algorithm and an empirical binding free energy function. *J. Comput. Chem.* **1998**, *19*, 1639–1662. [CrossRef]
79. Waterhouse, A.; Bertoni, M.; Bienert, S.; Studer, G.; Tauriello, G.; Gumienny, R.; Heer, F.T.; de Beer, T.A.P.; Rempfer, C.; Bordoli, L. SWISS-MODEL: Homology modelling of protein structures and complexes. *Nucleic Acids Res.* **2018**, *46*, W296–W303. [CrossRef]
80. Bienert, S.; Waterhouse, A.; de Beer, T.A.; Tauriello, G.; Studer, G.; Bordoli, L.; Schwede, T. The SWISS-MODEL Repository—New features and functionality. *Nucleic Acids Res.* **2017**, *45*, D313–D319. [CrossRef]
81. Schultz, D.; Mikala, G.; Yatani, A.; Engle, D.B.; Iles, D.E.; Segers, B.; Sinke, R.J.; Weghuis, D.O.; Klockner, U.; Wakamori, M.; et al. Cloning, chromosomal localization, and functional expression of the alpha 1 subunit of the L-type voltage-dependent calcium channel from normal human heart. *Proc. Natl. Acad. Sci. USA* **1993**, *90*, 6228–6232. [CrossRef] [PubMed]
82. Cabral, J.H.M.; Lee, A.; Cohen, S.L.; Chait, B.T.; Li, M.; Mackinnon, R. Crystal Structure and Functional Analysis of the HERG Potassium Channel N Terminus: A Eukaryotic PAS Domain. *Cell* **1998**, *95*, 649–655. [CrossRef]
83. Morais-Cabral, J.H.; Robertson, G.A. The enigmatic cytoplasmic regions of KCNH channels. *J. Mol. Biol.* **2015**, *427*, 67–76. [CrossRef]
84. Rayevsky, A.; Samofalova, D.O.; Maximyuk, O.; Platonov, M.; Hurmach, V.; Ryabukhin, S.; Volochnyuk, D. Modelling of an autonomous Nav1. 5 channel system as a part of in silico pharmacology study. *J. Mol. Model.* **2021**, *27*, 1–9. [CrossRef] [PubMed]
85. Ahmed, M.; Hasani, H.J.; Ganesan, A.; Houghton, M.; Barakat, K. Modeling the human Nav1. 5 sodium channel: Structural and mechanistic insights of ion permeation and drug blockade. *Drug Des. Dev. Ther.* **2017**, *11*, 2301. [CrossRef] [PubMed]

86. Hering, S.; Zangerl-Plessl, E.-M.; Beyl, S.; Hohaus, A.; Andranovits, S.; Timin, E. Calcium channel gating. *Pflügers Arch. Eur. J. Physiol.* **2018**, *470*, 1291–1309. [CrossRef]
87. Findeisen, F.; Minor, J.; Daniel, L. Progress in the structural understanding of voltage-gated calcium channel (CaV) function and modulation. *Channels* **2010**, *4*, 459–474. [CrossRef]
88. Al-Owais, M.; Bracey, K.; Wray, D. Role of intracellular domains in the function of the herg potassium channel. *Eur. Biophys. J.* **2009**, *38*, 569–576. [CrossRef] [PubMed]
89. Stansfeld, P.J.; Gedeck, P.; Gosling, M.; Cox, B.; Mitcheson, J.S.; Sutcliffe, M.J. Drug block of the hERG potassium channel: Insight from modeling. *Proteins Struct. Funct. Bioinform.* **2007**, *68*, 568–580. [CrossRef]

molecules MDPI

Article

Development of Halogenated Pyrazolines as Selective Monoamine Oxidase-B Inhibitors: Deciphering via Molecular Dynamics Approach

Aathira Sujathan Nair [1,†], Jong-Min Oh [2,†], Vishal Payyalot Koyiparambath [1], Sunil Kumar [1], Sachithra Thazhathuveedu Sudevan [1], Opeyemi Soremekun [3], Mahmoud E. Soliman [3], Ahmed Khames [4], Mohamed A. Abdelgawad [5,6], Leena K. Pappachen [1,*], Bijo Mathew [1,*,†] and Hoon Kim [2,*]

1 Department of Pharmaceutical Chemistry, Amrita School of Pharmacy, AIMS Health Sciences Campus, Amrita Vishwa Vidyapeetham, Kochi 682 041, India; sujuaathira@gmail.com (A.S.N.); vishalpk11@gmail.com (V.P.K.); solankimedchem@gmail.com (S.K.); sachithrasudevan22@gmail.com (S.T.S.)
2 Department of Pharmacy, Research Institute of Life Pharmaceutical Sciences, Sunchon National University, Suncheon 57922, Korea; ddazzo005@naver.com
3 Molecular Bio-computation and Drug Design Laboratory, School of Health Sciences, Westville Campus, University of KwaZulu-Natal, Durban 4001, South Africa; opeyemisoremekun@gmail.com (O.S.); soliman@ukzn.ac.za (M.E.S.)
4 Department of Pharmaceutics and Industrial Pharmacy, College of Pharmacy, Taif University, P.O. Box-11099, Taif 21944, Saudi Arabia; a.khamies@tu.edu.sa
5 Department of Pharmaceutical Chemistry, College of Pharmacy, Jouf University, Sakaka 72341, Saudi Arabia; hmdgwd@ju.edu.sa
6 Department of Pharmaceutical Organic Chemistry, Faculty of Pharmacy, Beni-Suef University, Beni Suef 62514, Egypt
* Correspondence: leenabijudaniel@gmail.com (L.K.P.); bijomathew@aims.amrita.edu or bijovilaventgu@gmail.com (B.M.); hoon@sunchon.ac.kr (H.K.)
† These authors contributed equally to this work.

Citation: Nair, A.S.; Oh, J.-M.; Koyiparambath, V.P.; Kumar, S.; Sudevan, S.T.; Soremekun, O.; Soliman, M.E.; Khames, A.; Abdelgawad, M.A.; Pappachen, L.K.; et al. Development of Halogenated Pyrazolines as Selective Monoamine Oxidase-B Inhibitors: Deciphering via Molecular Dynamics Approach. *Molecules* **2021**, *26*, 3264. https://doi.org/10.3390/molecules26113264

Academic Editors: Alicja Nowaczyk and Grzegorz Grześk

Received: 29 April 2021
Accepted: 27 May 2021
Published: 28 May 2021

Abstract: Halogens have been reported to play a major role in the inhibition of monoamine oxidase (MAO), relating to diverse cognitive functions of the central nervous system. Pyrazoline/halogenated pyrazolines were investigated for their inhibitory activities against human monoamine oxidase-A and -B. Halogen substitutions on the phenyl ring located at the fifth position of pyrazoline showed potent MAO-B inhibition. Compound 3-(4-ethoxyphenyl)-5-(4-fluorophenyl)-4,5-dihydro-1*H*-pyrazole (**EH7**) showed the highest potency against MAO-B with an IC_{50} value of 0.063 μM. The potencies against MAO-B were increased in the order of –F (in **EH7**) > –Cl (**EH6**) > –Br (**EH8**) > –H (**EH1**). The residual activities of most compounds for MAO-A were > 50% at 10 μM, except for **EH7** and **EH8** (IC_{50} = 8.38 and 4.31 μM, respectively). **EH7** showed the highest selectivity index (SI) value of 133.0 for MAO-B, followed by **EH6** at > 55.8. **EH7** was a reversible and competitive inhibitor of MAO-B in kinetic and reversibility experiments with a Ki value of 0.034 ± 0.0067 μM. The molecular dynamics study documented that **EH7** had a good binding affinity and motional movement within the active site with high stability. It was observed by MM-PBSA that the chirality had little effect on the overall binding of **EH7** to MAO-B. Thus, **EH7** can be employed for the development of lead molecules for the treatment of various neurodegenerative disorders.

Keywords: halogenated pyrazolines; monoamine oxidase inhibitors; kinetics; reversibility; molecular dynamics

1. Introduction

Monoamine oxidases (MAOs) are the principal metabolizing enzymes responsible for the oxidative degradation of various biogenic amines that are related to diverse cognitive functions of the central nervous system (CNS) [1]. Considering the difference in the structure, substrate specificity, biological functions, and catalytic mechanism of MAOs, two types of isoforms are available, namely, MAO-A and MAO-B [2]. Ammonia, aldehyde, and hydrogen peroxide are the major intermediate products formed during MAO-based catalyzed oxidative deamination [3]. These can produce substantial issues, such as astrocyte swelling, unbalancing of the signaling process in the neurotransmission, neuronal loss, and mitochondrial dysfunctions [4]. Eventually, these toxic by-products can lead to numerous neurodegenerative disorders, such as Alzheimer's disease (AD) and Parkinson's disease (PD) [5]. Selegiline is a selective/irreversible MAO-B inhibitor used as an adjuvant therapy with L-DOPA, which is considered a safe therapy for PD [6,7]. The latest research has also documented that potent, reversible dual targeted MAO-B/AChE inhibitors can decrease the production of β-amyloid peptide levels in AD-related neurons [8]. In 2017, safinamide, as the first selective and reversible MAO-B inhibitor approved by the USFDA for PD treatment, along with levodopa, has promising neuroprotective effects on MPTP-treated mice [9,10].

In the exploration of novel, selective, and reversible MAO-B inhibitors, a general blueprint of drug design has been widely accepted recently, and it consists of a molecular framework of two hydrophobic rings of phenyl/heteroaryl, which are separated by an electron-rich and flexible short spacer unit (Figure 1) [11]. Many of the molecules from this diverse class, such as pyrazolines, enamides, carboxamides, and α, β-unsaturated ketones, were identified as potent MAO-B inhibitors [12–21]. The presence of a rotatable bond and electron-rich Michael acceptor unit in the spacer can efficiently make appropriate orientations and binding affinities in the entrance and substrate cavity of MAO-B. The flexibility of the molecules provides good recognition of aromatic systems of the ligand to the hydrophobic cavity of the inhibitor binding cavity of MAO-B by Pi–Pi stacking or Pi–cation interactions. The binding requirements of the selective MAO-B inhibitors include one or more hydrophobic ring, preferably an aromatic or heteroaromatic nucleus with small lipophilic substituents, such as dimethylamino, ethoxy, methoxy, and halogens. The presence of a hydrogen bond acceptor (HBA) and hydrogen bond donor (HBD) linker with optimal rotatable bonds between these hydrophobic units had a pivotal role in the design of potent MAO-B inhibitors [22–26].

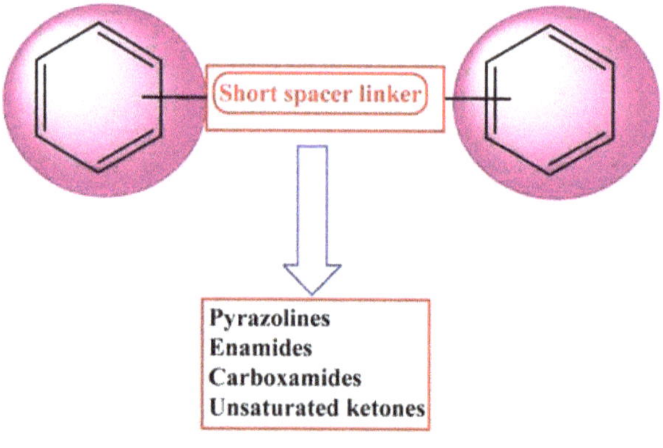

Figure 1. General blueprint of the design of MAO-B inhibitors.

Pyrazoline, or dihydropyrazole, is the partially reduced form of pyrazole, and 2-pyrazoline is the most stable tautomeric from in this class [27]. The presence of an asymmetric carbon atom at the C5 position of pyrazoline was revealed to be due to two epimers of the *R* and *S* forms [28]. The ring closure reaction of α, β-unsaturated ketones with hydrazine derivatives in the presence of basic medium is the commonly used synthetic methodology for 2-pyrazolines [29]. The separation of the *R* and *S* forms from the racemic mixture of 2-pyrazoline is a considerable task in the identification of biologically more active isomers [30]. Many studies of the literature have documented that the substitution of the 3rd and 5th position of pyrazolines with aryl/heteroaryl units can favor MAO-B inhibition [31]. At the same time, the length and bulkiness of the groups anchoring from the N1 position of pyrazolines can shift the selectivity from MAO-B to MAO-A. The presence of lipophilic groups, such as halogens, hydroxyl, and methoxy groups, on the phenyl ring of the third and fifth positions of the pyrazoline nucleus, can cause significant MAO-B inhibition [32–35].

Regarding the role of halogens in MAO inhibition, it is generally known that FDA-approved MAO inhibitors like clorgyline, moclobemide, safinamide, and lazabemide are chlorine-containing drugs [36]. The evidence shows that more than 40% of drugs in FDA-approved or clinical trials are in the halogenated form [37]. Recently, our group emphasized the presence and orientation of various halogens on chemical scaffolds, such as chalcones, chromones, coumarins, hydrazothiazoles, and pyrazolines, thereby providing in-depth knowledge on MAO inhibition and B isoform selectivity. It was noted that this can have a new type of impact on the drug–target interaction of these MAO inhibitors in order to fill the small lipophilic pockets in the inhibitor binding cavity (IBC) of MAOs [38].

The objective of the present study was focused on the in vitro evaluation of MAO-A and MAO-B inhibitions of pyrazoline/halogenated pyrazoline derivatives. The lead molecules were further studied for kinetics, reversibility, and blood–brain barrier (BBB) permeation. Detailed molecular dynamics established precisely the protein–ligand binding interactions of the halogenated molecules in their respective active sites of enzyme targets and the role of chirality towards MAO-B inhibition.

2. Results and Discussion

2.1. *Inhibitory Activities against MAO Enzymes*

At 10 μM, all derivatives in the **EH** sequence had potent inhibitory action against MAO-B, with residual activities of about 50% (Table 1). Fluorine-containing compound **EH7** showed the greatest inhibitory activities against MAO-B with an IC_{50} value of 0.063 μM, followed by chlorine-containing **EH6** (IC_{50} = 0.40 μM), and bromine-containing **EH8** (IC_{50} = 0.69 μM). Comparing **EH1** (IC_{50} = 5.38 μM) with **EH7**, the potencies for MAO-B greatly increased, i.e., by 85.4 times, based on their IC_{50} values, with the presence of –F instead of –H. Most of the compounds weakly inhibited MAO-A at 10 μM, with residual activities of >50%, except **EH7** and **EH8**. Among them, **EH7** showed the highest selectivity index (SI) value for MAO-B with 133.0, followed by **EH6** with 55.8.

Table 1. Inhibitions of recombinant human MAO enzymes by compounds of the **EH** series [a].

Compounds	Residual Activity at 10 μM (%)			IC_{50} (μM)			SI [b]
	MAO-A	MAO-B	AChE	MAO-A	MAO-B	AChE	
EH1	99.1 ± 0.27	33.7 ± 0.96	81.0 ± 6.21	>40	5.38 ± 0.16	>40	>7.43
EH6	68.1 ± 0.18	19.4 ± 1.01	63.5 ± 4.99	22.3 ± 0.12	0.40 ± 0.051	>40	55.8
EH7	46.9 ± 1.25	4.03 ± 0.53	74.0 ± 0.71	8.38 ± 0.88	0.063 ± 0.0042	>40	133.0
EH8	33.5 ± 0.65	11.3 ± 0.13	53.7 ± 2.15	4.31 ± 0.013	0.69 ± 0.017	10.8 ± 0.15	6.3
Toloxatone				1.08 ± 0.0025	-	-	
Lazabemide				-	0.11 ± 0.016	-	
Clorgyline				0.0070 ± 0.00070	-	-	
Pargyline				-	0.14 ± 0.0059	-	
Tacrine				-	-	0.27 ± 0.019	

[a] Results are expressed as the means ± standard errors of duplicate or triplicate experiments. [b] SI values are expressed for IC_{50} of MAO-B/IC_{50} of MAO-A. Values for reference compounds were determined after preincubation for 30 min with enzymes.

The enzyme inhibition results obtained in the current study revealed that all of the halogenated pyrazoline derivatives showed good selective MAO-B inhibitory activity. The study mainly confirmed the effect of halogens on the *para*-position of the **B** ring of ethoxylated pyrazolines. Among the halogens, fluorine had the greatest impact on MAO-B inhibition with a sub-micromolar level range. It is worth noting that a highly electronegative fluorine atom-containing compound is two times more potent than marketed drugs for the inhibition of MAO-B, such as reversible-type lazabemide (IC_{50} = 0.11 μM) and irreversible pargyline (IC_{50} = 0.14 μM). Recent reports state that the anisotropy of charge circulation around the fluorine atom, which is the reason for the directional and stabilizing property of the active site, proves that halogen enhances the analogy of drugs of new molecules [38].

Recently, we evaluated MAO-B inhibitory activities for ethoxylated head of chalcone derivatives and found that chlorine-, fluorine-, or bromine-containing chalcones had good IC_{50} values of 0.57, 0.053, and 2.01 μM, respectively [39]. Cyclization with hydrazine hydrate of the same halogenated molecules retained higher MAO-B inhibitory activities than the unsubstituted one. This finding clearly shows the importance of halogen incorporation both in ethoxylated chalcones and their pyrazolines moieties for MAO-B inhibition. Interestingly, in both series, fluorine-containing compounds showed dominant MAO-B inhibition profiles. For the purpose of the development of compounds with good MAO-B inhibitory activity, the bonding of fluorine to the molecule was an auspicious lead.

2.2. Kinetics of MAO Inhibition

Kinetic studies on MAO-A and MAO-B inhibitions by **EH6** and **EH7** were performed. Lineweaver–Burk plots and secondary plots showed that **EH6** was a competitive inhibitor of MAO-A and MAO-B (Figure 2A,C), with K_i values of 10.8 ± 1.03 and 0.19 ± 0.016 μM, respectively (Figure 2B,D). Lineweaver–Burk plots and secondary plots exhibited that **EH7** was a competitive inhibitor of MAO-A and MAO-B (Figure 3A,C), with K_i values of 3.64 ± 0.18 and 0.034 ± 0.0067 μM, respectively (Figure 3B,D). These results suggest that **EH6** and **EH7** are selective and competitive inhibitors of MAO-B.

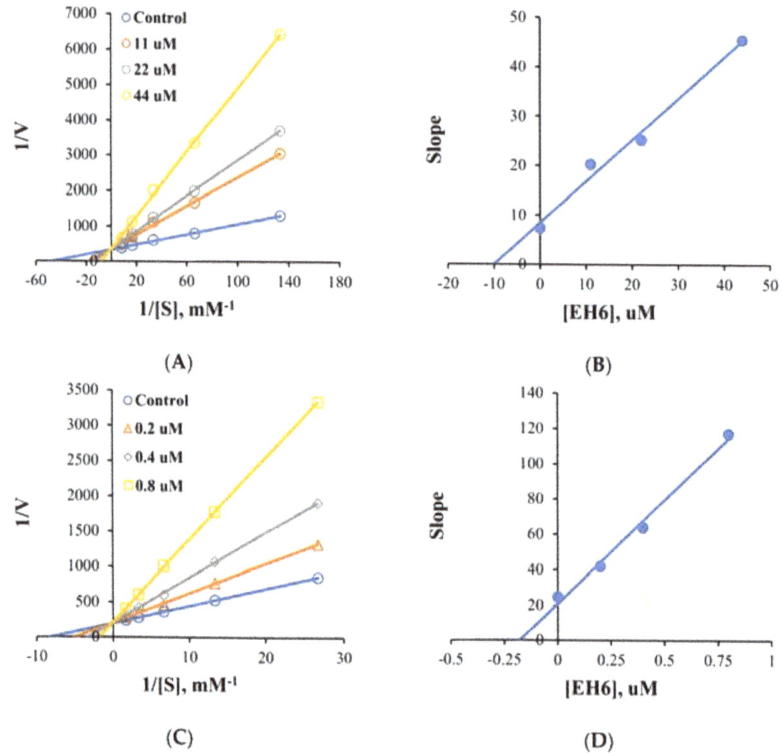

Figure 2. Lineweaver–Burk plots for MAO-A and MAO-B inhibitions by **EH6** (**A**,**C**) and their respective secondary plots (**B**,**D**) of slopes vs. inhibitor concentrations.

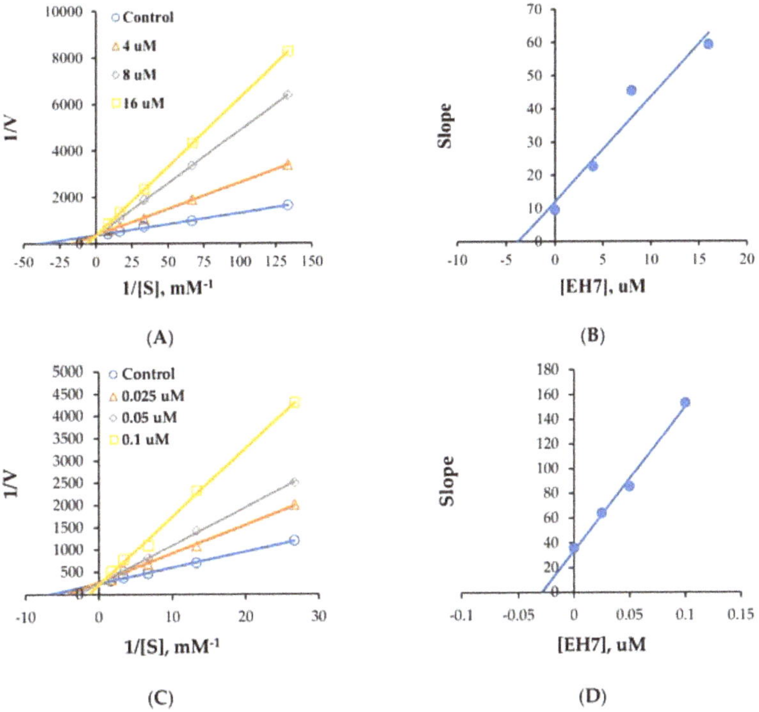

Figure 3. Lineweaver–Burk plots for MAO-A and MAO-B inhibitions by **EH7** (**A**,**C**) and their respective secondary plots (**B**,**D**) of slopes vs. inhibitor concentrations.

2.3. Reversibility Study

Reversibility studies on MAO-B inhibition were carried out on **EH7**. In these experiments, inhibition of MAO-B by **EH7** was recovered from 12.5% (value of A_U) to 89.5% (value of A_D). The recovery value was similar to that of the reversible reference lazabemide (from 35.3% to 75.7%); however, it was different from that of the irreversible inhibitor pargyline (from 41.3% to 44.9%), which was not recovered (Figure 4). Similar to the reversible reference level, inhibition of MAO-B by **EH7** was reversed in these experiments, indicating that **EH7** is a reversible inhibitor of MAO-B.

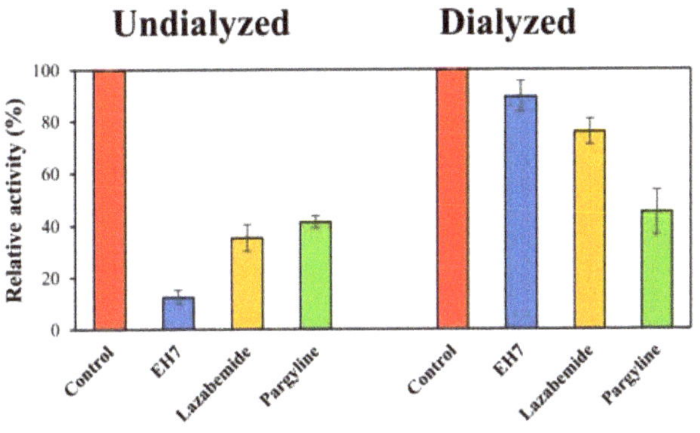

Figure 4. Recovery of MAO-B inhibition by **EH7**, using dialysis experiments. The concentrations used were **EH7** at 0.15 μM, lazabemide (a reversible reference inhibitor) at 0.20 μM, and pargyline (an irreversible reference inhibitor) at 0.30 μM.

2.4. Blood–Brain Barrier (BBB) Permeation Studies

The CNS bioavailability of the molecules was confirmed by a parallel artificial membrane permeability assay (PAMPA) [40]. From the assay, highly effective permeabilities and high CNS bioavailabilities were observed for the halogenated pyrazolines with Pe ranges of 14.13 ~ 14.56 × 10^{-6} cm/s (Table 2). All halogenated substituted derivatives showed higher CNS permeabilities than unsubstituted ones.

Table 2. BBB assay of standard and **EH** compounds.

Compounds	Bibliography Pe (×10^{-6} cm/s) [a]	Experimental Pe (×10^{-6} cm/s)	Prediction
Progesterone	9.3	9.02 ± 0.11	CNS+
Verapamil	16.0	15.53 ± 0.24	CNS+
Piroxicam	2.5	2.43 ± 0.30	CNS+/−
Lomefloxacin	1.1	1.12 ± 0.01	CNS−
Dopamine	0.2	0.22 ± 0.01	CNS−
EH1		10.34 ± 0.33	CNS+
EH6		14.26 ± 0.80	CNS+
EH7		14.13 ± 0.71	CNS+
EH8		14.56 ± 0.26	CNS+

CNS+ (high): Pe (10^{-6} cm/s) > 4.00; CNS− (low): Pe (10^{-6} cm/s) < 2.00; CNS± (uncertain): Pe (10^{-6} cm/s) from 4.00 to 2.00. [a] From [40].

2.5. Molecular Dynamics Studies

2.5.1. **EH1**, **EH6**, **EH7**, and **EH8** Exert Differential Impacts on the Stability of MAO-A and MAO-B

The root mean square deviation (RMSD) can be used to estimate the conformational stability of a system during a production run [41]. The differential structural perturbatory effect of the ligands on the structure of MAO-B relative to MAO-A was first explored. MAO-B_**EH6**, MAO-B_**EH7**, and MAO-B_**EH8** attained equilibration at around 20 ns (Figure 5). However, MAO-B_**EH1** achieved convergence earlier in the simulation run but eventually elicited a somewhat high structural movement at around 45 ns. In comparison, **EH1**, **EH6**, **EH7**, and **EH8** did not elicit similar stabilizing effects on the MAO-A protein; this could be due to the IC_{50} values experimentally reported, suggesting their low inhibitory potential towards MAO-A. The superior stabilizing effect elicited by the ligands against MAO-B when compared to MAO-A binding points to the high selective targeting of the ligands for MAO-B. As indicated by the IC_{50}, **EH7** had the highest stabilizing impact on MAO-B with an average RMSD value of 1.49 Å, while **EH1**, **EH6**, and **EH8** had 2.29, 1.61, and 1.79 Å, respectively (Table 3).

Table 3. Average RMSD, RMSD_AS, RMSF, and IC_{50} of the Apo and bound systems.

Complexes	RMSD	RMSD_AS	RMSF	IC_{50} (μM)
MAO-A_EH1	3.35 (0.73)	1.93 (0.18)	1.47 (1.28)	>40
MAO-A_EH6	2.63 (0.72)	1.44 (0.27)	1.15 (1.04)	22.3
MAO-A_EH7	2.74 (0.59)	2.09 (0.29)	1.07 (0.96)	8.38
MAO-A_EH8	3.26 (0.74)	1.96 (0.34)	1.40 (1.28)	4.31
MAO-B_EH1	2.29 (0.34)	2.85 (0.37)	0.88 (0.59)	5.38
MAO-B_EH6	1.61 (0.22)	1.54 (0.14)	0.83 (0.60)	0.40
MAO-B_EH7	1.49 (0.26)	1.60 (0.16)	0.68 (0.72)	0.063
MAO-B_EH8	1.79 (0.24)	1.70 (0.25)	0.75 (0.61)	0.69

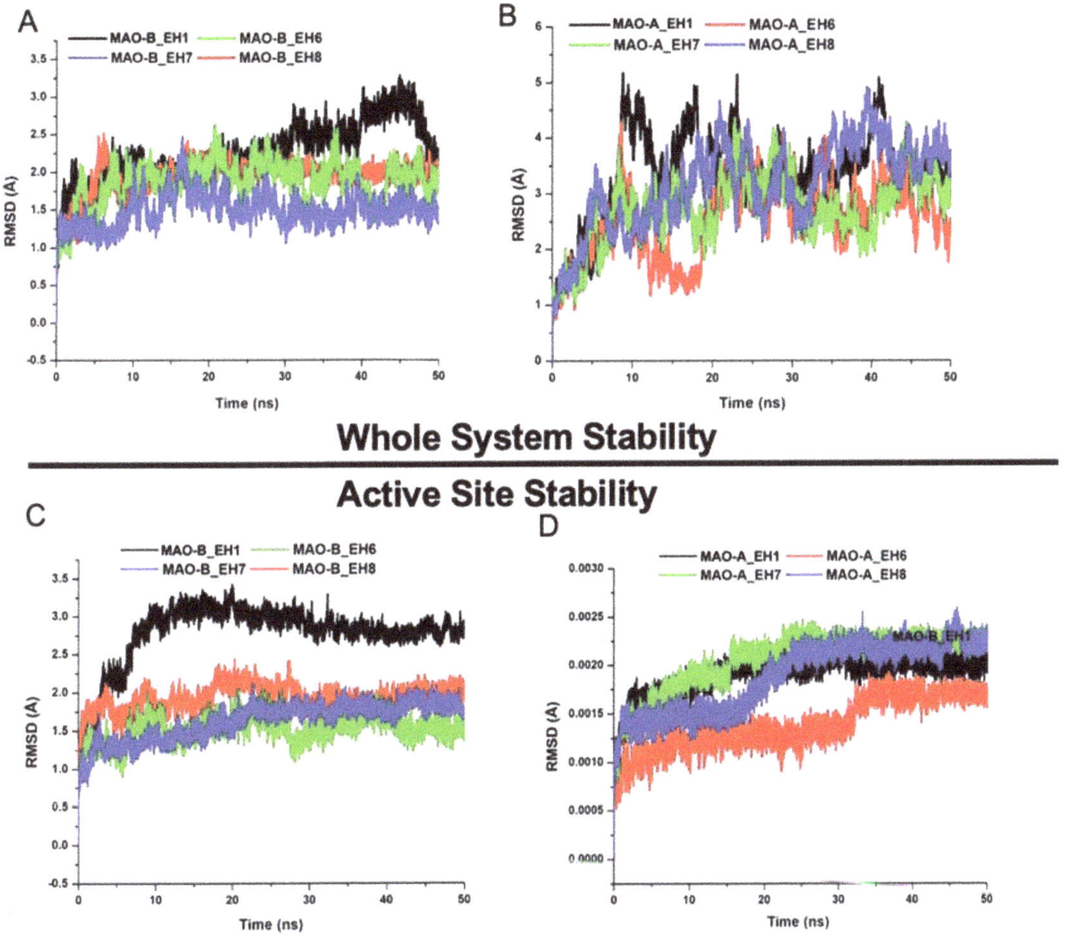

Figure 5. Comparative root mean square deviations (RMSDs) of the Cα carbon atoms of the compounds in whole systems for MAO-B (**A**) and MAO-A (**B**) and in active sites for MAO-B (**C**) and for MAO-A (**D**). (**A**,**C**) **EH1**, black; **EH6**, green; **EH7**, blue; and **EH8** red. (**B**,**D**) **EH1**, black; **EH6**, red; **EH7**, green; and **EH8**, blue.

Zeroing on structural influence of the ligands on the mechanistic behavior of the active site could provide more clues regarding their activity. The RMSD of the MAO-A and MAO-B active sites upon **EH1**, **EH6**, **EH7**, and **EH8** binding revealed that **EH6** and **EH7** had the highest active site-stabilizing effect on MAO-B, with overall average RMSD_AS values of 1.61 and 1.49 Å, respectively.

The orientation and position of a ligand are considerably indicative of how reactive the ligands can be within the active site. The characteristics of the ligands were therefore investigated. Interestingly, while **EH7** elicited some motional movement within the active site, which made it flexible enough to interact with crucial amino acid residues, it also exhibited good stability—just enough to be adequately anchored for overall binding (Figure 6).

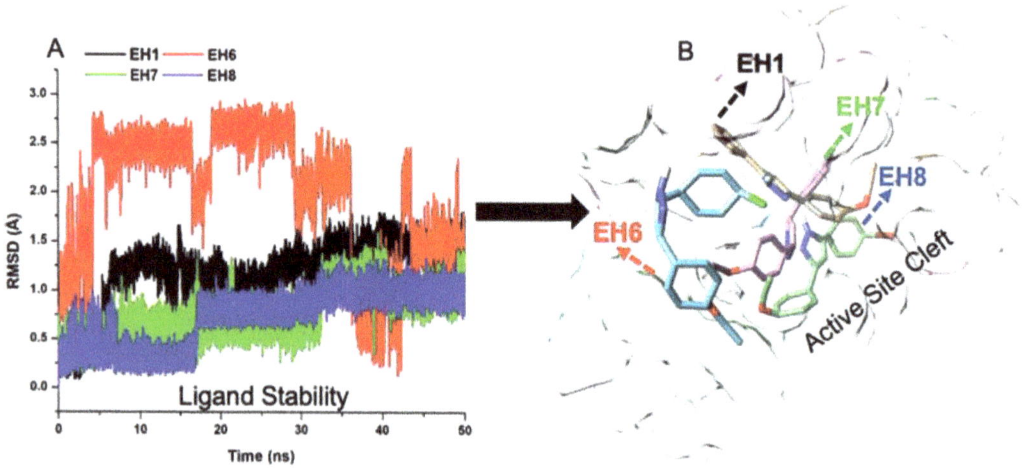

Figure 6. Stability plot of compounds **EH1**, **EH6**, **EH7**, and **EH8**.

2.5.2. **EH7** Exhibited Low Residual Motion and Trajectory Movement upon Binding to MAO-A and MAO-B

Principal component analysis (PCA) is a common molecular dynamic simulation analysis used in the estimation of the essential production run of a system when computed on a low-dimensional free energy space [42]. This estimation is associated with correlated vibrational modes; the translation of the MD trajectory towards the geometric center abolishes the initial rotational and translational movements of the atoms. The decomposition of the trajectory along PC1 and PC2 reveals that upon **EH7** binding to MAO-B, the system exhibits very low diagonalization when compared with other systems (Figure 7A). This further corroborates the results discussed above in the stability section, which attest to the superior activity of **EH7** over other ligands in the series. In contrast, due to the low specificity of **EH1**, **EH6**, **EH7**, and **EH8** towards MAO-A, less high trajectory motion was observed in the ligand-bound MAO-A (Figure 7B).

The root mean square fluctuation (RMSF) computes the residual deviation of a protein over a period of time using a reference position, such as the averaged residual position. RMSF estimates the level of fluctuation of residue from its original position [43]. As depicted in the RMSF plot, the average RMSF values of MAO-B_**EH1**, MAO-B_**EH6**, MAO-B_**EH7**, and MAO-B_**EH8** were 0.88, 0.83, 0.68, and 0.75 Å, respectively (Figure 7C), while those of MAO-A_**EH1**, MAO-A_**EH6**, MAO-A_**EH7**, and MAO-A_**EH8** were 1.47, 1.15, 1.07, and 1.40 Å, respectively (Figure 7D).

2.5.3. Estimation of Free Binding Energies of **EH1**, **EH6**, **EH7**, and **EH8** on MAO-A and MAO-B

The estimation of free binding energy using an MM/PBSA protocol can be employed to gain insight into the models and further obtain the semiquantitative values of their stability. We therefore used a representative snapshot and active site residue decomposition to further explore the time-wise bond interaction occurring between major residues in the active sites of MAO-A/MAO-B and the ligands. MM/PBSA has found useful application in the drug design space used in the estimation of binding affinity between ligands and biomolecules [44].

As indicated in Table 4, **EH7** had higher binding affinity (−36.29 kcal/mol) towards MAO-B than the other ligands, while the binding of **EH1**, **EH6**, and **EH8** was recorded to be −4.11, −11.5, and −5.48 kcal/mol, respectively. Of note is the surprising high binding affinity (−32.55 kcal/mol) of **EH7** for MAO-A. This could be due to the high electronegativity potential of fluorine, which is characteristic of compound **EH7**. In agreement with the IC_{50}, the binding affinity of the compounds also followed the same trend.

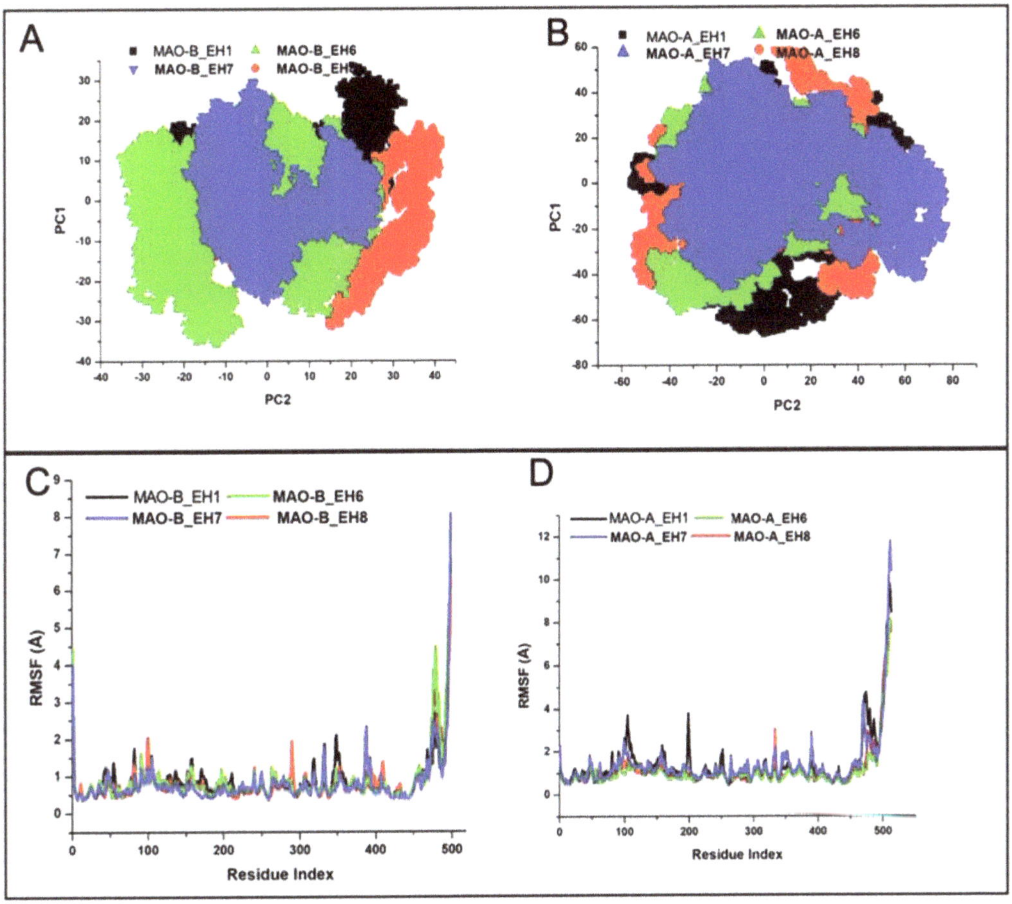

Figure 7. Principal component analysis of the compounds bound to MAO-B (**A**) and to MAO-A (**B**), and root mean square fluctuation (RMSF) of the compounds bound to MAO-B (**C**) and to MAO-A (**D**). (**A**,**B**) **EH1**, black; **EH6**, green; **EH7**, blue; and **EH8**, red. (**C**,**D**) **EH1**, black; **EH6**, green; **EH7**, blue; and **EH8**, red.

The individual energy contributions of the active sites were determined using the MM/PBSA per residue energy decomposition protocol [45]. The high binding energy exhibited by **EH7** was contributed by electrostatic interactions of Arg42, Arg87, Arg98, Lys296, and Lys386, with energy values of −28.4, −12.8, −15.3, −41.9, and −20.6 kcal/mol, respectively (Figure 8C). In the interaction between compound **EH6** and MAO-B, residues Arg42, Gly58, Tyr60, Arg87, Pro98, and Arg100 contributed an electrostatic energy of −2.68, −0.04, −0.12, −15.17, −0.14, and −17.27 kcal/mol, respectively (Figure 8B). Despite the electrostatic interactions and other favorable bonds elicited by **EH1**, **EH6**, and **EH8**, compound **EH7** still had the best binding energy and highest contribution of electrostatic interactions. This behavior may not be unrelated to the impact of fluorine found on compound **EH7**. Furthermore, the energetically favored disposition assumed by **EH7** could be attributed to the hydrogen bond formed between the fluorine of **EH7** and hydrogen of Trp386 (Figure 9C). The ligand interaction profile of the interaction of **EH1** (A), **EH6** (B), **EH7** (C), and **EH8** (D) with MAO-B is shown in Figure 9.

Table 4. The total free binding energy contributions of **EH**, **EH6**, **EH7**, and **EH8**.

Complexes	Energy (kcal/mol)						
	ΔE_{vdW}	ΔE_{ele}	ΔG_{gas}	ΔG_{GB}	ΔG_{SA}	ΔG_{sol}	ΔG_{bind}
MAO-B_**EH1**	−6.68 (±0.19)	−34.66 (±4.28)	−35.32 (±4.20)	35.91 (±3.99)	−1.68 (±0.01)	35.74 (±3.98)	−4.11 (±0.36)
MAO-B_**EH6**	−25.46 (±0.15)	−94.22 (±2.01)	−96.77 (±2.06)	108.35 (±2.64)	−4.28 (±0.01)	107.92 (±2.63)	−11.15 (±0.88)
MAO-B_**EH7**	−36.79 (±0.15)	−32.46 (±0.54)	−85.96 (±0.53)	55.09 (±0.50)	−5.12 (±0.01)	49.67 (±0.50)	−36.29 (±0.13)
MAO-B_**EH8**	−36.79 (±0.15)	−101.78 (±1.73)	−105.46 (±1.74)	106.54 (±1.56)	− 5.35 (±0.01)	106 (±1.56)	−5.48 (±0.37)
MAO-A_**EH1**	−33.17 (±0.22)	−12.98 (±4.07)	−13.31 (±4.20)	−12.85 (±2.86)	−4.65 (±0.01)	12.81 (±2.85)	−5.06 (±1.49)
MAO-A_**EH6**	−36.75 (±0.18)	−14.50 (±2.36)	−14.88 (±2.39)	13.78 (±1.61)	−4.86 (±0.01)	13.73 (±1.61)	−11.33 (±0.97)
MAO-A_**EH7**	−32.75 (±0.15)	−13.21 (±2.06)	−13.54 (±2.06)	−36.79 (±0.15)	−4.85 (±0.01)	13.21 (±1.36)	−32.55 (±1.07)
MAO-A_**EH8**	−7.52 (±0.15)	−12.07 (±2.49)	−12.14 (±2.56)	12.92 (±2.30)	−2.61 (±0.01)	12.89 (±0.15)	−7.48 (±0.15)

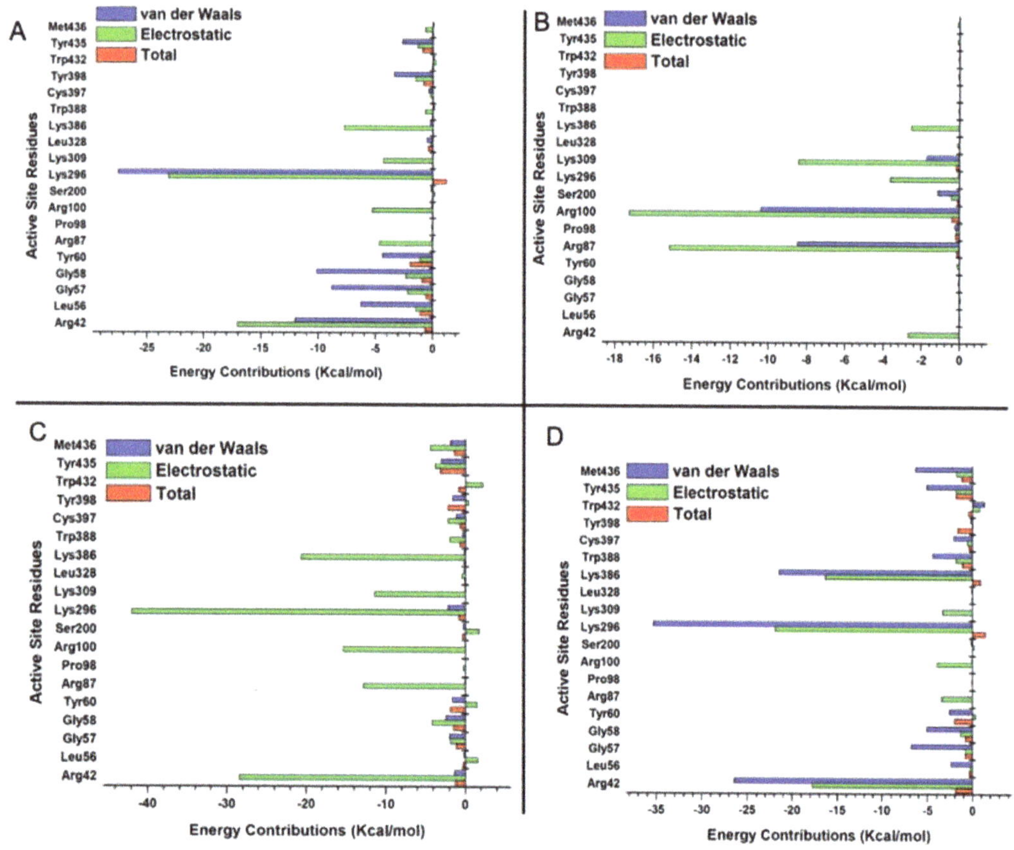

Figure 8. Per residue decomposition of **EH1** bound to MAO-B (**A**), **EH6** bound to MAO-B (**B**), **EH7** bound to MAO-B (**C**), and **EH8** bound to MAO-B (**D**) systems.

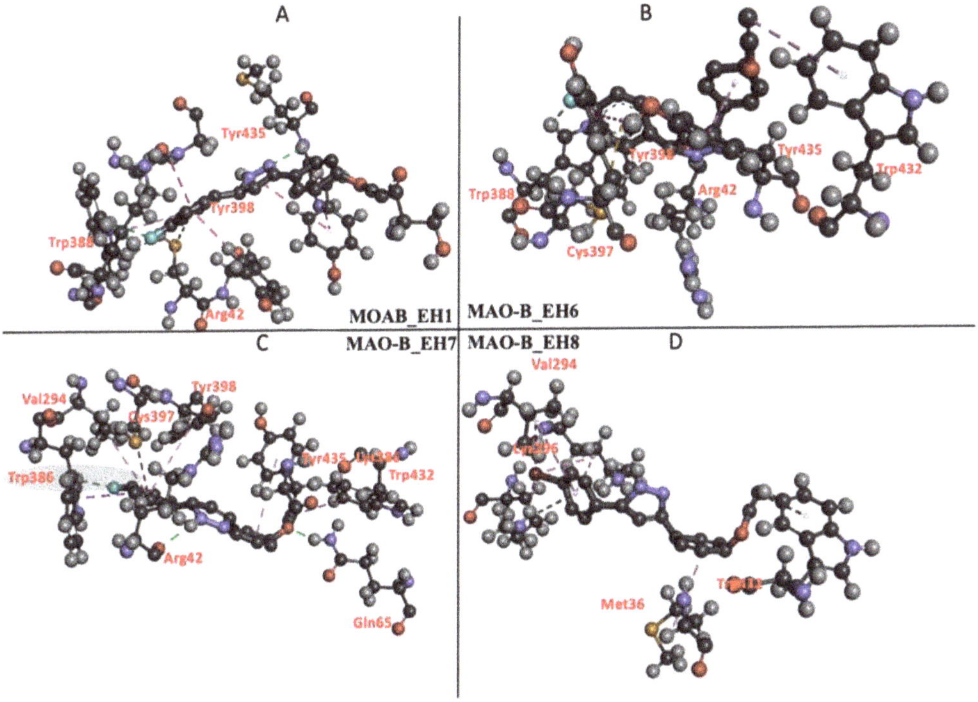

Figure 9. Ligand interaction profile of the interaction of **EH1** (**A**), **EH6** (**B**), **EH7** (**C**), and **EH8** (**D**) with MAO-B.

2.5.4. Estimation of Free Binding Energies of **EH1**, **EH6**, **EH7**, and **EH8** on MAO-A and MAO-B

Since our compounds contain a pyrazoline moiety, it is assumed that they possess an asymmetric carbon atom and, hence, exist as enantiomers. We therefore generated the R and S enantiomers of **EH7** as a representative structure of the compounds, taking into consideration the fact that it has the best IC_{50} and total free energy values. We explored the differential binding and estimated the total free binding energy of the R isomeric form of **EH7** (MAO-B_**EH7**R) and its S counterpart (MAO-B_**EH7**S) using MM/PBSA calculations. Our calculations revealed that MAO-B_**EH7**R and MAO-B_**EH7**S possess binding energies of −36.29 and −36.17 kcal/mol (Table 5). This suggests that the chirality does not change considerably in the overall binding of **EH7** to MAO-B. However, MAO-B_**EH7**S has more van der Waals interactions than MAO-B_**EH7**R. Despite having total free binding energy values that are close, dissimilar residues present in the active sites are responsible for the binding interactions. Chiefly among the residues are Tyr435, Tyr398, and Leu328 (jointly shared by MAO-B_**EH7**R), which contribute van der Waals binding energies of −2.93, −1.58, and −1.00 kcal/mol, respectively (Figure 10).

2.6. Target Predicition and ADME Analysis

The biological target and ADME predictions of the lead molecule of **EH7** were assessed by the online web-based program SwissTarget. The lead molecule showed good prediction results on biological targets of MAO and AChE (Figure 11A). The bioavailability radar gave saturation, size, flexibility, insolubility, and polarity of the molecule, which provided a quick judgement of the drug-likeness of the molecule. The lead molecule was recognized to be within the pink region (optimal ranges) and could be considered a compound endowed with drug-like characteristics (Figure 11B). The BOILED-Egg model also predicted the passive human BBB permeation and gastrointestinal absorption (HIA) for the compound

(Figure 11C). The results revealed that **EH7** had comparatively higher probability of BBB and HIA.

Table 5. The differential free binding energy of MAO-B_**EH7**R and MAO-B_**EH7**S enantiomers.

	Energy (kcal/mol)						
Complexes	ΔE_{vdW}	ΔE_{ele}	ΔG_{gas}	ΔG_{GB}	ΔG_{SA}	ΔG_{sol}	ΔG_{bind}
MAO-B_**EH7**R	−36.79 (±0.15)	−32.46 (±0.54)	−85.96 (±0.53)	55.09 (±0.50)	−5.12 (±0.01)	49.67 (±0.50)	−36.2 (±0.13)
MAO-B_**EH7**S	−53.42 (±0.08)	−17.59 (±1.56)	−22.93 (±0.50)	19.88 (±1.49)	−5.62 (±0.01)	19.31 (±0.47)	−36.17 (±0.12)

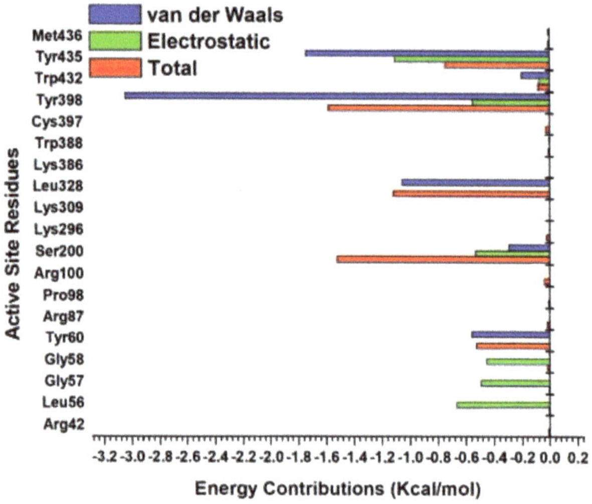

Figure 10. Per residue decomposition of MAO-B_**EH7**S enantiomer.

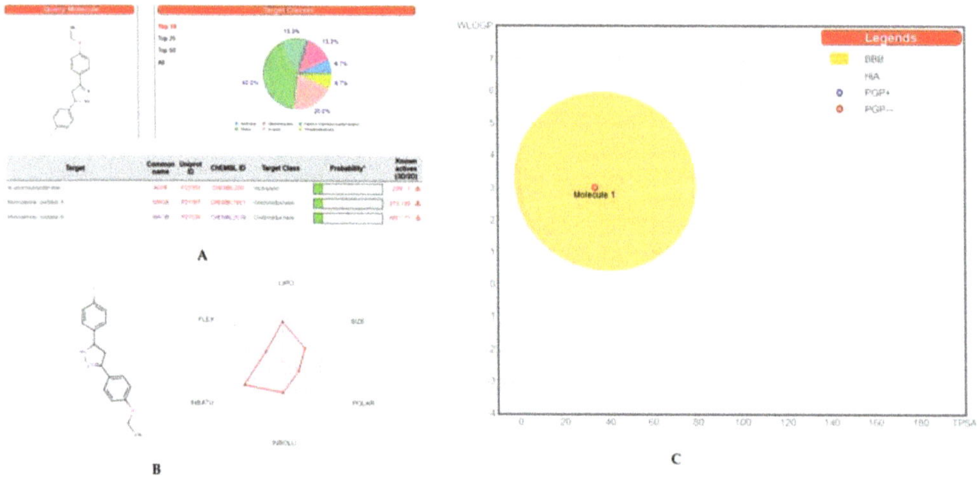

Figure 11. Swiss target/ADME prediction: (**A**) Biological target prediction of lead molecule **EH7**; (**B**) bioavailability radar of **EH7**; (**C**) the BOILED-Egg construction of **EH7**.

3. Materials and Methods

3.1. Synthesis

A series of ethoxylated chalcone (0.0078 M) was refluxed with (0.0629 M) hydrazine hydrate under ethanol medium. After 14–16 h of reflux, the product was cooled, acidified with dil. HCl, washed thoroughly with water, filtered, dried, and recrystallized from ethanol. The progress of the formation of pyrazoline product was monitored by thin-layer chromatography (TLC; ethylacetate–hexane = 1:9). The synthetic route is depicted in Scheme 1.

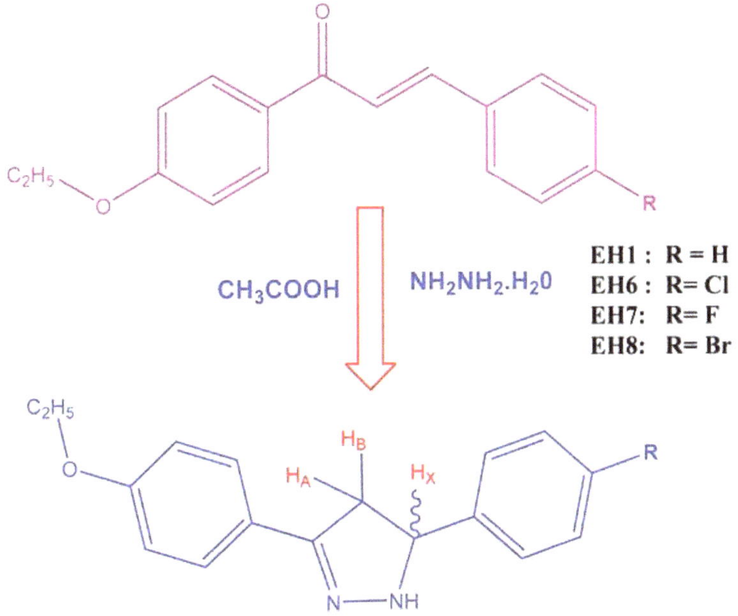

Scheme 1. Synthetic route of the compounds under the present study.

*3-(4-ethoxyphenyl)-5-phenyl-4,5-dihydro-1H-pyrazole (**EH1**)*: ^{1}H NMR (400 MHz, $CDCl_3$) δ: 1.47–1.45 (t, 3H, J = 8.0 Hz, CH_3), 4.15–4.13 (d, 2H, J = 8.0 Hz, CH_2), 3.76 (d, 1H, HA), 4.02 (d, 1H, HB), 5.51 (d, 1H, HX), 7.89–7.10 (d, 9H, ArH), 9.21(S, NH). MS (ESI) m/z calcd. for $C_{17}H_{18}N_2O$: 266.3376, found 266.3345.

*5-(4-chlorophenyl)-3-(4-ethoxyphenyl)-4,5-dihydro-1H-pyrazole (**EH6**)*: ^{1}H NMR (400 MHz, $CDCl_3$) δ: 1.47–1.45 (t, 3H, *J* = 8.0 Hz, CH_3), 4.14–4.12 (D, 2H, *J* = 8.0 Hz, CH_2), 3.75 (d, 1H, HA), 4.01 (d, 1H, HB), 5.51 (d, 1H, HX), 7.99–7.08 (d, 8H, ArH) 9.24 (S, NH). MS (ESI) m/z calcd. for $C_{17}H_{17}N_2OCl$: 284.3280, found 284.3276.

*3-(4-ethoxyphenyl)-5-(4-fluorophenyl)-4,5-dihydro-1H-pyrazole (**EH7**)*: ^{1}H NMR (400 MHz, $CDCl_3$) δ: 1.47–1.45 (t, 3H, *J* = 8.0 Hz, CH_3), 4.15–4.13 (d, 2H, *J* = 8.0 Hz, CH_2), 3.72 (d, 1H, HA), 4.04 (d, 1H, HB), 5.51 (d, 1H, HX), 7.96–7.03 (d, 8H, ArH) 9.23 (S, NH). MS (ESI) m/z calcd. for $C_{17}H_{17}N_2OF$: 266.3376, found 266.3345.

*5-(4-bromophenyl)-3-(4-ethoxyphenyl)-4,5-dihydro-1H-pyrazole (**EH8**)*: ^{1}H NMR (400 MHz, $CDCl_3$) δ: 1.47–1.45 (t, 3H, *J* = 8.0 Hz, CH_3), 4.15–4.13 (q, 2H, *J* = 8.0 Hz, CH_2), 3.76 (d, 1H, HA), 4.02 (d, 1H, HB), 5.51 (d, 1H, HX), 7.89–7.70 (d, 8H, ArH), 9.24(S, NH). $C_{17}H_{17}N_2OBr$: 345.2336, found 345.2340.

3.2. Enzyme Assays

MAO activities were assayed as described previously, using recombinant human MAO-A and MAO-B and kynuramine (0.06 mM) and benzylamine (0.3 mM) as substrates, respectively; both substrate concentrations were 1.5 × K_m (K_m = 0.041 and 0.20 mM, respectively). The enzymes and chemicals were purchased from Sigma-Aldrich (St. Louis, MO, USA) [17].

3.3. Analysis of Enzyme Inhibitions and Kinetics

The inhibitory activities of the four compounds against MAO-A and MAO-B were first observed at a concentration of 10 μM. IC_{50} values for MAO-B by compounds showing residual activities of <50% were determined. Kinetic studies were performed on the most potent inhibitors, i.e., **EH6** and **EH7** for MAO-A and MAO-B, at five concentrations of the substrates and three inhibitor concentrations, as previously described [18].

3.4. Analysis of Inhibitor Reversibilities

Reversibilities of **EH7** were analyzed using a dialysis method after preincubating with MAO-B for 30 min, as previously described. The concentrations used were **EH7** at 0.15 μM, lazabemide (a reversible MAO-B reference inhibitor) at 0.20 μM, and pargyline (an irreversible MAO-B reference inhibitor) at 0.30 μM. The relative activities for undialyzed (A_U) and dialyzed (A_D) samples were compared to determine the reversibility patterns [19].

3.5. Molecular Dynamics Study

The 3D structures of MAO-A (PDB ID: 2Z5X and MAO-B: 2V5Z), hereafter referred to as MAO-A and MAO-B, respectively, were retrieved from the Protein Data Bank (PDB) [46,47]. Molecules that were co-crystallized with MAO-A and MAO-B were deleted with the exception of the co-enzyme FAD. Missing residues were filled with the aid of MODELLER tools found in the graphic user interface of Chimera [48,49]. Marvin Sketch was employed to draw the 2D structures of **EH1**, **EH6**, **EH7**, and **EH8**; afterwards, geometrical and structural optimizations of these ligands were carried out using B3LYP/6-311 ++G (d,p) and the UFF forcefield of Gaussian 16, respectively [50]. Active site identification was achieved by centering the grid box around a co-crystallized ligand found on the MAO-A and MAO-B proteins downloaded from PDB. Molecular docking was then carried out using AutoDock Vina [51]. The systems were then subjected to a simulation run of 50 ns using Amber18 software (San Francisco, CA, USA) [52]. Eight systems were set up for simulation (MAO-A:**EH1**, MAO-A:**EH6**, MAO-A:**EH7**, MAO-A:**EH8**, MAO-B:**EH1**, MAO-B:**EH6**, MAO-B:**EH7**, and MAO-B:**EH8**). The simulation process was carried out in accordance with an in-house protocol. The CPPTRAJ module of Amber18 software was used to analyze the trajectories emanating from the simulation process [53,54].

3.6. Target Predicition and ADME Analysis

The biological target and ADME predictions of the lead molecule of **EH7** were assessed at http://www.swisstargetprediction.ch (access on 23 May 2021) [55,56].

4. Conclusions

A series of four halogenated pyrazolines with ethoxylated heads (**EH1**, **EH6**, **EH7**, and **EH8**) was synthesized from their corresponding chalcones. All four compounds were explored for their MAO-A and MAO-B inhibitory activities. On the basis of previous studies regarding the role of halogens in various scaffolds with MAO inhibition activities, we mainly focused on the effect of various halogens on the pyrazoline core with the ethoxylated head. According to the results of this study, the synthesized halogenated pyrazolines exhibited good selective MAO-B inhibition. Fluorine-containing pyrazoline (**EH7**) exhibited an improved selectivity profile against the MAO-B isoform. Kinetics and reversibility studies revealed that **EH7** is a selective and competitive inhibitor of MAO-B, with a recovery value similar to that of the reversible reference drug lazabemide.

Pyrazolines are said to be optically active compounds, and, from the MM/PBSA values obtained, it can be clearly observed that chirality has minimal influence on the binding of the compound to MAO-B. It may be suggested that the absence of bulky groups on the N1 position of pyrazoline limited the role of chirality in the binding mode of the lead molecule in the current study.

Author Contributions: Conceptualization: L.K.P., B.M., and H.K.; biological activity: J.-M.O., A.K., and M.A.A.; kinetics: J.-M.O.; molecular dynamics: O.S. and M.E.S.; synthesis: A.S.N., V.P.K., S.K., S.T.S., and B.M.; data curation: B.M. and J.-M.O.; writing—original draft preparation: J.-M.O. and B.M.; writing—review and editing: L.K.P., B.M., and H.K.; supervision: H.K.; funding acquisition: H.K. All authors have read and agreed to the published version of the manuscript.

Funding: This study was supported by the National Research Foundation of Korea (NRF) grant provided by the Korean Government (NRF-2019R1A2C1088967 to H. Kim), Republic of Korea, and by a grant from Amrita Vishwa Vidyapeetham University (Seed Grant Number K-PHAR-20-628 to B. Mathew).

Institutional Review Board Statement: Not applicable.

Informed Consent Statement: Not applicable.

Acknowledgments: Authors acknowledge Taif University Researchers Supporting Project number (TURSP-2020/68), Taif University, Taif, Saudi Arabia.

Conflicts of Interest: The authors have no conflict of interest to declare.

Sample Availability: Samples of the compounds are available from the authors.

References

1. Carradori, S.; Petzer, J.P. Novel monoamine oxidase inhibitors: A patent review (2012−2014). *Expert Opin. Ther. Pat.* **2015**, *25*, 91–110. [CrossRef]
2. Youdim, M B.; Bakhle, Y.S. Monoamine oxidase: Isoforms and inhibitors in Parkinson´s disease and depressive illness. *Br. J. Pharm.* **2006**, *147*, S287–S296. [CrossRef]
3. Ramsay, R.R. Inhibitor design for monoamine oxidases. *Curr. Pharm. Des.* **2013**, *19*, 2529–2539. [CrossRef]
4. Tripathi, R.K.P.; Ayyannan, S.R. Monoamine oxidase-B inhibitors as potential neurotherapeutic agents: An overview and update. *Med. Res. Rev.* **2019**, *39*, 1603–1706. [CrossRef] [PubMed]
5. Guglielmi, P.; Carradori, S.; Ammazzalorso, A.; Secci, D. Novel approaches to the discovery of selective human monoamine oxidase-B inhibitors: Is there room for improvement? *Expert Opin. Drug Discov.* **2019**, *14*, 995–1035. [CrossRef] [PubMed]
6. Kumar, B.; Sheetal, S.; Mantha, A.K.; Kumar, V. Recent developments on the structure-activity relationship studies of MAO inhibitors and their role in different neurological disorders. *RSC Adv.* **2016**, *6*, 42660–42683. [CrossRef]
7. Kumar, B.; Gupta, V.P.; Kumar, V. A perspective on monoamine oxidase enzyme as drug target. Challenges and opportunities. *Curr. Drug Targets* **2017**, *18*, 87–97. [CrossRef] [PubMed]
8. Tipton, K. 90 years of monoamine oxidase: Some progress and some confusion. *J. Neural Transm.* **2018**, *125*, 1519–1551. [CrossRef]
9. Leuratti, C.; Sardina, M.; Ventura, P.; Assandri, A.; Muller, M.; Brunner, M. Disposition and metabolism of safinamide, a novel drug for Parkinson's disease, in healthy male volunteers. *Pharmacology* **2013**, *92*, 7–16. [CrossRef]
10. Mao, Q.; Qin, W.; Zhang, A.; Ye, N. Recent advances in dopaminergic strategies for the treatment of Parkinson's disease. *Acta Pharmacol. Sin.* **2020**, *41*, 471–482. [CrossRef]
11. Hagenow, J.; Hagenow, S.; Grau, K.; Khanfar, M.; Hefke, L.; Proschak, E.; Stark, H. Reversible small molecule inhibitors of MAO A and MAO B with anilide motifs. *Drug Des. Dev. Ther.* **2020**, *14*, 371–393. [CrossRef] [PubMed]
12. Mathew, B.; Suresh, J.; Anbazhagan, S.; Mathew, G.E. Pyrazoline. A promising scaffold for the inhibition of monoamine oxidase. *Cent. Nerv. Syst. Agents Med. Chem.* **2013**, *13*, 195–206. [CrossRef] [PubMed]
13. Matos, M.J.; Vina, D.; Vazquez-Rodriquez, S.; Uriarte, E.; Santana, L. Focusing on new monoamine oxidase inhibitors. Differently substituted coumarins as an interesting scaffold. *Curr. Top. Med. Chem.* **2012**, *12*, 2210–2233. [CrossRef] [PubMed]
14. Kavully, F.S.; Oh, J.M.; Dev, S.; Kaipakasseri, S.; Palakkathondi, A.; Vengamthodi, A.; Azeez, R.F.A.; Tondo, A.R.; Nicolotti, O.; Kim, H.; et al. Design of enamides as new selective monoamine oxidase-B inhibitors. *J. Pharm. Pharmacol.* **2020**, *72*, 916–926. [CrossRef] [PubMed]
15. Chimenti, F.; Secci, D.; Bolasco, A.; Chimenti, P.; Bizzarri, B.; Granese, A.; Carradori, S.; Yáñez, M.; Orallo, F.; Ortuso, F.; et al. Synthesis, molecular modeling, and selective inhibitory activity against human monoamine oxidases of 3-carboxamido-7-substituted coumarins. *J. Med. Chem.* **2009**, *52*, 1935–1942. [CrossRef]

16. Gaspar, A.; Texeira, F.; Uriarte, E.; Milhazes, N.; Melo, A.; Cordeiro, M.N.D.S.; Ortuso, F.; Alcaro, S.; Borges, F. Towards the discovery of novel class of monoamine oxidase inhibitors: Structure property activity and docking studies on chromones amides. *Chem. Med. Chem.* **2011**, *6*, 628–632. [CrossRef] [PubMed]
17. Parambi, D.G.T.; Oh, J.M.; Baek, S.C.; Lee, J.P.; Tondo, A.R.; Nicolotti, O.; Hoon, K.; Mathew, B. Design, synthesis and biological evaluation of oxygenated chalcones as potent and selective MAO-B inhibitors. *Bioorg. Chem.* **2019**, *93*, 103335. [CrossRef]
18. Reeta; Baek, S.C.; Lee, J.P.; Rangarajan, T.M.; Ayushee; Singh, R.P.; Singh, M.; Mangiatordi, G.F.; Nicolotti, O.; Kim, H.; et al. Ethyl acetohydroxamate incorporated chalcones: Unveiling a novel class of chalcones for multitarget monoamine oxidase-B inhibitors against Alzheimer's disease. *CNS Neurol. Disord. Drug Targets* **2019**, *8*, 643–654. [CrossRef]
19. Oh, J.M.; Rangarajan, T.M.; Chaudhary, R.; Singh, R.P.; Singh, M.; Singh, R.P.; Tondo, A.R.; Gambacorta, N.; Nicolotti, O.; Mathew, B.; et al. Novel class of chalcone oxime ethers as potent monoamine oxidase-B and acetylcholinesterase inhibitors. *Molecules* **2020**, *25*, 2356. [CrossRef]
20. Mathew, B.; Baek, S.C.; Parambi, D.G.T.; Lee, J.P.; Mathew, G.E.; Jayanthi, S.; Devaraji, D.; Raphael, C.; Vinod, D.; Kondarath, S.S.; et al. Potent and highly selective dual-targeting monoamine oxidase-B inhibitors: Fluorinated chalcones of morpholine versus imidazole. *Arch. Pharm.* **2019**, *352*, e1800309. [CrossRef]
21. Guglielmi, P.; Mathew, B.; Secci, D.; Carradori, S. Chalcones: Unearthing their therapeutic possibility as monoamine oxidase B inhibitors. *Eur. J. Med. Chem.* **2020**, *205*, 112650. [CrossRef] [PubMed]
22. Mathew, B.; Parambi, D.G.T.; Mathew, G.E.; Uddin, M.S.; Inasu, S.T.; Kim, H.; Marathakam, A.; Unnikrishnan, M.K.; Carradori, S. Emerging therapeutic potentials of dual-acting MAO and AChE inhibitors in Alzheimer's and Parkinson's diseases. *Arch. Pharm.* **2019**, *352*, e1900177. [CrossRef] [PubMed]
23. Finberg, J.P.M.; Rabey, J.M. Inhibitors of MAO-A and MAO-B in Psychiatry and Neurology. *Front. Pharmacol.* **2016**, *7*, 340. [CrossRef] [PubMed]
24. Carradori, S.; Silvestri, R. New frontiers in selective human MAO-B inhibitors. *J. Med. Chem.* **2015**, *58*, 6717–6732. [CrossRef] [PubMed]
25. Gaspar, A.; Silva, T.; Yáñez, M.; Viña, D.; Orallo, F.; Ortuso, F.; Uriarte, E.; Alcaro, S.; Borges, F. Chromone, a privileged scaffold for the development of monoamine oxidase inhibition. *J. Med. Chem.* **2011**, *54*, 5165–5173. [CrossRef]
26. Reis, J.; Cagide, F.; Chavarria, D.; Silva, T.B.; Fernandes, C.; Gaspar, A.; Uriarte, E.; Remiao, F.; Alcaro, S.; Ortuso, F.; et al. Discovery of new chemical entities of old targets. Insight on the lead optimization of chromones based monoamine oxidase B inhibitors. *J. Med. Chem.* **2016**, *59*, 5879–5893. [CrossRef]
27. Shaaban, M.R.; Mayhoub, A.S.; Farag, A.M. Recent advances in the therapeutic applications of pyrazolines. *Expert Opin. Ther. Patents* **2012**, *22*, 253–291. [CrossRef]
28. Bansal, R.; Singh, R. Steroidal pyrazolines as a promising scaffold in drug discovery. *Future Med. Chem.* **2020**, *12*, 949–959. [CrossRef]
29. Badavath, V.N.; Baysal, I.; Ucar, G.; Sinha, B.N.; Jayaprakash, V. Monoamine oxidase inhibitory activity of novel pyrazoline analogues: Curcumin based design and synthesis. *ACS Med. Chem. Lett.* **2016**, *7*, 56–61. [CrossRef] [PubMed]
30. Goksen, U.S.; Sarigul, S.; Bultinck, P.; Herrebout, W.; Dogan, I.; Yelekci, K.; Ucar, G.; Gokhan Kelekci, N. Absolute configuration and biological profile of pyrazoline enantiomers as MAO inhibitory activity. *Chirality* **2019**, *31*, 21–33. [CrossRef] [PubMed]
31. Vishnu Nayak, B.; Ciftci-Yabanoglu, S.; Jadav, S.S.; Jagrat, M.; Sinha, B.N.; Ucar, G.; Jayaprakash, V. Monoamine oxidase inhibitory activity of 3,5-biaryl-4,5-dihydro-1H-pyrazole-1-carboxylate derivatives. *Eur. J. Med. Chem.* **2013**, *69*, 762–767. [CrossRef]
32. Tong, X.; Chen, R.; Zhang, T.T.; Han, Y.; Tang, W.J.; Liu, X.H. Design and synthesis of novel 2-pyrazoline-1-ethanone derivatives as selective MAO inhibitors. *Bioorg. Med. Chem.* **2015**, *23*, 515–525. [CrossRef] [PubMed]
33. Evranos-Aksoz, B.; Ucar, G.; Tas, S.T.; Aksoz, E.; Yelekci, K.; Erikci, A.; Sara, Y.; Iskit, A.B. New Human Monoamine Oxidase A Inhibitors with Potential Anti- Depressant Activity: Design, Synthesis, Biological Screening and Evaluation of Pharmacological Activity. *Comb. Chem. High Throughput Screen* **2017**, *20*, 461–473. [CrossRef] [PubMed]
34. Guglielmi, P.; Carradori, S.; Poli, G.; Secci, D.; Cirilli, R.; Rotondi, G.; Chimenti, P.; Petzer, A.; Petzer, J.P. Design, Synthesis, Docking Studies and Monoamine Oxidase Inhibition of a Small Library of 1-acetyl- and 1-thiocarbamoyl-3,5-diphenyl-4,5-dihydro-(1H)-pyrazoles. *Molecules* **2019**, *24*, 484. [CrossRef] [PubMed]
35. Hitge, R.; Smit, S.; Petzer, A.; Petzer, J.P. Evaluation of nitrocatechol chalcone and pyrazoline derivatives as inhibitors of catechol-O-methyltransferase and monoamine oxidase. *Bioorg. Med. Chem. Lett.* **2020**, *30*, 127188. [CrossRef]
36. Bolasco, A.; Carradori, S.; Fioravanti, R. Focusing on new monoamine oxidase inhibitors. *Expert Opin. Ther. Patents* **2010**, *20*, 909–939. [CrossRef]
37. Fang, W.Y.; Ravindar, L.; Rakesh, K.P.; Manukumar, H.M.; Shantharam, C.S.; Alharbi, N.S.; Qin, H.L. Synthetic approaches and pharmaceutical application of chlorine containing molecules for drug discovery: A critical review. *Eur. J. Med. Chem.* **2019**, *173*, 117–153. [CrossRef]
38. Mathew, B.; Carradori, S.; Guglielmi, P.; Uddin, M.S.; Kim, H. New aspects of monoamine oxidase B inhibitors. The key role of halogens to open the golden door. *Curr. Med. Chem.* **2021**, *28*, 266–283. [CrossRef]
39. Lakshminarayanan, B.; Baek, S.C.; Lee, J.P.; Kannappan, N.; Mangiatordi, G.F.; Nicolotti, O.; Subburaju, T.; Kim, H.; Mathew, B. Ethoxylated head of chalcones as a new class of multi-targeted MAO inhibitors. *ChemistrySelect* **2019**, *4*, 6614–6619. [CrossRef]
40. Di, L.; Kerns, E.H.; Fan, K.; McConnell, O.J.; Carter, G.T. High throughput artificial membrane permeability assay for blood-brain barrier. *Eur. J. Med. Chem.* **2003**, *38*, 223–232. [CrossRef]

41. Pitera, J.W. Expected distributions of root-mean-square positional deviations in proteins. *J. Phys. Chem. B.* **2014**, *118*, 6526–6530. [CrossRef]
42. David, C.C.; Jacobs, D.J. Principal component analysis: A method for determining the essential dynamics of proteins. *Methods Mol. Biol.* **2014**, *1084*, 193–226.
43. Martínez, L. Automatic identification of mobile and rigid substructures in molecular dynamics simulations and fractional structural fluctuation analysis. *PLoS ONE* **2015**, *10*, e0119264. [CrossRef]
44. Soremekun, O.S.; Olotu, F.A.; Agoni, C.; Soliman, M.E.S. Drug promiscuity: Exploring the polypharmacology potential of 1, 3, 6-trisubstituted 1, 4-diazepane-7-ones as an inhibitor of the 'god father' of immune checkpoint. *Comput. Biol. Chem.* **2019**, *80*, 433–440. [CrossRef] [PubMed]
45. Tubert-Brohman, I.; Sherman, W.; Repasky, M.; Beuming, T. Improved docking of polypeptides with glide. *J. Chem. Inf. Model.* **2013**, *53*, 1689–1699. [CrossRef]
46. Son, S.Y.; Ma, J.; Kondou, Y.; Yoshimura, M.; Yamashita, E.; Tsukihara, T. Structure of human monoamine oxidase A at 2.2-Å resolution: The control of opening the entry for substrates/inhibitors. *Proc. Natl. Acad. Sci. USA* **2008**, *105*, 5739–5744. [CrossRef] [PubMed]
47. Binda, C.; Wang, J.; Pisani, L.; Caccia, C.; Carotti, A.; Salvati, P.; Edmondson, D.E. Structures of human monoamine oxidase B complexes with selective noncovalent inhibitors: Safinamide and coumarin analogs. *J. Med. Chem.* **2007**, *50*, 5848–5852. [CrossRef]
48. Berman, H.M.; Westbrook, J.; Feng, Z.; Gilliland, G.; Bhat, T.N.; Weissig, H.; Shindyalov, I.N.; Bourne, P.E. The protein data bank. *Nucleic Acids Res.* **2000**, *28*, 235–242. [CrossRef] [PubMed]
49. Pettersen, E.F.; Goddard, T.D.; Huang, C.C.; Couch, G.S.; Greenblatt, D.M.; Meng, E.C.; Ferrin, T.E. UCSF Chimera—A visualization system for exploratory research and analysis. *J. Comput. Chem.* **2004**, *25*, 1605–1612. [CrossRef] [PubMed]
50. Weedbrook, C.; Pirandola, S.; García-Patrón, R.; Cerf, N.J.; Ralph, T.C.; Shapiro, J.H.; Lloyd, S. Gaussian Quantum Information. *Rev. Mod. Phys.* **2012**, *84*, 621. [CrossRef]
51. Morris, G.M.; Goodsell, D.S.; Pique, M.E.; Lindstrom, L.; Heuy, R.; Forli, S.; Hart, W.E.; Halliday, S.; Belew, R.; Olson, A.J. AutoDock Version 4.2. User Guide. 2009, pp. 1–49. Available online: http://autodock.scripps.edu/faqs-help/manual/autodock-4-2-user-guide/AutoDock4.2_UserGuide.pdf (accessed on 27 May 2021).
52. Lee, T.S.; Cerutti, D.S.; Mermelstein, D.; Lin, C.; LeGrand, S.; Giese, T.J.; Roitberg, A.; Case, D.A.; Walker, R.C.; York, D.M. GPU-Accelerated Molecular Dynamics and Free Energy Methods ion Amber18: Performance Enhancements and New Features. *J. Chem. Inf. Model.* **2018**, *58*, 2043–2050. [CrossRef] [PubMed]
53. Soremekun, O.S.; Olotu, F.A.; Agoni, C.; Soliman, M.E.S. Recruiting monomer for dimer formation: Resolving the antagonistic mechanisms of novel immune check point inhibitors against Programmed Death Ligand-1 in cancer immunotherapy. *Mol. Simul.* **2019**, *45*, 777–789. [CrossRef]
54. Soremekun, O.S.; Soliman, M.E.S. From genomic variation to protein aberration: Mutational analysis of single nucleotide polymorphism present in ULBP6 gene and implication in immune response. *Comput. Biol. Med.* **2019**, *111*, 103354. [CrossRef] [PubMed]
55. Daina, A.; Michielin, O.; Zoete, V. SwissTargetPrediction: Updated data and new features for efficient prediction of protein targets of small molecules. *Nucleic Acids Res.* **2019**, *47*, W357–W364. [CrossRef] [PubMed]
56. Daina, A.; Zoete, V. A boiled-egg too predict gastrointestinal absorption and brain penetration of small molecules. *Chem. Med. Chem.* **2016**, *11*, 1117–1121. [CrossRef] [PubMed]

molecules

Article

Cardiometabolic Risk Factors in Rosuvastatin-Treated Men with Mixed Dyslipidemia and Early-Onset Androgenic Alopecia

Robert Krysiak *, Marcin Basiak and Bogusław Okopień

Department of Internal Medicine and Clinical Pharmacology, Medical University of Silesia, 40-752 Katowice, Poland; mbasiak@sum.edu.pl (M.B.); mbkdokop@mp.pl (B.O.)
* Correspondence: r.krysiak@interia.pl; Tel./Fax: +48-322-523-902

Abstract: Men with early-onset androgenetic alopecia are characterized by hormonal profiles similar to those observed in women with polycystic ovary syndrome. The purpose of this research was to investigate levels of cardiometabolic risk factors in 3-hydroxy-3-methylglutaryl coenzyme A (HMG-CoA)-treated men with early-onset androgenic alopecia. We studied two matched rosuvastatin-treated groups of men with mixed dyslipidemia: subjects with early-onset androgenic alopecia (group A) and subjects with normal hair growth (group B). Plasma lipids, glucose homeostasis markers, and levels of sex hormones, uric acid, hsCRP, homocysteine, fibrinogen, and 25-hydroxyvitamin D were measured before entering the study and six months later. Both groups differed in insulin sensitivity and levels of calculated bioavailable testosterone, dehydroepiandrosterone-sulfate, uric acid, hsCRP, fibrinogen, and 25-hydroxyvitamin D. Though observed in both study groups, treatment-induced reductions in total cholesterol, LDL cholesterol, hsCRP, and fibrinogen were more pronounced in group B than group A. Moreover, only in group A did rosuvastatin deteriorate insulin sensitivity, and only in group B did the drug affect uric acid, homocysteine, and 25-hydroxyvitamin D. The impact of rosuvastatin on cardiometabolic risk factors correlated with insulin sensitivity, calculated bioavailable testosterone, and dehydroepiandrosterone-sulfate. The obtained results suggest that men with early-onset androgenic alopecia may benefit to a lesser degree from rosuvastatin treatment than their peers.

Keywords: androgenetic alopecia; 3-hydroxy-3-methylglutaryl coenzyme A reductase inhibitors; mixed dyslipidemia; risk factors

Citation: Krysiak, R.; Basiak, M.; Okopień, B. Cardiometabolic Risk Factors in Rosuvastatin-Treated Men with Mixed Dyslipidemia and Early-Onset Androgenic Alopecia. *Molecules* **2021**, *26*, 2844. https://doi.org/10.3390/molecules26102844

Academic Editors: Alicja Nowaczyk and Grzegorz Grześk

Received: 17 April 2021
Accepted: 10 May 2021
Published: 11 May 2021

1. Introduction

The presence of polycystic ovary syndrome (PCOS) in women is associated with an increased arterial stiffness, increased carotid intima-media thickness, endothelial dysfunction, thrombotic complications, cerebrovascular events, and possibly also cardiovascular events [1]. Compared with brothers of healthy women, brothers of women with PCOS are characterized by increased levels of two-hours post-challenge glucose, increased values of insulin resistance markers, and higher values of systolic blood pressure, as well as higher prevalences of impaired glucose tolerance, metabolic syndrome, and type 2 diabetes [2–8]. Brothers of PCOS probands are also characterized by elevated levels of dehydroepiandrosterone-sulfate (DHEA-S) levels and lower concentrations of bioavailable testosterone [5–7]. Therefore, it is reasonable to assume that male relatives of PCOS probands should be screened, identified, and appropriately treated [9,10].

Interestingly, a very similar hormonal profile to that observed in male siblings of women with PCOS was reported in men with early-onset androgenic alopecia. The prevalence of androgenic alopecia increases with age, and it is estimated that up 30% of Caucasian men have androgenic alopecia by the age of 30, and 80% of Caucasian men are affected by this disorder in the course of their life [11,12]. The classic male-pattern of hair loss involves the temporal and vertex region while leaving a rim of hair at the sides and sparing the occipital region [12]. Male pattern hair loss probably results from both genetic susceptibility and excessive androgen action [13]. The estimated heritability of early-onset androgenic alopecia in men is about 80%, while genetic variability in the androgen receptor gene and ectodysplasin A2 receptor gene is a prerequisite for the development of this disorder [9,13]. Compared with control subjects, men with early androgenetic alopecia have shown increased levels of testosterone, DHEA-S, LH, and prolactin; decreased levels of FSH and sex hormone-binding globulin; and increased values of the free androgen index and the LH/FSH ratio [14]. In comparison with healthy subjects, the risk of metabolic syndrome was found to be 2.3 times higher in men with early-onset androgenetic alopecia [15]. There is also evidence that early-onset androgenic alopecia is associated with obesity, insulin resistance, dyslipidemia, hypertension, and atherosclerosis [10]. Genetic, hormonal, and metabolic similarities to PCOS mean that early-onset androgenic alopecia is regarded as a male equivalent of PCOS [16].

The results of a recent study indicated that cardiometabolic effects of atorvastatin are less pronounced in brothers of women with polycystic ovary syndrome than in the male siblings of unaffected women [17]. Moreover, high-dose treatment with rosuvastatin, the latest and the most potent statin that is currently available on the market and frequently used in clinical practice, was found to reduce circulating testosterone levels but not to affect levels of DHEA-S in men with coronary artery disease [18]. Because no previous study has investigated statin action in subjects with male-pattern hair loss, the purpose of this study was to investigate whether early-onset androgenic alopecia determines the impact of rosuvastatin therapy on cardiometabolic risk factors in men with mixed dyslipidemia.

2. Results

At study entry, there were no differences between both groups in age, smoking, body mass index, and blood pressure, as well as in the plasma levels of total cholesterol, LDL cholesterol, HDL cholesterol, triglycerides, glucose, estradiol, and homocysteine. Both groups differed in HOMA1-IR and levels of calculated bioavailable testosterone, DHEA-S, uric acid, hsCRP, and fibrinogen, which were higher in group A than in group B, as well as in 25-hydroxyvitamin D, which was higher in group B than in group A (Tables 1 and 2).

Table 1. Baseline characteristics of patients.

Variable	Group A [a]	Group B [b]	*p*-Value (Group A vs. Group B)
Number (n)	25	25	-
Age (years; mean (SD))	30 (5)	31 (5)	0.4829
Smokers (%)	32	28	-
Body mass index (kg/m^2; mean (SD))	28.9 (4.3)	28.7 (4.6)	0.8745
Systolic blood pressure (mmHg; mean (SD))	131 (14)	129 (15)	0.62828
Systolic blood pressure (mmHg; mean (SD))	85 (6)	84 (6)	0.5585

[a] Men with early-onset androgenic alopecia. [b] Control men.

Rosuvastatin did not result in serious adverse events, and all patients completed the study. Body mass index and blood pressure remained at a similar level throughout the study.

In both study groups, rosuvastatin decreased the levels of total cholesterol, LDL-cholesterol, hsCRP, and fibrinogen. Treatment-induced changes in total and LDL cholesterol, hsCRP, and fibrinogen were more pronounced in group B than group A. Rosuvastatin increased HOMA1-IR exclusively in group A, while the drug only reduced levels of triglycerides, uric acid and homocysteine and increased levels of HDL cholesterol, and 25-hydroxyvitamin D only in group B. Rosuvastatin treatment did not affect glucose, DHEA-S, total testosterone, bioavailable testosterone, estradiol, and the estimated glomerular filtration rate. After six months of treatment, there were differences between both groups in total cholesterol, LDL cholesterol, HOMA1-IR, DHEA-S, calculated bioavailable testosterone, uric acid, hsCRP, homocysteine, fibrinogen, and 25-hydroxyvitamin (Table 2).

Table 2. The effect of rosuvastatin on plasma lipids, glucose homeostasis markers, hormones, and the investigated cardiometabolic risk factors in young men with mixed dyslipidemia.

Variable	Group A [a]	Group B [b]	*p*-Value (Group A vs. Group B)
Total cholesterol (mg/dL; mean (SD))			
At the beginning of the study	262 (32)	267 (35)	0.6005
At the end of the study	216 (28)	196 (25) *	0.0105
p-value (post-treatment vs. baseline)	<0.0001	<0.0001	-
LDL cholesterol (mg/dL; mean (SD))			
At the beginning of the study	167 (23)	171 (26)	0.5672
At the end of the study	124 (20)	103 (15) *	0.0001
p-value (post-treatment vs. baseline)	<0.0001	<0.0001	-
HDL cholesterol (mg/dL; mean (SD))			
At the beginning of the study	43 (7)	42 (7)	0.6158
At the end of the study	46 (8)	48 (8) *	0.3812
p-value (post-treatment vs. baseline)	0.1647	0.0069	-
Triglycerides (mg/dL; mean (SD))			
At the beginning of the study	240 (62)	252 (58)	0.4832
At the end of the study	218 (51)	195 (43) *	0.0912
p-value (post-treatment vs. baseline)	0.177	0.0003	-
Glucose (mg/dl; mean (SD))			
At the beginning of the study	95 (10)	93 (12)	0.5251
At the end of the study	97 (11)	93 (8)	0.148
p-value (post-treatment vs. baseline)	0.5044	1	-
HOMA1-IR (mean (SD))			
At the beginning of the study	3.4 (0.7)	3.0 (0.6)	0.035
At the end of the study	3.9 (0.8) *	2.8 (0.7)	< 0.0001
p-value (post-treatment vs. baseline)	0.0228	0.2835	-
DHEA-S (μmol/L; mean (SD))			
At the beginning of the study	4.8 (0.9)	4.1 (1.0)	0.0123
At the end of the study	5.0 (1.2)	4.2 (1.1)	0.0177
p-value (post-treatment vs. baseline)	0.5082	0.7381	-
Total testosterone (nmol/L; mean (SD))			
At the beginning of the study	20.8 (6.4)	17.9 (6.0)	0.1049
At the end of the study	20.4 (7.2)	16.8 (5.8)	0.0574
p-value (post-treatment vs. baseline)	0.8364	0.5131	-
Calculated bioavailable testosterone			
(nmol/L; mean (SD))	8.09 (2.11)	6.31 (1.98)	0.0035
At the beginning of the study	8.26 (2.28)	6.02 (2.06)	0.0007
At the end of the study	0.7856	0.6141	-
p-value (post-treatment vs. baseline)			
Estradiol (pmol/L; mean (SD))			
At the beginning of the study	140 (29)	148 (32)	0.359
At the end of the study	135 (25)	143 (34)	0.348
p-value (post-treatment vs. baseline)	0.5169	0.5982	-
Uric acid (mg/dL; mean (SD))			
At the beginning of the study	4.9 (1.3)	4.2 (1.0)	0.038
At the end of the study	4.7 (1.2)	3.6 (1.0) *	0.001
p-value (post-treatment vs. baseline)	0.1641	0.0391	-
hsCRP (mg/L; mean (SD))			
At the beginning of the study	3.4 (0.9)	2.8 (0.8)	0.0162
At the end of the study	2.8 (0.9)	1.8 (0.7) *	0.0001
p-value (post-treatment vs. baseline)	0.0225	< 0.0001	-
Fibrinogen (mg/dL; mean (SD))			
At the beginning of the study	375 (82)	329 (64)	0.0318
At the end of the study	324 (70)	260 (59) *	0.001
p-value (post-treatment vs. baseline)	0.0221	0.0002	-
Homocysteine (μmol/L; mean (SD))			
At the beginning of the study	24 (8)	25 (9)	0.6798
At the end of the study	20 (7)	15 (6) *	0.0093
p-value (post-treatment vs. baseline)	0.0661	<0.0001	-

Table 2. *Cont.*

Variable	Group A [a]	Group B [b]	*p*-Value (Group A vs. Group B)
25-hydroxyvitamin D (ng/mL; mean (SD))			
At the beginning of the study	25 (10)	32 (10)	0.0169
At the end of the study	27 (8)	38 (9) *	<0.0001
p-value (post-treatment vs. baseline)	0.6446	0.0305	-
Estimated glomerular filtration rate (ml/min/1.73 m^2; mean (SD))			
At the beginning of the study	92 (15)	93 (16)	0.8206
At the end of the study	92 (13)	94 (14)	0.6031
p-value (post-treatment vs. baseline)	1	0.8151	-

[a] Men with early-onset androgenic alopecia. [b] Control men. * The impact of rosuvastatin (percent changes from baseline after adjustment for baseline values) stronger than in the second group.

At entry, total cholesterol and LDL cholesterol correlated with levels of uric acid, hsCRP, homocysteine, and fibrinogen (group A: r values between 0.24 ($p = 0.0499$) and 0.40 ($p = 0.0011$); group B: r values between 0.30 ($p = 0.0345$) and 0.47 ($p = 0.0001$)), and there were inversely correlated with levels of 25-hydroxyvitamin D (group A: r = −0.32 ($p = 0.0285$) and r = −0.41 ($p = 0.0007$); group B: r = −0.35 ($p = 0.0122$) and r = −0.44 ($p = 0.0002$)). Moreover, there were positive correlations between HDL cholesterol and 25-hydroxyvitamin D (group A: r = 0.48 ($p < 0.0001$); group B: r = 0.50 ($p < 0.0001$), triglycerides or HOMA1-IR and hsCRP and fibrinogen (group A: r values between 0.26 ($p = 0.0385$) and 0.47 ($p = 0.0001$); group B: r values between 0.29 ($p = 0.0403$) and 0.49 ($p = 0.0001$)), and there were inverse correlations between triglycerides or HOMA1-IR and 25-hydroxyvitamin D (group A: r = −0.35 ($p = 0.0071$) and r = −0.43 ($p = 0.0008$); group B: r = −0.41 ($p = 0.0014$) and r = −0.49 ($p < 0.0001$)), as well as between HDL cholesterol and hsCRP and fibrinogen (group A: r = −0.34 ($p = 0.0087$) and r = −0.40 ($p = 0.0025$); group B: r = −0.39 ($p = 0.0037$) and r = −0.47 ($p = 0.0001$)). Treatment-induced changes in uric acid, hsCRP, fibrinogen, homocysteine, and 25-hydroxyvitamin D inversely correlated with calculated bioavailable testosterone levels (group A: r values between −0.32 ($p = 0.0298$) and −0.42 ($p = 0.0006$); group B: r values between −0.35 ($p = 0.0281$) and −0.48 ($p < 0.0001$)) and DHEA-S (group A: r values between -0.24 ($p = 0.0488$) and −0.37 ($p = 0.0046$); group B: r values between −0.31 ($p = 0.0011$) and −0.47 ($p < 0.0001$)). All other correlations were not significant.

3. Discussion

In comparison with the control subjects, men with androgenic alopecia had increased plasma concentrations of DHEA-S and increased levels of calculated bioavailable testosterone. Because of the exclusion criteria and selection procedure, these findings could not be attributed to differences in body mass index, blood pressure, plasma lipids, concomitant disorders, or drug interactions. The hormonal profile of individuals with early-onset alopecia differed from that observed in the male siblings of PCOS probands, in whom elevated concentrations of DHEA-S coexisted with lower levels of calculated bioavailable testosterone [17]. Unlike bioavailable testosterone, in both studies, mean total testosterone levels were similar to those observed in control groups. This discrepancy may be explained by the fact that bioavailable testosterone (denoting the sum of the free and free weakly bound testosterone) calculated by Vermeulen's formula (used in the current study) correlates with free testosterone levels when assessed by equilibrium dialysis [19,20]. Because only unbound testosterone binds the androgen receptor in target tissues in order to exert its activity, the obtained results seem clinically relevant. Under physiological conditions, DHEA-S is converted to testosterone by three enzymes: steroid sulfatase, 3β-hydroxysteroid dehydrogenase, and 17β-hydroxysteroid dehydrogenase type 3 [21,22]. Therefore, it is possible that in brothers of PCOS women, but not in men with early-onset androgenic alopecia, the activity of at least one these enzymes is slightly disturbed. In addition to increased levels of HOMA1-IR, uric acid, and hsCRP and a decreased concentration of 25-hydroxyvitamin D, as observed in both brothers of PCOS probands and men with early-onset alopecia, individuals with early-onset alopecia were characterized by elevated levels of fibrinogen. Interestingly, fibrinogen levels were found to correlate with the incidence rates of myocardial infarction and stroke and with cardiovascular mortality, while the risk of coronary artery disease in individuals with hyperfibrinogenemia was comparable to or higher than that in subjects with elevated total cholesterol levels [23]. Based on the obtained results, at least three conclusions may be drawn. Firstly, from the phenotype point of view, men with early-onset androgenic alopecia and male siblings of women with PCOS represent different clinical entities or constitute different spectra of the same entity. Secondly, they may differ in cardiometabolic risk, which seems to be higher in subjects with alopecia. Finally, because men with early-onset androgenic alopecia were more insulin-resistant than body mass index-, plasma lipid- and blood pressure-matched peers, this state may predispose subjects to type 2 diabetes, metabolic syndrome, and other conditions associated with insulin resistance.

The current study also showed that subjects with alopecia differed from the control group in the impact of rosuvastatin on lipids, insulin sensitivity, and levels of cardiometabolic risk factors. Individuals with early-onset alopecia were characterized by less pronounced changes in plasma lipids and cardiometabolic risk factors, as well as by a potentially unfavorable effect on insulin sensitivity. These findings indicate that men with early-onset male-pattern hair loss may benefit to a lesser degree from rosuvastatin therapy than subjects with normal hair growth, at least in the primary prevention of cardiovascular disease. This observation is of clinical significance because early-onset androgenic alopecia can be easily diagnosed based on anamnesis and basic clinical signs.

There are different possible explanations for dimorphism in rosuvastatin action between both study groups. Some our observations seemed to indicate that they are probably partially related to differences in insulin sensitivity. Both groups differed in baseline HOMA1-IR and in the impact of rosuvastatin on HOMA1-IR, present only in men with alopecia. Moreover, treatment-induced changes in circulating levels of uric acid, hsCRP, fibrinogen, homocysteine, and 25-hydroxyvitamin D levels correlated with HOMA1-IR. If this explanation is accurate, non-pharmacological treatment or metformin may restore the pleiotropic effects of rosuvastatin in subjects with early-onset androgenic alopecia, and we intend to verify this hypothesis in our future studies. Despite numerous clinical cardiovascular benefits of 3-hydroxy-3-methylglutaryl coenzyme A (HMG-CoA) reductase inhibitors in type 2 diabetes, statin therapy is associated with a slightly increased risk of developing new-onset diabetes [24]. Considering the results of our study, this risk may be higher in men with early-onset androgenic alopecia than in other groups of patients with indications for treatment with HMG-CoA reductase inhibitors.

According to another explanation, dimorphism in the lipid-lowering and extra-lipid effects of statins may be associated with differences in the baseline levels of endogenous androgens, particularly testosterone. Over the entire study period, the levels of DHEA-S and calculated bioavailable testosterone were higher in subjects with early-onset androgenic alopecia than in individuals without it, while the impact of rosuvastatin on all assessed cardiometabolic risk factors correlated with calculated bioavailable testosterone and, though to a lesser extent, with DHEA-S. Because HMG-CoA reductase inhibitors do not affect androgen levels [18], except for high-dose statin therapy, between-group differences in the impact of rosuvastatin cannot be attributed to their effect on plasma androgens. They are also not associated with differences in the conversion of androgens to estrogens because estradiol levels were similar in both study groups. It is much more probable that statins and testosterone may interact at the level of conversion of HMG-CoA to mevalonate. The pleiotropic properties of statins result from their inhibitory effect on the biosynthesis of some isoprenoids, particularly farnesyl pyrophosphate and geranylgeranyl pyrophosphate, that play essential roles in the posttranslational modification of numerous key proteins that act as molecular switches (especially Ras, Rac, and Rho) [25]. This mechanism may be attenuated by high testosterone levels. Even a single dose of exogenous testosterone was found to induce the expression of HMG-CoA reductase [26]. Moreover, testosterone has recently been shown to increase levels of key enzymes of the mevalonate pathway, and its high levels may stimulate the posttranslational prenylation and farnesylation of numerous small signaling proteins [27].

This study had some study limitations that require consideration. The study population exceeded the required sample size, but due to a relatively small number of participants, our findings should be verified in a large prospective study. We did not investigate hard clinical endpoints, such as morbidity and mortality rates. The study design did not allow us to conclude whether the obtained results may be explained by a "class effect" of HMG-CoA reductase inhibitors or only characterize rosuvastatin or some statins. Finally, because the study included only men with normal glucose homeostasis or prediabetes, it cannot be totally ruled out that the impact of rosuvastatin is different in individuals with coexisting type 2 diabetes.

In conclusion, compared with age-, body mass index-, and blood pressure-matched subjects with isolated mixed dyslipidemia, men with early-onset androgenic alopecia were characterized by impaired insulin sensitivity; elevated levels of DHEA-S, calculated bioavailable testosterone, uric acid, hsCRP, and fibrinogen; and lower levels of 25-hydroxyvitamin D. In addition to less expressed lipid-lowering properties, men with early-onset androgenic alopecia were characterized by less pronounced cardiometabolic effects of rosuvastatin. Contrary to the control subjects, the rosuvastatin treatment of men with alopecia deteriorated insulin sensitivity. The obtained results suggest that men with early-onset androgenic alopecia may benefit from rosuvastatin treatment to a lesser degree than other subjects with mixed dyslipidemia.

4. Materials and Methods

The study was conducted in accordance with the 1964 Helsinki Declaration and its later amendments. The experimental protocol was reviewed and approved by the Institutional Review Board. All participants provided written informed consent prior to enrolment in the study.

4.1. Patients

We studied two groups of young men (aged 18–35 years) with mixed dyslipidemia, defined as total cholesterol levels above 200 mg/dL, low-density lipoprotein (LDL) cholesterol levels above 115 mg/dL, and triglyceride levels of more than 150 mg/dL, despite complying with the lifestyle modification for more than 3 months before entering the study. Group A included 25 individuals with early-onset androgenic alopecia, while group B (which was a control group) included 25 matched men with isolated mixed dyslipidemia. Early-onset androgenic alopecia was defined as grade 3 vertex or more alopecia on the Hamilton and Norwood scale, which is used to classify the stages of male pattern baldness as diagnosed before the age of 30 years [28,29].

The study population was selected among a larger group of subjects with mixed dyslipidemia (n = 112), diagnosed and treated in our department. A power calculation using 80% power and a type I error of 0.05 indicated that at least 23 individuals would need to be enrolled in each group to detect a 20% difference in the effects of treatment on the measured cardiometabolic risk factors between the groups. The selection procedure, performed using the freely available PEPI-for-Windows computer program, was intended to obtain two groups matched for age, blood pressure, and body mass index. To minimize the impact of seasonal fluctuations in the study outcomes, similar numbers of participants were included in January or February (n = 26) and in July and August (n = 24).

The exclusion criteria were as follows: cardiovascular disease (with the exception of mild arterial hypertension), impaired renal or hepatic function, diabetes, thyroid disorders or other endocrine disorders, acute and chronic inflammatory processes, malabsorption syndromes, any other serious disorder, and any pharmacotherapy.

4.2. Study Design

Rosuvastatin was administered at a dose of 10 mg once daily at bedtime for 6 months. All participants were also given detailed advice about how to achieve the goals of lifestyle modification, which were a total fat intake of less than 30% of total energy intake, a saturated fat intake of less than 7% of energy consumed, a cholesterol intake of less than 200 mg per day, and an increase in fiber intake to 15 g per 1000 kcal. They were also recommended to do at least 150 min of moderate-intensity aerobic physical activity per week, as well as muscle-strengthening activities that were of moderate intensity and involved all major muscle groups on two or more days a week. Medication adherence was assessed every 6 weeks by means of a four-item Morisky–Green test and by pill count.

4.3. Laboratory Assays

All laboratory assays were carried out at baseline and 6 months later. Venous blood samples for laboratory were collected between 7.00 and 8.00 a.m. after 12-h overnight fasting in a quiet and air-conditioned room (constant temperature of 23–24 °C), and they were assessed in duplicate. Standard laboratory techniques were used to measure plasma glucose levels, plasma lipids (total cholesterol, LDL cholesterol, HDL cholesterol, and triglycerides), uric acid, and creatinine (Roche Diagnostics, Basel, Switzerland). The plasma levels of insulin, DHEA-S, total testosterone, estradiol, sex-hormone binding globulin, homocysteine, and 25-hydroxyvitamin D were assayed by direct chemiluminescence using acridinium ester technology (ADVIA Centaur XP Immunoassay System, Siemens Healthcare Diagnostics, Munich, Germany). The plasma levels of high-sensitivity C-reactive protein (hsCRP) were measured using an immunoassay with chemiluminescent detection (Immulite 2000XPi, Siemens Healthcare, Warsaw, Poland), while fibrinogen levels were measured by the Clauss technique using an automated BCS XP analyzer (Siemens Healthcare, Warsaw, Poland). The homeostasis model assessment 1 of insulin resistance index (HOMA1-IR) was calculated by multiplying plasma insulin (mIU/L) by plasma glucose (mg/dL) and dividing that by 405. Bioavailable testosterone was calculated on the basis of total testosterone and sex hormone-binding globulin levels using a freely available online calculator (www.issam.ch/freetesto.htm). The estimated glomerular filtration rate was calculated using the Modification of Diet in Renal Disease equation.

4.4. Statistical Analysis

Outcome variables were log-transformed for analysis to obtain a better approximation of the normal distribution, and they were transformed back for reporting in the tables. All analyses were adjusted for age, smoking, body mass index, and blood pressure as potential confounding factors. Both groups and differences between percent changes from baseline after adjustment for baseline values (reflecting rosuvastatin action) were compared by Student's *t*-tests for independent samples. The differences between the means of variables within the same group were analyzed using Student's paired *t*-test. Qualitative data were compared using the $\chi 2$ test. Correlations were assessed using Pearson's correlation coefficient (r). Two-tailed *p*-values corrected for multiple testing below 0.05 were considered statistically significant.

Author Contributions: R.K. conceived of the study, participated in its design, performed the statistical analysis, and drafted and edited the manuscript. M.B. conducted the literature search, carried out the assays, and performed the statistical analysis. B.O. participated in its design and coordination and provided critical input during manuscript preparations. All authors read and approved the final manuscript.

Funding: The study was supported by the statutory grant of the Medical University of Silesia (PCN-1-185/N/9/O).

Institutional Review Board Statement: The study was conducted according to the guidelines of the Declaration of Helsinki and approved by the Institutional Review Board (the Bioethical Committee of the Medical University of Silesia [KNW/0022/KB/188/16]; 19 October 2016).

Informed Consent Statement: Informed consent was obtained from all subjects involved in the study.

Data Availability Statement: The data that support the findings of this study are available from the corresponding author upon reasonable request.

Conflicts of Interest: The authors declare no conflict of interest.

Sample Availability: Samples of the compounds are not available from authors.

Abbreviations

DHEA-S: dehydroepiandrosterone-sulfate; HDL: high-density lipoproteins; HMG-CoA: 3-hydroxy-3-methylglutaryl coenzyme A; FSH: follicle-stimulating hormone; HOMA1-IR: the homeostasis model assessment 1 of insulin resistance index; hsCRP: high sensitivity C-reactive protein; LDL: low-density lipoproteins; LH: luteinizing hormone; PCOS: polycystic ovary syndrome; SD: standard deviation

References

1. Azziz, R. Polycystic ovary syndrome. *Obstet. Gynecol.* **2018**, *132*, 321–336. [CrossRef] [PubMed]
2. Yilmaz, B.; Vellanki, P.; Ata, B.; Yildiz, B.O. Metabolic syndrome, hypertension, and hyperlipidemia in mothers, fathers, sisters, and brothers of women with polycystic ovary syndrome: A systematic review and meta-analysis. *Fertil. Steril.* **2018**, *109*, 356–364. [CrossRef] [PubMed]
3. Baillargeon, J.P.; Carpentier, A.C. Brothers of women with polycystic ovary syndrome are characterised by impaired glucose tolerance, reduced insulin sensitivity and related metabolic defects. *Diabetologia* **2007**, *50*, 2424–2432. [CrossRef]
4. Sam, S.; Coviello, A.D.; Sung, Y.A.; Legro, R.S.; Dunaif, A. Metabolic phenotype in the brothers of women with polycystic ovary syndrome. *Diabetes Care* **2008**, *31*, 1237–1241. [CrossRef] [PubMed]
5. Karthik, S.; Vipin, V.P.; Kapoor, A.; Tripathi, A.; Shukla, M.; Dabadghao, P. Cardiovascular disease risk in the siblings of women with polycystic ovary syndrome. *Hum. Reprod.* **2019**, *34*, 1559–1566. [CrossRef]
6. Subramaniam, K.; Tripathi, A.; Dabadghao, P. Familial clustering of metabolic phenotype in brothers of women with polycystic ovary syndrome. *Gynecol. Endocrinol.* **2019**, *35*, 601–603. [CrossRef]
7. Coviello, A.D.; Sam, S.; Legro, R.S.; Dunaif, A. High prevalence of metabolic syndrome in first-degree male relatives of women with polycystic ovary syndrome is related to high rates of obesity. *J. Clin. Endocrinol. Metab.* **2009**, *94*, 4361–4366. [CrossRef]
8. Yilmaz, B.; Vellanki, P.; Ata, B.; Yildiz, B.O. Diabetes mellitus and insulin resistance in mothers, fathers, sisters, and brothers of women with polycystic ovary syndrome: A systematic review and meta-analysis. *Fertil. Steril.* **2018**, *110*, 523–533. [CrossRef]
9. Kurzrock, R.; Cohen, P.R. Polycystic ovary syndrome in men: Stein-Leventhal syndrome revisited. *Med. Hypotheses* **2007**, *68*, 480–483. [CrossRef]
10. Cohen, P.R.; Kurzrock, R. Polycystic ovary syndrome in men. *Med. Hypotheses* **2017**, *103*, 64. [CrossRef]
11. Lolli, F.; Pallotti, F.; Rossi, A.; Fortuna, M.C.; Caro, G.; Lenzi, A.; Sansone, A.; Lombardo, F. Androgenetic alopecia: A review. *Endocrine* **2017**, *57*, 9–17. [CrossRef] [PubMed]
12. Kelly, Y.; Blanco, A.; Tosti, A. Androgenetic alopecia: An update of treatment options. *Drugs* **2016**, *76*, 1349–1364. [CrossRef]
13. Lie, C.; Liew, C.F.; Oon, H.H. Alopecia and the metabolic syndrome. *Clin. Dermatol.* **2018**, *36*, 54–61. [CrossRef] [PubMed]
14. Sanke, S.; Chander, R.; Jain, A.; Garg, T.; Yadav, P. A comparison of the hormonal profile of early androgenetic alopecia in men with the phenotypic equivalent of polycystic ovarian syndrome in women. *JAMA Dermatol.* **2016**, *152*, 986–991. [CrossRef] [PubMed]
15. Wu, D.X.; Wu, L.F.; Yang, Z.X. Association between androgenetic alopecia and metabolic syndrome: A meta-analysis. *Zhejiang Da Xue Xue Bao Yi Xue Ban* **2014**, *43*, 597–601.
16. Roth, M.M.; Leader, N.; Kroumpouzos, G. Gynecologic and andrologic dermatology and the metabolic syndrome. *Clin. Dermatol.* **2018**, *36*, 72–80. [CrossRef] [PubMed]
17. Krysiak, R.; Szkróbka, W.; Okopień, B. The impact of atorvastatin on cardiometabolic risk factors in brothers of women with polycystic ovary syndrome. *Pharmacol. Rep.* **2021**, *73*, 261–268. [CrossRef]
18. Krysiak, R.; Okopień, B. The effect of aggressive rosuvastatin treatment on steroid hormone production in men with coronary artery disease. Basic Clin. *Pharmacol. Toxicol.* **2014**, *114*, 330–335.
19. Diver, M. Laboratory measurement of testosterone. *Front. Horm. Res.* **2009**, *37*, 21–31.
20. Ho, C.K.; Stoddart, M.; Walton, M.; Anderson, R.A.; Beckett, G.J. Calculated free testosterone in men: Comparison of four equations and with free androgen index. *Ann. Clin. Biochem.* **2006**, *43*, 389–397. [CrossRef]
21. George, M.M.; New, M.I.; Ten, S.; Sultan, C.; Bhangoo, A. The clinical and molecular heterogeneity of 17βHSD-3 enzyme deficiency. *Horm. Res. Paediatr.* **2010**, *74*, 229–240. [CrossRef] [PubMed]
22. Longcope, C. Dehydroepiandrosterone metabolism. *J. Endocrinol.* **1996**, *150*, S125–S127. [CrossRef] [PubMed]
23. Krysiak, R.; Okopień, B.; Herman, Z. Effects of HMG-CoA reductase inhibitors on coagulation and fibrinolysis processes. *Drugs* **2003**, *63*, 1821–1854. [CrossRef] [PubMed]

24. Laakso, M.; Kuusisto, J. Diabetes secondary to treatment with statins. *Curr. Diab. Rep.* **2017**, *17*, 10. [CrossRef]
25. Greenwood, J.; Steinman, L.; Zamvil, S.S. Statin therapy and autoimmune disease: From protein prenylation to immunomodulation. *Nat. Rev. Immunol.* **2006**, *6*, 358–370. [CrossRef]
26. Gårevik, N.; Skogastierna, C.; Rane, A.; Ekström, L. Single dose testosterone increases total cholesterol levels and induces the expression of HMG CoA reductase. *Subst. Abuse Treat. Prev. Policy* **2012**, *7*, 12. [CrossRef]
27. Mokarram, P.; Alizadeh, J.; Razban, V.; Barazeh, M.; Solomon, C.; Kavousipour, S. Interconnection of estrogen/testosterone metabolism and mevalonate pathway in breast and prostate cancers. *Curr. Mol. Pharmacol.* **2017**, *10*, 86–114.
28. Hamilton, J.B. Patterned loss of hair in man; types and incidence. *Ann. N Y Acad Sci.* **1951**, *53*, 708–728. [CrossRef]
29. Norwood, O.T. Male pattern baldness: Classification and incidence. *South. Med. J.* **1975**, *68*, 1359–1365. [CrossRef]

molecules

MDPI

Article

Serotonergic Neurotransmission System Modulator, Vortioxetine, and Dopaminergic D_2/D_3 Receptor Agonist, Ropinirole, Attenuate Fibromyalgia-Like Symptoms in Mice

Kinga Sałat * and Anna Furgała-Wojas

Department of Pharmacodynamics, Faculty of Pharmacy, Jagiellonian University Medical College, 9 Medyczna St., 30-688 Krakow, Poland; anna.furgala@student.uj.edu.pl
* Correspondence: kinga.salat@uj.edu.pl

Abstract: Fibromyalgia is a disease characterized by lowered pain threshold, mood disorders, and decreased muscular strength. It results from a complex dysfunction of the nervous system and due to unknown etiology, its diagnosis, treatment, and prevention are a serious challenge for contemporary medicine. Impaired serotonergic and dopaminergic neurotransmission are regarded as key factors contributing to fibromyalgia. The present research assessed the effect of serotonergic and dopaminergic system modulators (vortioxetine and ropinirole, respectively) on the pain threshold, depressive-like behavior, anxiety, and motor functions of mice with fibromyalgia-like symptoms induced by subcutaneous reserpine (0.25 mg/kg). By depleting serotonin and dopamine in the mouse brain, reserpine induced symptoms of human fibromyalgia. Intraperitoneal administration of vortioxetine and ropinirole at the dose of 10 mg/kg alleviated tactile allodynia. At 5 and 10 mg/kg ropinirole showed antidepressant-like properties, while vortioxetine had anxiolytic-like properties. None of these drugs influenced muscle strength but reserpine reduced locomotor activity of mice. Concluding, in the mouse model of fibromyalgia vortioxetine and ropinirole markedly reduced pain. These drugs affected emotional processes of mice in a distinct manner. Hence, these two repurposed drugs should be considered as potential drug candidates for fibromyalgia. The selection of a specific drug should depend on patient's key symptoms.

Keywords: reserpine-induced fibromyalgia model; vortioxetine; ropinirole; serotonin and dopamine in fibromyalgia; mouse

Citation: Sałat, K.; Furgała-Wojas, A. Serotonergic Neurotransmission System Modulator, Vortioxetine, and Dopaminergic D_2/D_3 Receptor Agonist, Ropinirole, Attenuate Fibromyalgia-Like Symptoms in Mice. *Molecules* **2021**, *26*, 2398. https://doi.org/10.3390/molecules26082398

Academic Editors: Alicja Nowaczyk and Grzegorz Grześk

Received: 13 March 2021
Accepted: 19 April 2021
Published: 20 April 2021

1. Introduction

According to the American College of Rheumatology, fibromyalgia (FM) is a common neurological health problem that causes widespread musculoskeletal pain accompanied by fatigue, sleep, memory, and mood issues [1–4]. The development of FM results from a complex dysfunction of the nervous system, and therefore, not only its diagnosis but also treatment and prevention based on combined pharmacological, alternative medicine [5,6], and educational methods [7] are a serious challenge for contemporary medicine [8].

FM affects 2–4% of the population and it is more prevalent in the population of people from urban than rural areas [8–13]. Other risk factors comprise female sex, stress, genetic factors, and comorbid inflammatory diseases (e.g., osteoarthritis, rheumatoid arthritis, lupus, and ankylosing spondylitis) [8,14–16]. Clinical symptoms of FM arise from the central sensitization [17] due to the neuroendocrine dysfunction and fluctuations in the concentration of neurotransmitters, namely decreased levels of biogenic amines, accompanied by cytokine abnormalities, increased concentrations of excitatory neurotransmitters, and substance P. Impaired functions of the hypothalamic–pituitary–adrenal axis and the autonomic nervous system are also observed in FM patients [18,19].

On the molecular level, the development of FM is based on the impaired serotonin-, noradrenaline-, and dopamine-mediated neurotransmission [20]. This dysregulated neurotransmission is likely to be responsible not only for painful symptoms of FM but also mood control deficits, sleep dysregulation, and cognitive dysfunction as these neurotransmitters serve as neurochemical substrates for a wide range of central nervous system activities [21–23].

In view of potential neurochemical mechanisms underlying FM, for years many attempts have been made to search for effective therapies for FM and drugs targeting at serotonergic, noradrenergic, and dopaminergic neurotransmission systems, including serotonin/noradrenaline reuptake inhibitors (duloxetine and desvenlafaxine) [24–27], or ligands of the α_2-δ subunit of voltage-gated calcium channels [7,8] have been recommended for FM treatment but their efficacy seems to be modest [25,28]. On the other hand, selective serotonin reuptake inhibitors turned out to be ineffective in the treatment of other than depression symptoms of FM [29].

In the present study we focused on the assessment of two potential drug candidates for FM treatment. The first one affects serotonergic signaling in the brain, while the second one stimulates dopaminergic neurotransmission in the central nervous system. We used a mouse model of FM, i.e., the reserpine (RES) model, and we compared the effects of vortioxetine (VORT), a serotonin transporter (SERT) inhibitor, a 5-HT_3, 5-HT_7 receptor antagonist, and a 5-HT_{1A} receptor agonist [30], and ropinirole (ROP), a dopaminergic D_2 and D_3 receptor agonist [31], on the pain threshold, depressive-like and anxiety-like responses, locomotor activity and muscle strength of mice exposed to RES to assess if these drugs are able to attenuate the key symptoms resembling those of human FM. The anti-FM effectiveness of multitarget serotonergic agents (e.g., VORT) has not been established, yet. Additionally, the effectiveness of dopamine-mimetics in FM patients requires further confirmation [32] because at present, such compounds are mainly used in the treatment of Parkinson's disease and restless legs syndrome [33,34]. ROP, because of its previously shown significant impact on decreasing tenderness without causing side effects [35], and pramipexole, which affects muscle pressure and tactile allodynia [36], seem to be promising drugs for FM, even though their therapeutic potential in FM has never been thoroughly investigated.

2. Results

The experimental design for in vivo tests is presented in Figure 1. A general procedure used for the induction of FM-like symptoms (Figure 1A) and the behavioral testing protocol used in this study (Figure 1B) are described in Sections 4.3 and 4.4.

Since this set of experiments, which focused on the assessment of the influence of VORT and ROP on FM-like symptoms, was the first-in-animal study, we investigated pharmacological activities of both drugs at only one time point of testing and we did not carry out time-effect studies. In our study only one route of drug administration was used. Available literature indicates that in pain tests utilizing mechanical and thermal stimulation the maximum effect of oral VORT can be achieved 60–240 min after its administration [37], and oral ROP reaches its peak concentration within approximately 60–120 min [38]. Therefore, in this study we chose 60 min after drug administration as the time point for behavioral testing. We used the intraperitoneal route because the pharmacokinetics of substances administered intraperitoneally resembles that seen after oral administration [39].

2.1. *Effect on Tactile Allodynia (Von Frey Test)*

In the von Frey test repeated-measures ANOVA revealed an overall effect of treatment ($F[5, 108] = 62.72$, $p < 0.0001$). Time effect and drug × time interaction were also significant ($F[1, 108] = 38.25$, $p < 0.0001$ and $F[5, 108] = 10.98$, $p < 0.0001$, respectively).

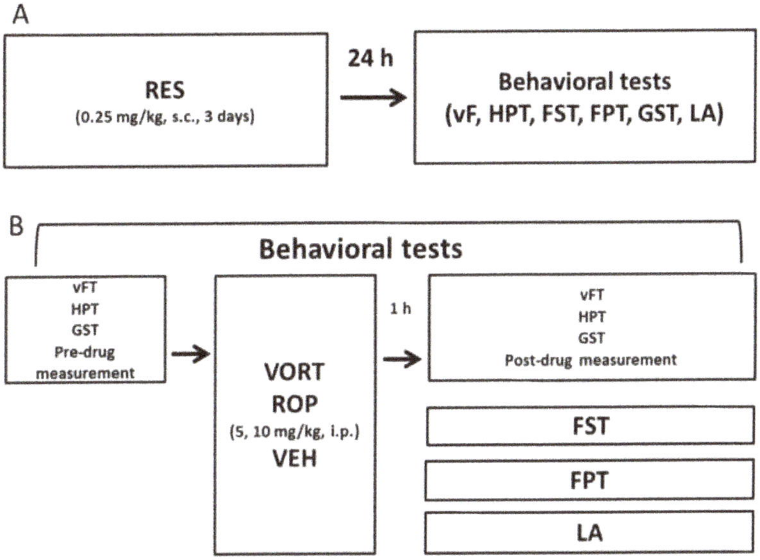

Figure 1. Experimental design used in the present study. FM-like model was induced in mice by a 3-day administration of subcutaneous reserpine (RES; 0.25 mg/kg). Twenty-four hours after the last administration of RES, behavioral tests were carried out (**A**). Vortioxetine (VORT) and ropinirole (ROP) were injected intraperitoneally at doses 5 and 10 mg/kg (**B**). Before test compound administration and 1 h later, the effects of test drugs on tactile allodynia and heat hyperalgesia were measured in the von Frey test (vFT) and the hot plate test (HPT), respectively. Antidepressant-like and anxiolytic-like activities of VORT and ROP were measured in the forced swim test (FST) and the four-plate test (FPT), respectively. Effects of test drugs on the muscle strength were measured using the grip strength test (GST), while the effects of VORT and ROP on the locomotor activity of mice were measured using the locomotor activity test (LA).

In this assay (Figure 2A), Tukey's post hoc analysis showed that RES significantly lowered the mechanical nociceptive threshold in mice ($p < 0.0001$ vs. predrug paw withdrawal of VEH group). VORT and ROP influenced the paw withdrawal threshold of mice treated with RES and compared to RES + VEH group a statistically significant ($p < 0.001$) elevation of the mechanical nociceptive threshold was noted in RES + VORT 10 mg/kg and RES + ROP 10 mg/kg groups. The dose 5 mg/kg of VORT or ROP did not affect the mechanical nociceptive threshold of mice treated with RES (Figure 2A).

2.2. *Effect on Heat Hyperalgesia (Hot Plate Test)*

Repeated measures ANOVA did not reveal an effect of treatment on the hot plate test results ($F[5, 108] = 1.994$, $p > 0.05$). Time effect was significant ($F[1, 108] = 6.455$, $p < 0.05$) but the drug × time interaction was not ($F[5, 108] = 0.3449$, $p > 0.05$). Post hoc analysis did not reveal statistically significant antihyperalgesic properties of VORT or ROP in this assay (Figure 2B).

2.3. *Effect on Depressive-Like Symptoms (Forced Swim Test; FST)*

In the FST one-way ANOVA showed an overall effect of treatment on the duration of immobility in mice ($F[5, 51] = 25.00$, $p < 0.0001$).

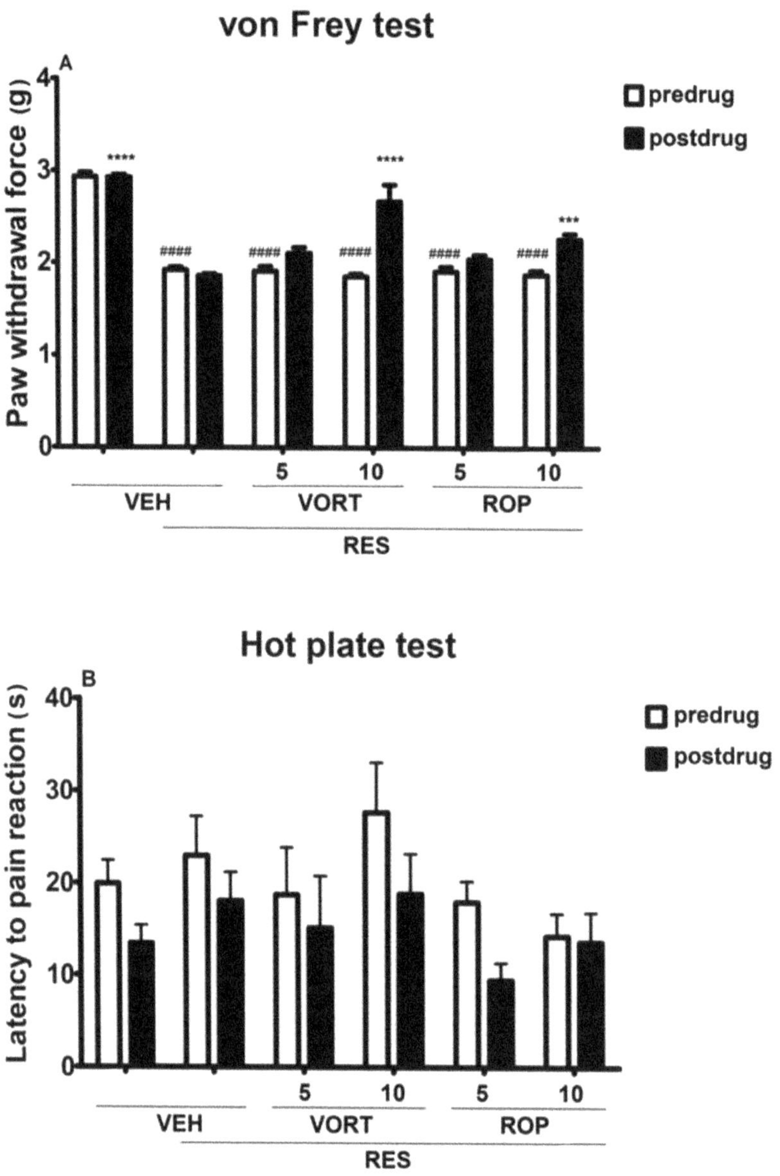

Figure 2. Antiallodynic and antihyperalgesic activities of intraperitoneally administered vortioxetine (VORT; 5 and 10 mg/kg) and ropinirole (ROP; 5 and 10 mg/kg) in the mouse FM-like model induced by a 3-day administration of subcutaneous reserpine (RES; 0.25 mg/kg). The effect of test drugs on tactile allodynia was measured in the von Frey test (**A**) and their effect on heat hyperalgesia was measured in the hot plate test (**B**) 1 h after drug administration. Results are shown as the mean paw withdrawal threshold (g) (**A**), or the mean latency to pain reaction (s) (**B**) ± SEM for n = 10. Statistical analysis: repeated measures analysis of variance, followed by Tukey's post hoc comparison. Significance vs. predrug paw withdrawal of VEH group: #### $p < 0.0001$ and significance vs. postdrug paw withdrawal of RES + VEH group: *** $p < 0.001$, **** $p < 0.0001$.

In the FST Dunnett's post hoc test revealed that although RES prolonged immobility in mice this effect was not specific, i.e., the effect of RES on the duration of immobility compared to that of VEH was not statistically significant (Figure 3). In contrast to this, in mice treated with RES, both doses of ROP significantly reduced the duration of immobility ($p < 0.001$ vs. RES + VEH group; Figure 3). In this test, VORT did not influence immobility of animals, which were previously treated with RES (Figure 3).

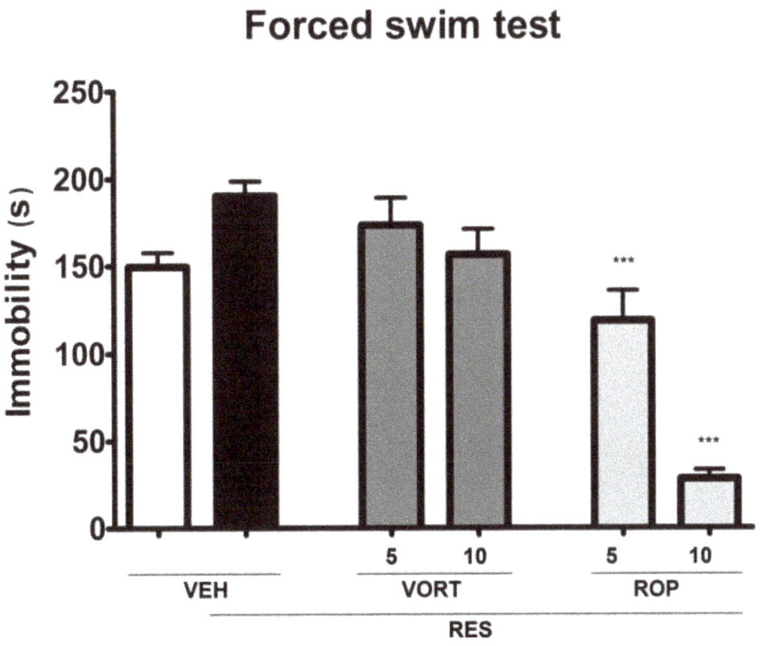

Figure 3. Antidepressant-like properties of intraperitoneally administered vortioxetine (VORT; 5 and 10 mg/kg) and ropinirole (ROP, 5 and 10 mg/kg) in the mouse FM-like model induced by a 3-day administration of subcutaneous reserpine (RES; 0.25 mg/kg). The effect of test drugs on the duration of immobility was measured in the FST carried out 1 h after drug administration. Results are shown as the mean duration of immobility (s) ± SEM for $n = 8$–10. Statistical analysis: one-way analysis of variance, followed by Dunnett's post hoc test. Significance vs. RES + VEH group: *** $p < 0.001$.

2.4. *Effect on Anxiety-Like Symptoms (Four-Plate Test; FPT)*

One-way ANOVA demonstrated a statistically significant overall effect of treatment on the number of punished crossings in the FPT ($F[5, 52] = 7.953$, $p < 0.0001$).

Dunnett's post hoc analysis revealed that the number of punished crossings in the RES + VEH group was significantly lower as compared to the VEH group ($p < 0.05$), RES + VORT 5 mg/kg ($p < 0.01$), and RES + VORT 10 mg/kg groups ($p < 0.0001$, Figure 4). ROP at doses 5 and 10 mg/kg did not show anxiolytic-like properties in the mouse FPT (Figure 4).

2.5. *Effect on Muscle Strength (Grip Strength Test)*

The grip strength test was carried out to assess if RES, VORT, or ROP affect muscle strength of mice. Repeated measures ANOVA showed that neither drug effect, time effect, nor the drug × time interaction were significant ($F[5, 108] = 0.4860$, $p > 0.05$, $F[1, 108] = 0.1589$, $p > 0.05$, and $F[5, 108] = 1.639$, $p > 0.05$. respectively) and none of the drugs used affected muscle strength of mice (Figure 5).

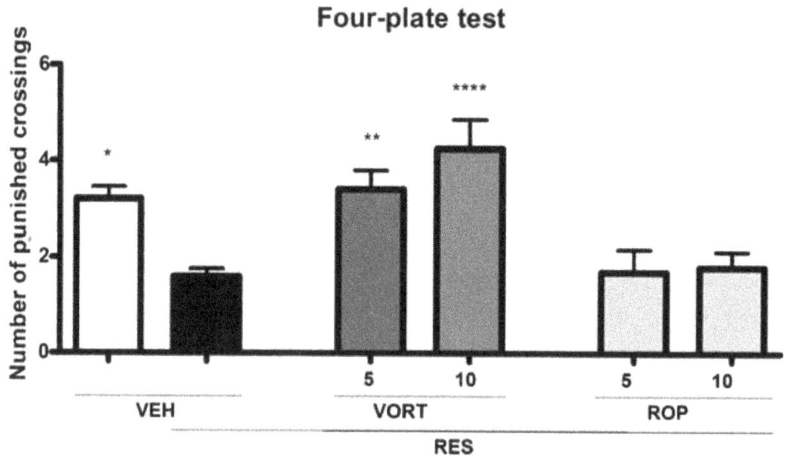

Figure 4. Anxiolytic-like properties of intraperitoneally administered vortioxetine (VORT; 5 and 10 mg/kg) and ropinirole (ROP; 5 and 10 mg/kg) in the mouse FM-like model induced by a 3-day administration of subcutaneous reserpine (RES; 0.25 mg/kg). The effect of test drugs on the number of punished crossings was measured in the FPT performed 1 h after drug administration. Results are shown as the mean number of punished crossings ± SEM for n = 8–10. Statistical analysis: one-way analysis of variance, followed by Dunnett's post hoc test. Significance vs. RES + VEH group: * $p < 0.05$, ** $p < 0.01$, and **** $p < 0.0001$.

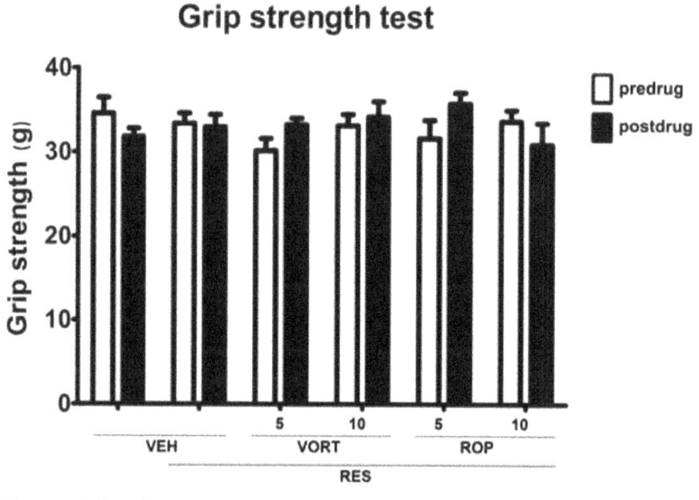

Figure 5. Effect of intraperitoneally administered vortioxetine (VORT; 5 and 10 mg/kg) and ropinirole (ROP; 5 and 10 mg/kg) on the muscle strength in the mouse FM-like model induced by a 3-day administration of subcutaneous reserpine (RES; 0.25 mg/kg). The effect of VORT and ROP was measured in the grip strength test carried out 1 h after drug administration. Results are shown as the mean force (expressed in (g)) that evoked the animal's reaction ± SEM for n = 10. Statistical analysis: repeated-measures analysis of variance, followed by Tukey's post hoc comparison. Significance vs. RES + VEH group at the respective time point of testing: $p > 0.05$.

2.6. *Effect on Locomotor Activity*

Repeated measures ANOVA demonstrated an overall effect of treatment on the locomotor activity of mice ($F[3, 84] = 9.104$, $p < 0.0001$). Time effect was also statistically significant (F[2, 84] = 78.90, $p < 0.0001$) but the drug × time interaction was not (F[6, 84] = 1.421, $p > 0.05$).

Locomotor activity did not differ in RES + VEH group compared to RES + VORT group or RES + ROP group. However, locomotor activity of RES + VEH group was significantly decreased as compared to the VEH group ($p < 0.01$ in the 5th min of the test, and $p < 0.001$ in the 6th min of the test, Figure 6).

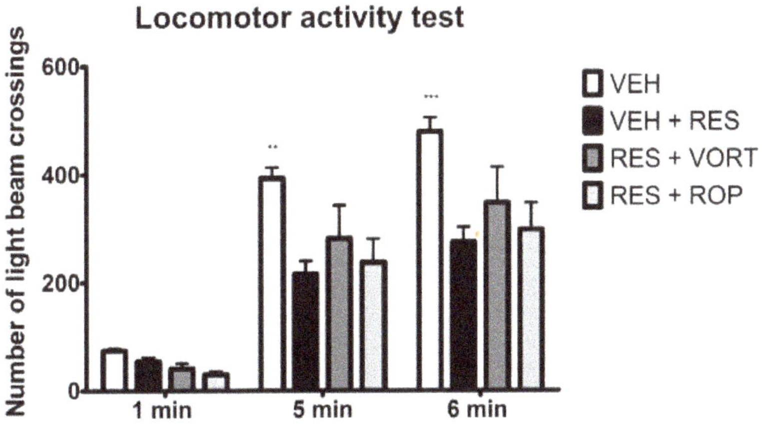

Figure 6. Effect of intraperitoneally administered vortioxetine (VORT; 10 mg/kg) and ropinirole (ROP; 10 mg/kg) on the locomotor activity of mice in the FM-like model induced by a 3-day administration of subcutaneous reserpine (RES; 0.25 mg/kg). The effect of test drugs on the number of light beam crossings was measured in the locomotor activity test carried out 1 h after drug administration. Results are shown as the mean number of light beam crossings ± SEM for $n = 8$. Statistical analysis: repeated-measures analysis of variance, followed by Tukey's post hoc comparison. Significance vs. RES + VEH group at the respective time point of testing: ** $p < 0.01$ and *** $p < 0.001$.

3. Discussion

FM is a disease that results from the impaired neurotransmission mediated by serotonin and catecholamines [40–42]. This altered neurotransmission underlies many symptoms of this disease, including chronic pain, mood and sleep disorders, and cognitive decline [43]. In FM dysregulated dopaminergic neurotransmission was shown and a strong correlation between dopamine metabolism and reduced gray matter density was reported. These phenomena contributed to the enhanced pain perception, cognitive deficits and abnormal stress reactivity [44]. Additionally, a disruption of presynaptic dopaminergic neurotransmission in those brain regions where dopamine plays a putative role in analgesia was shown in FM patients [45]. Recent human and animal studies have revealed that a decreased level of dopamine or the hypofunction of the dopaminergic system might lead to a significantly lowered pain threshold [46,47] and chronic pain intensification [48]. In patients suffering from FM, abnormal dopamine function may be associated with differential processing of pain perception [49,50]. It has also been shown that the polymorphism in the serotonergic 5-HT_3 receptor gene (HTR3) might modulate the striatal dopamine D_2/D_3 receptor availability in FM patients [15].

Considering this key role of the abnormal serotonergic and dopaminergic neurotransmission in the development of FM in humans, in the present research we investigated the influence of VORT and ROP on the pain threshold, depressive-like symptoms, anxiety, and motor functions in a rodent model of FM caused by RES.

In this mouse study we used RES, a natural alkaloid [51,52], which acts by inhibiting the sequestration of monoamine neurotransmitters, namely noradrenaline, dopamine, and serotonin into storage vesicles [53,54]. This action triggers increased metabolism of neurotransmitters resulting in their marked decrease in the brain and the spinal cord [55].

Peripheral administration of RES at doses 1–10 mg/kg produces a significant (70–95%) depletion of monoamine content in the central nervous system. This monoamine depletion occurs 30 min after RES injection and may last up to 2 weeks, finally returning to physiological levels after 21 days of retrieval [56].

As proposed by Nagakura and colleagues [36], repeated-dose RES-induced depletion of biogenic amines in the nervous system underlies the development of sensory hypersensitivity accompanied by depressive-like and anxiety-like behavior in rodents [57,58]. Behavioral studies also proved the effect of RES on sleep architecture [59], muscle strength [60], and cognitive impairment [61]. Hence, RES is regarded as a reliable tool compound to induce FM-like symptoms in laboratory animals. It offers good construct validity, face validity, and predictive validity [41] because its use mimics disease biochemistry, many symptoms that occur in FM patients and it is also useful in the search for new biologically active compounds with potential therapeutic effectiveness in FM.

It should be however emphasized that the RES-induced mouse model of FM used in this present study has several limitations, mainly because it is not entirely specific for this disease. Particular attention should be paid to the fact that RES is also used as a tool to model Parkinson's disease and similarities in behavioral changes in the FM model and the Parkinson's disease model are observed. As shown by Leal and colleagues [62] repeated administrations of low doses of RES can mimic the progressive nature of Parkinson's disease. This confirms the ability of RES to produce symptoms similar to those observed in the early stages of this disease, i.e., RES-treated animals show cognitive and emotional deficits in the early stages of this disorder, even before the onset of motor abnormalities. The non-motor symptoms typical for the RES-induced model of Parkinson's disease have been associated mainly to impairments in the serotonergic and noradrenergic neurotransmission pathways. In this sense, it is not fully understood, whether the model that we used in this present study more closely reflects the symptoms of FM, or rather those which are typical for the early stages of Parkinson's disease as behavioral changes present in both these disorders can be easily modeled with the use of RES. Due to this issue, future studies using another rodent model of FM should be carried out to confirm the results obtained in the present experiment [62], also considering that at concentrations similar to those used in this present research, RES has still been used in rodents to investigate the pathophysiology of Parkinson's disease and to demonstrate therapeutic efficacy of drugs and drug candidates for this neurodegenerative disorder [63,64], while its higher dosages varying from 1 to 10 mg/kg induce a wide range of motor impairments that resemble Parkinson's disease: akinesia, hypokinesia, catalepsy, limb rigidity, and oral tremor. Importantly, some of these motor deficits might influence locomotor activity measures [56,62] and they might be accompanied by memory deficits, anxiety-like behavior, depressive-like behavior, and nociceptive sensitization. Of note, anxiety-like behavior occurs in RES-treated animals in a dose range that does not produce motor impairment (0.1–0.5 mg/kg) and this dose range was used in our study. Moreover, the repeated treatment with low doses of RES (0.1 mg/kg) was suggested as a progressive model of Parkinson's disease in which motor impairments were preceded by cognitive decline, neuronal alterations compatible with the pathophysiology of Parkinson's disease, and emotional processing deficits. In this progressive model of Parkinson's disease, the observed immobility in the FST correlated well with nociceptive sensitization, anxiety, and depression, showing that RES induced non-motor symptoms comorbid with the motor ones [56,65]. Taken together, these data indicate that RES has good face validity for both FM and Parkinson's disease by inducing symptoms that are noted in both disorders, although for the latter condition, a longer period of RES administration (i.e., 3 weeks) is usually recommended [65]. Additionally, high predictive validity of RES as a tool to assess the efficacy of dopaminergic and non-dopaminergic drugs for both FM and Parkinson's disease seems to be another potential limitation of our study and the effectiveness of drugs such as ROP in the RES-based Parkinson's disease model (and FM) must be considered. For ROP increased locomotor activity and the ability to reverse hind limb rigidity were shown previously [64]. In addition to this, ROP at doses almost 2-fold higher than those used in our study was able to reduce catalepsy caused by RES [63].

Chronic and widespread pain is one of the most distressing symptoms of FM that often leads to a significant reduction in the normal physical activity, social, and professional exclusion and it is estimated that the use of both pharmacological and non-pharmacological methods to treat FM symptoms is inadequate in approximately 50% of FM patients [66]. In our present study, RES significantly lowered mechanical nociceptive threshold measured in the von Frey test. It induced anxiety-like symptoms in mice and it significantly reduced animals' locomotor activity measured in the locomotor activity test. RES also prolonged immobility in the FST, however this effect did not reach statistical significance. It did not affect thermal nociceptive threshold measured in the hot plate test. Muscle strength was not altered by RES, either. Taken together, the analysis of the effects of RES on FM-like symptoms revealed that it mainly influenced the mechanical nociceptive threshold and anxiety-like behavior of mice. Lowered pain threshold for mechanical stimulation [67] and increased anxiety due to RES administration [68] were also shown previously.

In our study we demonstrated that both VORT and ROP used at the dose of 10 mg/kg were able to elevate the mechanical nociceptive threshold and VORT was more efficacious than ROP in this assay. Previous studies revealed analgesic properties of VORT in various pain conditions in mice [37,69] and humans [70,71] and it was suggested that the analgesic properties of VORT in chronic pain conditions were due to the increased content of serotonin and noradrenaline in the brainstem of mice [37]. Our present study is the first one that shows that VORT might also be effective in pain in the course of FM.

In the von Frey test we also demonstrated that ROP, the dopaminergic D_2/D_3 receptor agonist was effective as an antiallodynic agent. The role of spinal D_2 receptor stimulation in the reduction of superficial dorsal horn neuron hyperexcitability has been recently shown [72] and it has been suggested that spinal D_2 receptors might be promising therapeutic targets for the treatment of pain symptoms in some chronic diseases [72,73]. Interestingly, the latter study used the von Frey test and it showed antiallodynic properties of ROP in a mouse model of Parkinson's disease. Potential analgesic efficacy of ROP resulting from its agonistic activity at D_2/D_3 receptors in FM patients was suggested previously based on results from clinical trials [74,75] and our present study confirmed antiallodynic properties of this drug in a mouse model of this disease.

In contrast to previously published results [55], in our present research RES did not induce heat hyperalgesia in mice. This difference is hard to explain. Specific strain differences or distinct temperature range used during testing might be potential explanation for this discrepancy between these two studies. On the other hand, there are also some studies that showed antinociceptive properties of RES in the hot plate test [76], which might be the explanation for the observed lack of hyperalgesia due to RES administration. In the hot plate test, neither VORT, nor ROP influenced the thermal pain threshold of mice treated with RES.

Acute stress is one of contributing factors to increased depressive symptomatology and anxiety [77]. Stress also plays an important role in the development of FM in humans [16] and for this reason some antidepressants, which act as inhibitors of serotonin and noradrenaline reuptake, were previously found to be effective in FM patients [24,78,79]. The FST is an assay for screening of compounds with potential antidepressant properties and it reveals compounds, even after their acute administration [80]. In this test, increased immobility of mice is not only a measure of depressive-like state but it also shows a coping strategy of a mouse exposed to an acute inescapable stress. Thus, the test provides some insight into the neural mechanisms of the stress response [81].

In our present research RES did not induce depressive-like behavior measured in the FST in mice. Although the 3-day administration of this alkaloid slightly prolonged the duration of immobility, this activity did not reach statistical significance. We can therefore conclude that the FM model based on repeated administrations of RES showed limited face validity for this disorder. Our finding is, however, in contrast with that previously reported by Klein and colleagues [55] who noted a prolongation of immobility of mice injected with RES in the FST.

Interestingly, in the FST we were not able to demonstrate antidepressant-like properties of VORT. In contrast to this, a statistically significant reduction of immobility time was shown for ROP-treated group. The FST results obtained for the antidepressant drug VORT might seem surprising, however the lack of antidepressant-like properties of VORT revealed in this test might be explained as follows: VORT is a drug that acts by modulating serotonergic neurotransmission and according to Cryan and colleagues [82] serotonergic compounds might not reveal their potential antidepressant properties in the classical FST, which was used in the present experiment. In contrast to this, antidepressant-like properties shown for ROP in the FST in a mouse model of FM are in line with the previous reports. They demonstrated that ROP possessed antidepressant-like properties in mice [83,84], which were due to ROP-induced altered functions of dopaminergic, serotonergic, or sigma receptors [83]. This activity of ROP was also confirmed in humans [85].

The above-mentioned previous study [84] showed that ROP significantly and dose-dependently decreased immobility time in experimental animals. Only at the dose of 10 mg/kg it increased swimming and climbing. Different active behaviors are related to different neurotransmitter systems [86]. Specifically, the serotonergic system has been implicated in swimming behavior, while climbing might be related to function of the noradrenergic system. Taken together these data demonstrated that ROP may affect serotoninergic neurotransmission, whereas noradrenergic neurotransmission might be affected only following high doses of this drug. Our present data are in accordance with previous findings, which indicated that ROP decreased duration of immobility time in rodents [83,87]. Those effects of ROP seem to be mediated by D_2-like receptors, because they were blocked by D_2-like receptor antagonists (e.g., haloperidole), but not by the D_1 receptor antagonists (e.g., SCH 23390) [83].

In our present research we also assessed potential anxiolytic-like properties of VORT and ROP in a mouse model of FM induced by RES. In the FPT, RES caused a statistically significant decrease in the number of punished crossings, which was a measure of anxiety-like behavior in this assay [88]. In contrast to the FST, the FPT revealed a significant anxiolytic-like activity of VORT, but not of ROP in mice treated with RES. Anxiolytic properties of VORT were also previously reported [89–92]. For ROP both anxiety [93,94] and anxiolytic-like properties [84,95] were demonstrated. A possible explanation for the observed lack of anxiolytic-like properties of the D_2/D_3 receptor agonist, ROP, in mice with FM-like symptoms shown in our present study might be related to the previously reported correlation between abnormally high D_2/D_3 receptor availability in the ventral striatum and enhanced anxiety symptoms in depressed subjects [96]. It should also be noted that an increased dopaminergic neurotransmission involving D_2 (and D_1) dopaminergic receptors is postulated as an underlying mechanism for anxiety-like behavior in mice [97].

Pain threshold of mice measured in the von Frey test and the hot plate test, immobility duration assessed in the FST or the number of punished crossings measured in the FPT might be influenced by compounds, which impair locomotor activity or other motor functions of animals used in behavioral tests [88]. This, in turn, can significantly reduce the translational value of the preclinical research. Having this in mind, in order to avoid false positive results in behavioral tests assessing the effect of VORT and ROP on key symptoms of FM, we additionally assessed their effects on the muscle strength and locomotor activity of mice. None of the test drugs altered muscle strength of mice measured in the grip strength test and only RES (but not VORT or ROP) reduced locomotor activity of mice. This finding is in line with previous studies, which showed that RES induced features of akinesia and hind limb rigidity in rats for up to 24 h [56,64]. This effect was dependent on striatal dopamine deficits and it was reversed by dopamine replenishment. In our study, locomotor activity of mice was investigated 24 h after the last RES injection and this might explain the observed decreased locomotor functions in the RES + VEH group. As for intraperitoneal ROP or VORT, we did not demonstrate their effects on the locomotor activity of mice.

This is in line with previous studies showing that ROP at doses 1–10 mg/kg showed the antidepressant-like effect in the FST without impairing locomotion in rats [84] or mice [83], and that VORT did not affect locomotor activity of mice [92]. Taken together, it can be concluded that the results obtained for VORT and ROP in pain tests, FST and FPT are not falsified by impaired motor functions of mice treated with these drugs. Additionally, it has to be noted that in mice treated with RES, neither VORT, nor ROP were able to restore motor activity of animals to levels observed in the VEH group.

4. Materials and Methods

4.1. Animals and Housing Conditions

In vivo experiments were performed at the Department of Pharmacodynamics, Faculty of Pharmacy, Jagiellonian University Medical College, Krakow, Poland. Behavioral tests were carried out between 9 am and 2 pm. All procedures for in vivo tests were performed in full accordance with ethical standards laid down in respective Polish and EU regulations (Directive No. 86/609/EEC and the 1st Local Ethics Committee's in Krakow approval No. 250/2019). In order to avoid potential bias in data recording the investigators who were involved behavioral assays were blinded to experimental groups.

In behavioral tests adult male CD-1 mice weighing 18–22 g were used. The animals were kept in groups of 10–15 mice in cages at standard laboratory conditions (room temperature of 22 ± 2 °C, light/dark (12:12) cycle, humidity 50% ± 10%, free access to food and water, and environmental enrichment before the experiments). The ambient temperature of the room and humidity were kept consistent throughout all the tests. For all experiments the animals were selected randomly. Each experimental group of mice consisted of 8–10 animals/dose. Immediately after the experiment the animals were euthanized.

4.2. Chemicals

RES, VORT, and ROP were purchased from Sigma Aldrich (Poznan, Poland). For in vivo tests, the solution of RES was prepared by dissolving an appropriate amount of this drug in the glacial acetic acid (Polskie Odczynniki Chemiczne, Gliwice, Poland) and diluted to a final concentration of 0.5% acetic acid with phosphate buffer (PBS, BioShop Canada Inc., Burlington, ON, Canada). VORT and ROP were suspended in 1% solution of Tween 80 (Pol-Aura, Zabrze, Poland). Test drugs were administered by the intraperitoneal route at a constant volume of 0.1 mL/10 g, 1 h before behavioral tests. Two fixed doses of VORT and ROP were used in this study. Dose selection was based on the previously published literature data [83,98,99]. Control mice received 1% Tween 80.

4.3. Induction of FM-Like Model in Mice

The mouse FM-like model induced by RES administration is based on causing a decrease in the concentration of biogenic amines, mostly dopamine and serotonin in the structures of the central nervous system, resulting in a decreased pain threshold and induction of depressive-like and anxiety-like responses. This model was established by Nagakura and colleagues [36] to be used in rats and then adapted for mice by de Souza and colleagues [57]. To induce symptoms mimicking human FM, mice were injected subcutaneously with RES (0.25 mg/kg) for the three consecutive days. Behavioral tests were carried out 24 h after the last RES administration (Figure 1).

4.4. Behavioral Tests

4.4.1. Effect on Pain Threshold

Pain threshold of RES-treated mice was assessed at two time points, i.e., before the test drug (VORT, ROP, or VEH) administration (referred to as 'predrug' measurement) and 60 min after its administration ('postdrug' measurement). Both mechanical and thermal nociceptive thresholds were assessed in each experimental group using the von Frey test and the hot plate test, respectively.

Influence on Tactile Allodynia (Von Frey Test)

The test was carried out according to a procedure previously described [100]. The electronic von Frey unit (Bioseb, Vitrolles, France) is a device supplied with a single flexible filament applying the increasing force (from 0 to 10 g) against the plantar surface of the hind paw of a mouse. In this assay the nocifensive paw withdrawal response automatically turned off the stimulus and the mechanical pressure that evoked the response was recorded. On the day of the experiment, the mice were placed individually in test compartments with a wire mesh bottom and were allowed to habituate for 1 h. After the habituation period, in order to obtain baseline (predrug) values of mechanical nociceptive threshold, each mouse was tested 3 times alternately in each hind paw, allowing at least 30 s between each measurement. Then, the mice received tested compounds or vehicle and 1 h later they were tested again and mean postdrug values were obtained for each mouse.

Influence on Thermal Hyperalgesia (Hot Plate Test)

The hot plate test evaluated the effect of compounds on thermally-induced pain. The assay was carried out as previously described [100]. Briefly, the mice were placed on a plate with a surface temperature of 55–56 °C (hot/cold plate analgesiameter, Bioseb, Vitrolles, France). The predrug latency to pain reaction, i.e., the hind paw licking or jumping was measured in all experimental groups. Then, the test compounds were injected and 1 h later the test was carried out again to obtain postdrug measurements. To prevent paw tissue damage, the cut-off time of 60 s was established and mice not responding within 60 s were removed from the apparatus and assigned a score of 60 s.

4.4.2. Assessment of Antidepressant-Like Activity (Forced Swim Test, FST)

The FST was carried out according to the method originally described by Porsolt and colleagues [101] with some modification [102]. Mice were dropped individually into glass cylinders (height: 25 cm, diameter: 10 cm) filled with water (maintained at 23–25 °C) to a height of 10 cm. The whole test lasted for 6 min, during which after an initial 2-min period of vigorous activity, each mouse assumed an immobile posture. The total duration of immobility was recorded during the final 4 min of the whole 6-min testing period and the results obtained were compared between control and drug-treated groups of mice. Animals were regarded to be immobile when they remained floating passively in the water, making only small movements to keep their heads above the water surface.

4.4.3. Assessment of Anxiolytic-Like Activity (Four-Plate Test, FPT)

The FPT test was carried out according to a previously described method [103]. The four-plate apparatus (Bioseb, Vitrolles, France) is a cage (25 cm × 18 cm × 16 cm) that is floored with four identical, rectangular plates (11 cm × 8 cm) separated from each other by 4-mm gaps. An electric stimulus transmitted to plates (0.6 mA, duration: 0.5 s) was produced by an electric shock generator. In this test, after a 15-s habituation period, each animal was subjected to an electric shock when crossing from one plate to another (two limbs on one plate and two on another) with a 3-s break between each shock. The total duration of this test was 60 s. The number of punished crossings were counted and compounds with anxiolytic-like properties were able to increase the number of punished passages.

4.4.4. Assessment of the Effect on Muscle Strength (Grip-Strength Test)

The grip-strength apparatus (TSE Systems, Bad Homburg, Germany) was supplied with a steel wire grid (8 cm × 8 cm) connected to anisometric force transducer. In this assay, each mouse was gently kept by its tail so that it could grasp the grid mounted to a high-precision force sensor of the grip-strength device with its forepaws. Then, the animal was pulled back gently by the tail until it released the grid and the maximal grip strength value (expressed in grams) was recorded for each animal. This procedure was repeated three times and the mean of three measurements for each mouse was calculated [104].

4.4.5. Assessment of the Effect on Locomotor Activity

The locomotor activity test was performed using activity cages (40 cm × 40 cm × 31 cm, Ugo Basile, Varese, Italy) supplied with I.R. beam emitters connected to a counter for the recording of light-beam interrupts [102]. Sixty minutes before the locomotor activity test, the mice were pretreated with VORT, ROP, or VEH. Then, they were individually placed in the activity cages for an adaptation period (30 min). The animals' locomotor activity (i.e., the number of light beam crossings) was counted during the next 6 min in 1-min intervals.

4.5. Data Analysis

Data analysis was performed using GraphPad Prism software (version 8.0, San Diego, CA, USA). Numerical results obtained in behavioral tests are expressed as the mean ± SEM. Statistical analysis was carried out using a one-way analysis of variance (ANOVA), followed by Dunnett's post hoc comparison to compare results obtained for drug-treated groups and the control group. Repeated measures ANOVA and Tukey's post hoc comparison were used for group comparisons made repeatedly at different time points. $p < 0.05$ was considered significant.

5. Conclusions

To sum up, the treatment of EM is a challenge for contemporary medicine and novel treatment options for this disorder are a serious medical demand. In the present study a mouse model of FM was used to assess if two drugs modulating serotonergic and dopaminergic neurotransmission, namely VORT and ROP, might be potentially useful in the treatment of key symptoms of FM in humans. Both drugs markedly reduced tactile allodynia caused by RES, but they affected emotional processes of mice in a distinct manner. VORT reduced anxiety-related behavior induced by RES in mice, while ROP showed an- tidepressant-like properties in RES-treated mice but these RES-exposed mice did not develop depressive-like phenotype. Hence, we concluded that these two repurposed drugs should be considered as potential drug candidates for FM patients, but the selection of a specific drug (i.e., either VORT or ROP) should depend on a careful analysis of the type of patient's key symptoms (severe anxiety or depressive state comorbid chronic pain).

The alterations of central nervous system neurotransmitter levels induced by RES used to develop the FM-like animal model, could be translated into psychiatric and neurological impairments typically observed in FM patients. However, it is worth noting that the model that was used in this present study has some limitations, of which the lack of full specificity for FM and the ability of this model to reflect symptoms typical for Parkinson's disease are of particular concern. Therefore, future studies should be focused on testing VORT and ROP in other FM models, such as the acid saline-induced pain model, sound, intermittent cold, and subchronic swimming stress models. As FM is a diverse syndrome that involves multiple etiologies and multiple subtypes, the combined use of these models may be relevant for the assessment of pathways and mechanisms underlying this disease. These combined models are able to mimic particular biomarkers and clinical conditions observed in FM patients and may contribute to a successful development of drugs and their combinations for FM [105].

Since we demonstrated that the RES model did not show signs of depressive-like behavior measured in the FST, and FST was not sensitive enough to measure this FM symptom, we also proposed using additional methods to study antidepressant-like potential of VORT and ROP. Such behavioral assays (e.g., the novelty-suppressed feeding test) were previously used for the validation of RES model of FM [106] but they also seem to be of interest in terms of their potential usefulness to develop drugs for FM. Other behavioral methods for measuring muscle strength deficits and heat hyperalgesia in mice exposed to RES should also be considered in future studies as the tests we used (grip strength test and hot plate test) did not reveal differences between animals treated and animals not treated with RES.

Author Contributions: Conceptualization, K.S.; Methodology, K.S., A.F.-W.; Software, K.S., A.F.-W.; Validation, A.F.-W. Formal Analysis, K.S.; Investigation, A.F.-W., K.S.; Data Curation, K.S., A.F.-W.; Writing—Original Draft Preparation, K.S., A.F.-W.; Writing—Review and Editing, K.S.; Visualization, K.S.; Supervision, K.S.; Project Administration, K.S., A.F.-W.; Funding Acquisition, A.F.-W. All authors have read and agreed to the published version of the manuscript.

Funding: This study was financially supported by the funds of Ministry of Science and Higher Education N42/DBS/000066.

Institutional Review Board Statement: The study was conducted according to the guidelines of the Directive 2010/63/EU, and approved by the 1st Local Ethics Committee of the Jagiellonian University, Krakow, Poland (protocol 250/2019).

Informed Consent Statement: Not applicable.

Data Availability Statement: The data presented in this study are available on request from the corresponding author.

Acknowledgments: The authors would like to thank Agnieszka Kaczkowska for her technical help during the research.

Conflicts of Interest: The authors declare no conflict of interest.

Sample Availability: Samples of the compounds tested in this study are available from the authors or can be purchased from the official suppliers.

Abbreviations

FM	Fibromyalgia
HTR3	Serotonergic 5-HT_3 receptor gene
HPT	Hot plate test
FST	Forced swim test
FPT	Four-plate test
GST	Grip strength test
LA	Locomotor activity test
SERT	Serotonin transporter
RES	Reserpine
ROP	Ropinirole
VEH	Vehicle
vFT	Von Frey test
VORT	Vortioxetine

References

1. Sallinen, M.; Kukkurainen, M.L.; Peltokallio, L.; Mikkelsson, M. "I'm tired of being tired"—Fatigue as experienced by women with fibromyalgia. *Adv. Physiother.* **2011**, *13*, 11–17. [CrossRef]
2. Hadlandsmyth, K.; Dailey, D.L.; Rakel, B.A.; Zimmerman, M.B.; Vance, C.G.T.; Merriwether, E.N.; Chimenti, R.L.; Geasland, K.M.; Crofford, L.J.; Sluka, K.A. Somatic symptom presentations in women with fibromyalgia are differentially associated with elevated depression and anxiety. *J. Health Psychol.* **2017**, *25*, 819–829. [CrossRef]
3. Wolfe, F.; Clauw, D.J.; Fitzcharles, M.A.; Goldenberg, D.L.; Katz, R.S.; Mease, P.; Russell, A.S.; Russell, I.J.; Winfield, J.B.; Yunus, M.B. The American College of Rheumatology preliminary diagnostic criteria for fibromyalgia and measurement of symptom severity. *Arthritis Care Res.* **2010**, *62*, 600–610. [CrossRef]
4. Aguilera, M.; Paz, C.; Compañ, V.; Medina, J.C.; Feixas, G. Cognitive rigidity in patients with depression and fibromyalgia. *Int. J. Clin. Health Psychol.* **2019**, *9*, 160–164. [CrossRef] [PubMed]
5. Häuser, W.; Jung, E.; Erbslöh-Möller, B.; Gesmann, M.; Kühn-Becker, H.; Petermann, F.; Langhorst, J.; Thoma, R.; Weiss, T.; Wolfe, F.; et al. The German fibromyalgia consumer reports—A cross-sectional survey. *BMC Musculoskelet. Disord.* **2012**, *13*, 74. [CrossRef]
6. Bennett, R.M.; Jones, J.; Turk, D.C.; Russell, I.J.; Matallana, L. An internet survey of 2596 people with fibromyalgia. *BMC Musculoskelet. Disord.* **2007**, *8*, 27. [CrossRef]
7. Ablin, J.; Fitzcharles, M.A.; Buskila, D.; Shir, Y.; Sommer, C.; Häuser, W. Treatment of fibromyalgia syndrome: Recommendations of recent evidence-based interdisciplinary guidelines with special emphasis on complementary and alternative therapies. *Evid. Based Complement. Altern. Med.* **2013**, *2013*. [CrossRef]

8. Available online: https://www.rheumatology.org/I-Am-A/Patient-Caregiver/Diseases-Conditions/Fibromyalgia (accessed on 24 February 2020).
9. Marques, A.P.; Santo, A.S.D.E.; Berssaneti, A.A.; Matsutani, L.A.; Yuan, S.L.K. Prevalence of fibromyalgia: Literature review update. *Rev. Bras. Reumatol.* **2017**, *57*, 356–363. [CrossRef]
10. Smith, S.B.; Maixner, D.W.; Fillingim, R.B.; Slade, G.; Gracely, R.H.; Ambrose, K.; Zaykin, D.V.; Hyde, C.; John, S.; Tan, K.; et al. Large candidate gene association study reveals genetic risk factors and therapeutic targets for fibromyalgia. *Arthritis Rheum.* **2012**, *64*, 584–593. [CrossRef] [PubMed]
11. Ruiz-Pérez, I.; Plazaola-Castaño, J.; Cáliz-Cáliz, R.; Rodríguez-Calvo, I.; García-Sánchez, A.; Ferrer-González, M.Á.; Guzmán-Ubeda, M.; del Río-Lozano, M.; López-Chicheri García, I. Risk factors for fibromyalgia: The role of violence against women. *Clin. Rheumatol.* **2009**, *28*, 777–786. [CrossRef] [PubMed]
12. Bradley, L.A. Pathophysiology of Fibromyalgia. *Am. J. Med.* **2009**, *122* (Suppl. 12), S22–S30. [CrossRef]
13. Goldenberg, D.L. Fibromyalgia Syndrome a Decade Later: What Have We Learned? *Arch. Intern. Med.* **1999**, *159*, 777–785. [CrossRef]
14. Gran, J.T. The epidemiology of chronic generalized musculoskeletal pain. *Best Pract. Res. Clin. Rheumatol.* **2003**, *17*, 547–561. [CrossRef]
15. Ledermann, K.; Hasler, G.; Jenewein, J.; Sprott, H.; Schnyder, U.; Martin-Soelch, C. 5′UTR polymorphism in the serotonergic receptor HTR3A gene is differently associated with striatal Dopamine D2/D3 receptor availability in the right putamen in Fibromyalgia patients and healthy controls-Preliminary evidence. *Synapse* **2020**, *74*, e22147. [CrossRef]
16. Van Houdenhove, B.; Egle, U.; Luyten, P. The role of life stress in fibromyalgia. *Curr. Rheumatol. Rep.* **2005**, *7*, 365–370. [CrossRef] [PubMed]
17. Desmeules, J.A.; Cedraschi, C.; Rapiti, E.; Baumgartner, E.; Finckh, A.; Cohen, P.; Dayer, P.; Vischer, T.L. Neurophysiologic evidence for a central sensitization in patients with fibromyalgia. *Arthritis Rheum.* **2003**, *48*, 1420–1429. [CrossRef] [PubMed]
18. Fitzcharles, M.A.; Boulos, P. Inaccuracy in the diagnosis of fibromyalgia syndrome: Analysis of referrals. *Rheumatology* **2003**, *42*, 263–267. [CrossRef] [PubMed]
19. Mease, P. Fibromyalgia syndrome: Review of clinical presentation, pathogenesis, outcome measures, and treatment. *J. Rheumatol. Suppl.* **2005**, *75*, 6–21.
20. Senba, E.; Kami, K. A new aspect of chronic pain as a lifestyle-related disease. *Neurobiol. Pain* **2017**, *1*, 6–15. [CrossRef] [PubMed]
21. Häuser, W. Fibromyalgiesyndrom Basiswissen, Diagnostik und Therapie [Fibromyalgia syndrome: Basic knowledge, diagnosis and treatment]. *Med. Monatsschr. Pharm.* **2016**, *39*, 504–511.
22. Olivier, B. Serotonin: A never-ending story. *Eur. J. Pharmacol.* **2015**, *753*, 2–18. [CrossRef]
23. Štrac, D.Š.; Pivac, N.; Mück-Šeler, D. The serotonergic system and cognitive function. *Transl. Neurosci.* **2016**, *7*, 35–49. [CrossRef] [PubMed]
24. Lian, Y.N.; Wang, Y.; Zhang, Y.; Yang, C.X. Duloxetine for pain in fibromyalgia in adults: A systematic review and a meta-analysis. *Int. J. Neurosci.* **2020**, *130*, 71–82. [CrossRef] [PubMed]
25. Welsch, P.; Üçeyler, N.; Klose, P.; Walitt, B.; Häuser, W. Serotonin and noradrenaline reuptake inhibitors (SNRIs) for fibromyalgia. *Cochrane Database Syst. Rev.* **2018**, *2*, CD010292. [CrossRef]
26. Shelton, R.C. Serotonin and Norepinephrine Reuptake Inhibitors. *Handb. Exp. Pharmacol.* **2019**, *250*, 145–180. [CrossRef]
27. Lawson, K. Tricyclic antidepressants and fibromyalgia: What is the mechanism of action? *Expert Opin. Investig. Drugs* **2002**, *11*, 1437–1445. [CrossRef] [PubMed]
28. Häuser, W.; Urrútia, G.; Tort, S.; Uçeyler, N.; Walitt, B. Serotonin and noradrenaline reuptake inhibitors (SNRIs) for fibromyalgia syndrome. *Cochrane Database Syst. Rev.* **2013**, CD010292. [CrossRef]
29. Walitt, B.; Urrútia, G.; Nishishinya, M.B.; Cantrell, S.E.; Häuser, W. Selective serotonin reuptake inhibitors for fibromyalgia syndrome. *Cochrane Database Syst. Rev.* **2015**, *2015*, CD011735. [CrossRef]
30. Gonda, X.; Sharma, S.R.; Tarazi, F.I. Vortioxetine: A novel antidepressant for the treatment of major depressive disorder. *Expert Opin. Drug Discov.* **2019**, *14*, 81–89. [CrossRef]
31. Okano, H.; Yasuda, D.; Fujimori, K.; Morimoto, S.; Takahashi, S. Ropinirole, a New ALS Drug Candidate Developed Using iPSCs. *Trends Pharmacol. Sci.* **2020**, *41*, 99–109. [CrossRef] [PubMed]
32. Albrecht, D.S.; MacKie, P.J.; Kareken, D.A.; Hutchins, G.D.; Chumin, E.J.; Christian, B.T.; Yoder, K.K. Differential dopamine function in fibromyalgia. *Brain Imaging Behav.* **2016**, *10*, 829–839. [CrossRef]
33. Garcia-Borreguero, D.; Silber, M.H.; Winkelman, J.W.; Högl, B.; Bainbridge, J.; Buchfuhrer, M.; Hadjigeorgiou, G.; Inoue, Y.; Manconi, M.; Oertel, W.; et al. Guidelines for the first-line treatment of restless legs syndrome/Willis-Ekbom disease, prevention and treatment of dopaminergic augmentation: A combined task force of the IRLSSG, EURLSSG, and the RLS-foundation. *Sleep Med.* **2016**, *1*, 1–11. [CrossRef] [PubMed]
34. Ellis, J.M.; Fell, M.J. Current approaches to the treatment of Parkinson's Disease. *Bioorg. Med. Chem. Lett.* **2017**, *27*, 4247–4255. [CrossRef] [PubMed]
35. Holman, A.J. Ropinirole, open preliminary observations of a dopamine agonist for refractory fibromyalgia. *J. Clin. Rheumatol.* **2003**, *9*, 277–279. [CrossRef]
36. Nagakura, Y.; Oe, T.; Aoki, T.; Matsuoka, N. Biogenic amine depletion causes chronic muscular pain and tactile allodynia accompanied by depression: A putative animal model of fibromyalgia. *Pain* **2009**, *146*, 26–33. [CrossRef]

37. Micov, A.M.; Tomić, M.A.; Todorović, M.B.; Vuković, M.J.; Pecikoza, U.B.; Jasnic, N.I.; Djordjevic, J.D.; Stepanović-Petrović, R.M. Vortioxetine reduces pain hypersensitivity and associated depression-like behavior in mice with oxaliplatin-induced neuropathy. *Prog. Neuropsychopharmacol. Biol. Psychiatry* **2020**, *103*, 109975. [CrossRef]
38. Available online: https://www.accessdata.fda.gov/drugsatfda_docs/label/2008/020658s018s020s021lbl.pdf (accessed on 1 April 2021).
39. Turner, P.V.; Brabb, T.; Pekow, C.; Vasbinder, M.A. Administration of substances to laboratory animals: Routes of administration and factors to consider. *J. Am. Assoc. Lab. Anim. Sci.* **2011**, *50*, 600–613. [PubMed]
40. Sumpton, J.E.; Moulin, D.E. Fibromyalgia. *Handb. Clin. Neurol.* **2014**, *119*, 513–527. [CrossRef] [PubMed]
41. Stahl, S.M. Fibromyalgia-pathways and neurotransmitters. *Hum. Psychopharmacol.* **2009**, *24* (Suppl. 1), S11–S17. [CrossRef] [PubMed]
42. Paredes, S.; Cantillo, S.; Candido, K.D.; Knezevic, N.N. An Association of Serotonin with Pain Disorders and Its Modulation by Estrogens. *Int. J. Mol. Sci.* **2019**, *20*, 5729. [CrossRef] [PubMed]
43. Maffei, M.E. Fibromyalgia: Recent Advances in Diagnosis, Classification, Pharmacotherapy and Alternative Remedies. *Int. J. Mol. Sci.* **2020**, *21*, 7877. [CrossRef]
44. Wood, P.B.; Glabus, M.F.; Simpson, R.; Patterson, J.C., 2nd. Changes in gray matter density in fibromyalgia: Correlation with dopamine metabolism. *J. Pain* **2009**, *10*, 609–618. [CrossRef]
45. Wood, P.B.; Patterson, J.C., 2nd; Sunderland, J.J.; Tainter, K.H.; Glabus, M.F.; Lilien, D.L. Reduced presynaptic dopamine activity in fibromyalgia syndrome demonstrated with positron emission tomography: A pilot study. *J. Pain* **2007**, *8*, 51–58. [CrossRef]
46. Sung, S.; Vijiaratnam, N.; Chan, D.W.C.; Farrell, M.; Evans, A.H. Pain sensitivity in Parkinson's disease: Systematic review and meta-analysis. *Park. Relat. Disord.* **2018**, *48*, 17–27. [CrossRef]
47. Valek, L.; Auburger, G.; Tegeder, I. Sensory neuropathy and nociception in rodent models of Parkinson's disease. *DMM Dis. Model. Mech.* **2019**, *12*, dmm039396. [CrossRef]
48. Wawrzczak-Bargieła, A.; Ziółkowska, B.; Piotrowska, A.; Starnowska-Sokół, J.; Rojewska, E.; Mika, J.; Przewłocka, B.; Przewłocki, R. Neuropathic Pain Dysregulates Gene Expression of the Forebrain Opioid and Dopamine Systems. *Neurotox. Res.* **2020**, *37*, 800–814. [CrossRef] [PubMed]
49. Wood, P.B.; Schweinhardt, P.; Jaeger, E.; Dagher, A.; Hakyemez, H.; Rabiner, E.A.; Bushnell, M.C.; Chizh, B.A. Fibromyalgia patients show an abnormal dopamine response to pain. *Eur. J. Neurosci.* **2007**, *25*, 3576–3582. [CrossRef] [PubMed]
50. Wood, P.B. Role of central dopamine in pain and analgesia. *Expert Rev. Neurother.* **2008**, *8*, 781–797. [CrossRef]
51. Kashyap, P.; Kalaiselvan, V.; Kumar, R.; Kumar, S. Ajmalicine and Reserpine: Indole Alkaloids as Multi-Target Directed Ligands towards Factors Implicated in Alzheimer's Disease. *Molecules* **2020**, *25*, 1609. [CrossRef]
52. Li, L.M.; Shi, S.D.; Liu, Y.; Zou, Q. Bioactivity-Guided Isolation and Identification of New and Immunosuppressive Monoterpenoid Indole Alkaloids from Rauvolfia yunnanensis Tsiang. *Molecules* **2019**, *24*, 4574. [CrossRef]
53. Celano, C.M.; Freudenreich, O.; Fernandez-Robles, C.; Stern, T.A.; Caro, M.A.; Huffman, J.C. Depressogenic effects of medications: A review. *Dialogues Clin. Neurosci.* **2011**, *13*, 109–125. [CrossRef]
54. Sulser, F.; Brodie, B.B. Is reserpine tranquilization linked to change in brain serotonin or brain norepinephrine? *Science* **1960**, *131*, 1440–1441. [CrossRef]
55. Klein, C.P.; Sperotto, N.D.; Maciel, I.S.; Leite, C.E.; Souza, A.H.; Campos, M.M. Effects of D-series resolvins on behavioral and neurochemical changes in a fibromyalgia-like model in mice. *Neuropharmacology* **2014**, *86*, 57–66. [CrossRef]
56. Leão, A.H.; Sarmento-Silva, A.J.; Santos, J.R.; Ribeiro, A.M.; Silva, R.H. Molecular, Neurochemical, and Behavioral Hallmarks of Reserpine as a Model for Parkinson's Disease: New Perspectives to a Long-Standing Model. *Brain Pathol.* **2015**, *25*, 377–390. [CrossRef]
57. De Souza, A.H.; Da Costa Lopes, A.M.; Castro, C.J.; Pereira, E.M.R.; Klein, C.P.; Da Silva, C.A.; Da Silva, J.F.; Ferreira, J.; Gomez, M.V. The effects of Phα1β, a spider toxin, calcium channel blocker, in a mouse fibromyalgia model. *Toxicon* **2014**, *81*, 37–42. [CrossRef]
58. Bisong, S.A.; Brown, R.; Osim, E.E. Comparative effects of Rauwolfia vomitoria and chlorpromazine on locomotor behaviour and anxiety in mice. *J. Ethnopharmacol.* **2010**, *132*, 334–339. [CrossRef]
59. Hernandez-Leon, A.; Fernández-Guasti, A.; Martínez, A.; Pellicer, F.; González-Trujano, M.E. Sleep architecture is altered in the reserpine-induced fibromyalgia model in ovariectomized rats. *Behav. Brain Res.* **2019**, *364*, 383–392. [CrossRef]
60. Fischer, S.P.M.; Brusco, I.; Brum, E.S.; Fialho, M.F.P.; Camponogara, C.; Scussel, R.; Machado-de-Ávila, R.A.; Trevisan, G.; Oliveira, S.M. Involvement of TRPV1 and the efficacy of α-spinasterol on experimental fibromyalgia symptoms in mice. *Neurochem. Int.* **2020**, *134*, 104673. [CrossRef]
61. Kaur, A.; Singh, L.; Singh, N.; Bhatti, M.S.; Bhatti, R. Ameliorative effect of imperatorin in chemically induced fibromyalgia: Role of NMDA/NFkB mediated downstream signaling. *Biochem. Pharmacol.* **2019**, *166*, 56–69. [CrossRef]
62. Leal, P.C.; Lins, L.C.; de Gois, A.M.; Marchioro, M.; Santos, J.R. Commentary: Evaluation of Models of Parkinson's Disease. *Front. Neurosci.* **2016**, *10*, 283. [CrossRef] [PubMed]
63. Fukuzaki, K.; Kamenosono, T.; Nagata, R. Effects of ropinirole on various parkinsonian models in mice, rats, and cynomolgus monkeys. *Pharmacol. Biochem. Behav.* **2000**, *65*, 503–508. [CrossRef]
64. Duty, S.; Jenner, P. Animal models of Parkinson's disease: A source of novel treatments and clues to the cause of the disease. *Br. J. Pharmacol.* **2011**, *164*, 1357–1391. [CrossRef]

65. Ikram, H.; Haleem, D.J. Repeated treatment with a low dose of reserpine as a progressive model of Parkinson's dementia. *Pak. J. Pharm. Sci.* **2019**, *32*, 555–562.
66. Leventhal, L.J. Management of Fibromyalgia. *Ann. Intern. Med.* **1999**, *131*, 850. [CrossRef] [PubMed]
67. Oe, T.; Tsukamoto, M.; Nagakura, Y. Reserpine causes biphasic nociceptive sensitivity alteration in conjunction with brain biogenic amine tones in rats. *Neuroscience* **2010**, *169*, 1860–1871. [CrossRef] [PubMed]
68. Sarwer-Foner, G.J.; Ogle, W. Psychosis and enhanced anxiety produced by reserpine and chlorpromazine. *Can. Med. Assoc. J.* **1956**, *74*, 526–532.
69. Zuena, A.R.; Maftei, D.; Alemà, G.S.; Dal Moro, F.; Lattanzi, R.; Casolini, P.; Nicoletti, F. Multimodal antidepressant vortioxetine causes analgesia in a mouse model of chronic neuropathic pain. *Mol. Pain* **2018**, *14*, 1744806918808987. [CrossRef]
70. Adamo, D.; Pecoraro, G.; Aria, M.; Favia, G.; Mignogna, M.D. Vortioxetine in the Treatment of Mood Disorders Associated with Burning Mouth Syndrome: Results of an Open-Label, Flexible-Dose Pilot Study. *Pain Med.* **2020**, *21*, 185–194. [CrossRef]
71. Adamo, D.; Pecoraro, G.; Coppola, N.; Calabria, E.; Aria, M.; Mignogna, M. Vortioxetine versus other antidepressants in the treatment of burning mouth syndrome: An open-label randomized trial. *Oral Dis.* **2020**. [CrossRef]
72. Tang, D.L.; Luan, Y.W.; Zhou, C.Y.; Xiao, C. D2 receptor activation relieves pain hypersensitivity by inhibiting superficial dorsal horn neurons in parkinsonian mice. *Acta Pharmacol. Sin.* **2021**, *42*, 189–198. [CrossRef]
73. van Reij, R.R.I.; Joosten, E.A.J.; van den Hoogen, N.J. Dopaminergic neurotransmission and genetic variation in chronification of post-surgical pain. *Br. J. Anaesth.* **2019**, *123*, 853–864. [CrossRef]
74. Holman, A.J. Treatment of fibromyalgia: A changing of the guard. *Womens Health* **2005**, *1*, 409–420. [CrossRef]
75. Okifuji, A.; Gao, J.; Bokat, C.; Hare, B.D. Management of fibromyalgia syndrome in 2016. *Pain Manag.* **2016**, *6*, 383–400. [CrossRef]
76. Ross, J.W.; Ashford, A. The effect of reserpine and alpha-methyldopa on the analgesic action of morphine in the mouse. *J. Pharm. Pharmacol.* **1967**, *19*, 709–713. [CrossRef]
77. Barber, B.A.; Kohl, K.L.; Kassam-Adams, N.; Gold, J.I. Acute stress, depression, and anxiety symptoms among English and Spanish speaking children with recent trauma exposure. *J. Clin. Psychol. Med. Settings* **2014**, *21*, 66–71. [CrossRef]
78. Ottman, A.A.; Warner, C.B.; Brown, J.N. The role of mirtazapine in patients with fibromyalgia: A systematic review. *Rheumatol. Int.* **2018**, *38*, 2217–2224. [CrossRef]
79. Arnold, L.M. Duloxetine and other antidepressants in the treatment of patients with fibromyalgia. *Pain Med.* **2007**, *8* (Suppl. 2), S63–S74. [CrossRef]
80. Kara, N.Z.; Stukalin, Y.; Einat, H. Revisiting the validity of the mouse forced swim test: Systematic review and meta-analysis of the effects of prototypic antidepressants. *Neurosci. Biobehav Rev.* **2018**, *84*, 1–11. [CrossRef]
81. Commons, K.G.; Cholanians, A.B.; Babb, J.A.; Ehlinger, D.G. The Rodent Forced Swim Test Measures Stress-Coping Strategy, Not Depression-like Behavior. *ACS Chem. Neurosci.* **2017**, *8*, 955–960. [CrossRef]
82. Cryan, J.; Markou, A.; Lucki, I. Assessing antidepressant activity in rodents: Recent developments and future needs. *Trends Pharmacol. Sci.* **2002**, *23*, 238–245. [CrossRef]
83. Dhir, A.; Kulkarni, S.K. Involvement of dopamine (DA)/serotonin (5-HT)/sigma (sigma) receptor modulation in mediating the antidepressant action of ropinirole hydrochloride, a D2/D3 dopamine receptor agonist. *Brain Res. Bull.* **2007**, *74*, 58–65. [CrossRef]
84. Mavrikaki, M.; Schintu, N.; Nomikos, G.G.; Panagis, G.; Svenningsson, P. Ropinirole regulates emotionality and neuronal activity markers in the limbic forebrain. *Int. J. Neuropsychopharmacol.* **2014**, *17*, 1981–1993. [CrossRef] [PubMed]
85. Benes, H.; Mattern, W.; Peglau, I.; Dreykluft, T.; Bergmann, L.; Hansen, C.; Kohnen, R.; Banik, N.; Schoen, S.W.; Hornyak, M. Ropinirole improves depressive symptoms and restless legs syndrome severity in RLS patients: A multicentre, randomized, placebo-controlled study. *J. Neurol.* **2011**, *258*, 1046–1054. [CrossRef] [PubMed]
86. Rénéric, J.P.; Lucki, I. Antidepressant behavioral effects by dual inhibition of monoamine reuptake in the rat forced swimming test. *Psychopharmacology* **1998**, *136*, 190–197. [CrossRef] [PubMed]
87. Ghorpade, S.; Tripathi, R.; Sonawane, D.; Manjrekar, N. Evaluation of antidepressant activity of ropinirole coadministered with fluoxetine in acute and chronic behavioral models of depression in rats. *J. Basic Clin. Physiol. Pharmacol.* **2011**, *22*, 109–114. [CrossRef]
88. Bourin, M. Animal models for screening anxiolytic-like drugs: A perspective. *Dialogues Clin. Neurosci.* **2015**, *17*, 295–303. [CrossRef]
89. Sowa-Kućma, M.; Pańczyszyn-Trzewik, P.; Misztak, P.; Jaeschke, R.R.; Sendek, K.; Styczeń, K.; Datka, W.; Koperny, M. Vortioxetine: A review of the pharmacology and clinical profile of the novel antidepressant. *Pharmacol. Rep.* **2017**, *69*, 595–601. [CrossRef] [PubMed]
90. Christensen, M.C.; Loft, H.; Florea, I.; McIntyre, R.S. Efficacy of vortioxetine in working patients with generalized anxiety disorder. *CNS Spectr.* **2019**, *24*, 249–257. [CrossRef] [PubMed]
91. Pae, C.U.; Wang, S.M.; Han, C.; Lee, S.J.; Patkar, A.A.; Masand, P.S.; Serretti, A. Vortioxetine, a multimodal antidepressant for generalized anxiety disorder: A systematic review and meta-analysis. *J. Psychiatr. Res.* **2015**, *64*, 88–98. [CrossRef]
92. Guilloux, J.P.; Mendez-David, I.; Pehrson, A.; Guiard, B.P.; Repérant, C.; Orvoën, S.; Gardier, A.M.; Hen, R.; Ebert, B.; Miller, S.; et al. Antidepressant and anxiolytic potential of the multimodal antidepressant vortioxetine (Lu AA21004) assessed by behavioural and neurogenesis outcomes in mice. *Neuropharmacology* **2013**, *73*, 147–159. [CrossRef]

93. Available online: https://www.mayoclinic.org/drugs-supplements/ropinirole-oral-route/side-effects/drg-20066810?p=1 (accessed on 1 March 2021).
94. Available online: https://parkinsonsnewstoday.com/forums/forums/topic/ropinirole-cause-of-shortness-of-breath-anxiety-like-symptoms-between-med-dose/ (accessed on 1 March 2021).
95. Rogers, D.C.; Costall, B.; Domeney, A.M.; Gerrard, P.A.; Greener, M.; Kelly, M.E.; Hagan, J.J.; Hunter, A.J. Anxiolytic profile of ropinirole in the rat, mouse and common marmoset. *Psychopharmacology* **2000**, *151*, 91–97. [CrossRef] [PubMed]
96. Peciña, M.; Sikora, M.; Avery, E.T.; Heffernan, J.; Peciña, S.; Mickey, B.J.; Zubieta, J.K. Striatal dopamine D2/3 receptor-mediated neurotransmission in major depression: Implications for anhedonia, anxiety and treatment response. *Eur. Neuropsychopharmacol.* **2017**, *27*, 977–986. [CrossRef]
97. Simon, P.; Panissaud, C.; Costentin, J. Anxiogenic-like effects induced by stimulation of dopamine receptors. *Pharmacol. Biochem. Behav.* **1993**, *45*, 685–690. [CrossRef]
98. Jiang, L.X.; Huang, G.D.; Su, F.; Wang, H.; Zhang, C.; Yu, X. Vortioxetine administration attenuates cognitive and synaptic deficits in 5×FAD mice. *Psychopharmacology* **2020**, *237*, 1233–1243. [CrossRef] [PubMed]
99. Witt, N.A.; Lee, B.; Ghent, K.; Zhang, W.Q.; Pehrson, A.L.; Sánchez, C.; Gould, G.G. Vortioxetine Reduces Marble Burying but Only Transiently Enhances Social Interaction Preference in Adult Male BTBR T+Itpr3tf/J Mice. *ACS Chem. Neurosci.* **2019**, *10*, 4319–4327. [CrossRef]
100. Sałat, K.; Gawlik, K.; Witalis, J.; Pawlica-Gosiewska, D.; Filipek, B.; Solnica, B.; Więckowski, K.; Malawska, B. Evaluation of antinociceptive and antioxidant properties of 3-[4-(3-trifluoromethyl-phenyl)-piperazin-1-yl]-dihydrofuran-2-one in mice. *Naunyn. Schmiedebergs Arch. Pharmacol.* **2013**, *386*, 493–505. [CrossRef]
101. Porsolt, R.D.; Bertin, A.; Jalfre, M. Behavioral despair in mice: A primary screening test for antidepressants. *Arch. Int. Pharmacodyn. Ther.* **1977**, *229*, 327–336.
102. Sałat, K.; Siwek, A.; Starowicz, G.; Librowski, T.; Nowak, G.; Drabik, U.; Gajdosz, R.; Popik, P. Antidepressant-like effects of ketamine, norketamine and dehydronorketamine in forced swim test: Role of activity at NMDA receptor. *Neuropharmacology* **2015**, *99*, 301–307. [CrossRef]
103. Bourin, M.; Masse, F.; Dailly, E.; Hascoët, M. Anxiolytic-like effect of milnacipran in the four-plate test in mice: Mechanism of action. *Pharmacol. Biochem. Behav.* **2005**, *81*, 645–656. [CrossRef]
104. Montilla-García, Á.; Tejada, M.Á.; Perazzoli, G.; Entrena, J.M.; Portillo-Salido, E.; Fernández-Segura, E.; Cañizares, F.J.; Cobos, E.J. Grip strength in mice with joint inflammation: A rheumatology function test sensitive to pain and analgesia. *Neuropharmacology* **2017**, *125*, 231–242. [CrossRef]
105. DeSantana, J.M.; da Cruz, K.M.; Sluka, K.A. Animal models of fibromyalgia. *Arthritis Res. Ther.* **2013**, *15*, 222. [CrossRef] [PubMed]
106. Blasco-Serra, A.; Escrihuela-Vidal, F.; González-Soler, E.M.; Martínez-Expósito, F.; Blasco-Ausina, M.C.; Martínez-Bellver, S.; Cervera-Ferri, A.; Teruel-Martí, V.; Valverde-Navarro, A.A. Depressive-like symptoms in a reserpine-induced model of fibromyalgia in rats. *Physiol. Behav.* **2015**, *151*, 456–462. [CrossRef] [PubMed]

molecules MDPI

Review

The Role of Serotonin Neurotransmission in Gastrointestinal Tract and Pharmacotherapy

Tomasz Guzel [1] and Dagmara Mirowska-Guzel [2,*]

[1] Department of General, Gastroenterology and Oncologic Surgery, Medical University of Warsaw, Banacha 1a, 02-097 Warsaw, Poland; tomasz.guzel@wum.edu.pl
[2] Department of Experimental and Clinical Pharmacology, Medical University of Warsaw, Banacha 1b, 02-097 Warsaw, Poland
* Correspondence: dagmara.mirowska-guzel@wum.edu.pl; Tel.: +48-50-132-21-71

Abstract: 5-Hydroxytryptamine (5-HT, serotonin) is a neurotransmitter in both the central nervous system and peripheral structures, acting also as a hormone in platelets. Although its concentration in the gut covers >90% of all organism resources, serotonin is mainly known as a neurotransmitter that takes part in the pathology of mental diseases. Serotonin modulates not only CNS neurons, but also pain transmission and platelet aggregation. In the periphery, 5-HT influences muscle motility in the gut, bronchi, uterus, and vessels directly and through neurons. Serotonin synthesis starts from hydroxylation of orally delivered tryptophan, followed by decarboxylation. Serotonin acts via numerous types of receptors and clinically plays a role in several neural, mental, and other chronic disorders, such as migraine, carcinoid syndrome, and some dysfunctions of the alimentary system. 5-HT acts as a paracrine hormone and growth factor. 5-HT receptors in both the brain and gut are targets for drugs modifying serotonin neurotransmission. The aim of the present article is to review the 5-HT receptors in the gastrointestinal (GI) tract to determine the role of serotonin in GI physiology and pathology, including known GI diseases and the role of serotonin in GI pharmacotherapy.

Keywords: serotonin; 5-HT receptors; gastrointestinal tract

Citation: Guzel, T.; Mirowska-Guzel, D. The Role of Serotonin Neurotransmission in Gastrointestinal Tract and Pharmacotherapy. *Molecules* **2022**, *27*, 1680. https://doi.org/10.3390/molecules27051680

Academic Editor: Marcello Leopoldo

Received: 12 February 2022
Accepted: 1 March 2022
Published: 3 March 2022

1. Introduction

Serotonin (5-hydroxytryptamine; 5-HT) and serotoninergic drugs have become popular in the treatment of depression, and this common use has contributed to a broad knowledge of serotoninergic neurotransmission in the central nervous system (CNS). However, serotonin is not found solely in the CNS, and its highest concentrations occur elsewhere. Though obtained from a normal diet, serotonin must be synthesized de novo from tryptophan at the destinations of its action because it is almost fully metabolized before being absorbed. Tryptophan (TRP) is a nutritional amino acid and precursor of many physiologically essential substances, including 5-HT, melatonin, and kynurenine. Only 1–2% of TRP is degraded into 5-HT and melatonin, as 95% goes into kynurenine, kynurenic acid, xanturenic acid, quinolinic acid, and picolinic acid through the kynurenine pathway [1]. TRP undergoes hydroxylation in neurons and chromaffin cells via the enzyme tryptophan hydroxylase (TPH), which exists as two isoforms: TPH1 localized in the gut and TPH2 found in CNS neurons, mainly the raphe nuclei of the brain stem, and some neurons in the enteric nervous system (ENS). 5-Hydroxytryptophan (5-HTP) is then decarboxylated by a non-specific aromatic L-amino acid decarboxylase (L-AADC) that also participates in histamine and catecholamine transformation. 5-HT compounded with chromogranin A (CGA) is stored in vesicular monoamine transporter 1 (VMAT1), which is expressed by granules/vesicles in enterochromaffin (EC) cells [2]. EC cells within the gastrointestinal (GI) mucosa synthesize and secrete up to 95% of total body serotonin, whereas the remaining 5% is synthesized by neurons, mostly in the CNS, but also in pancreatic islets, mammary glands, and adipose tissue [3]. These cells respond to chemical and mechanical stimulation, but also collect signals from gut microbiota to release serotonin [4]. 5-HT interacts with nerve terminals or other cells (immune, epithelial) or is transported into enterocytes by the serotonin reuptake transporter (SERT) or organic cation transporters and dopamine transporter when SERT does not work. Elimination occurs through deamination to 5-hydroxyindole acetaldehyde (5-HIAL), followed by oxidation to 5-hydroxyindoloacetic acid (5-HIAA), which is excreted by the kidneys. The urine concentration of 5-HIAA is clinically important as an indicator of 5-HT synthesis [5]. A scheme of serotonin production is presented on Figure 1 [6].

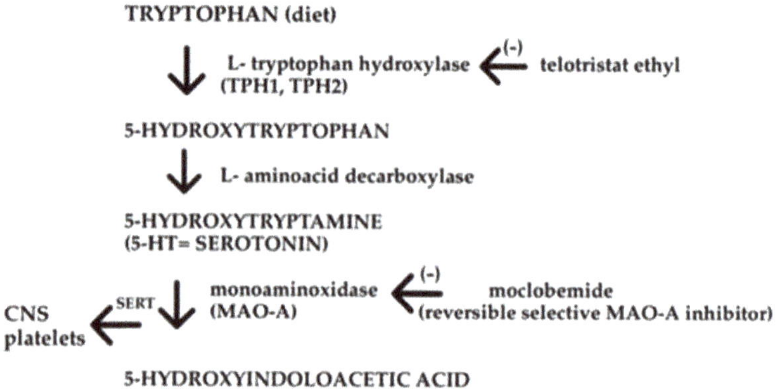

Figure 1. A scheme of serotonin production.

Serotonin was first discovered in the bowel and called "enteramine" by Vittorio Espramer in 1937 [7]. Further studies showed that "enteramine" has the same structure as the serum vasoconstrictor described by Rupport in 1947, which was called "serotonin" [8]. Serotonin and its receptors are part of the multimodal processes that affect homeostasis. 5-HT receptors are classified into seven families involving at least 15 subgroups of receptors [9]. Only the 5-HT3 receptor is a cation channel activated by a ligand; the others are coupled to a G protein, which is a membrane protein consisting of three subunits (alpha, beta, gamma), interacts with guanine nucleotides (GTP and GDP), and conjugates with different receptors that may result in several intracellular effects. The most common type of receptors in the GI tract are 5-HT3, 5-HT4, and 5-HT7. 5-HT receptors and their functions are presented in Table 1.

Table 1. Serotonin receptors and their functions in the gastrointestinal tract.

Receptor Family	Receptor or Subtype	Function
5-HT1	5-HT1A, 5HT1D	Gastric fundus relaxation
	5-HT1B/1D	Prokinetic intestinal stimulation
	5-HT1D	Contraction of intestinal circular muscle
	5-HT1B	Contraction of intestinal longitudinal muscle
	5-HT1P	Peristaltic and secretory reflexes
5-HT2	5-HT2A	Contraction of smooth muscles
	5-HT2B	Contraction of smooth muscles in stomach fundus, relaxation of longitudinal muscle in the intestine
5-HT3	5-HT3	Chloride secretion and serotonin release from EC cells
	5-HT3A	Increase intestinal motility
5-HT4	7 splice variants	Increase intestinal motility, contraction of esophagus, relaxation of colon, chloride secretion

Table 1. *Cont.*

Receptor Family	Receptor or Subtype	Function
5-HT5	-	Not known in gastrointestinal tract (essential solely in CNS)
5-HT6	-	Not known in gastrointestinal tract (essential solely in CNS)
5-HT7	5 splice variants	Excitatory effect, anti-inflammatory activity

CNS—central nervous system.

Serotonin increases the motility of the GI tract muscles, induces muscle constriction in the lungs and uterus, influences vessel muscles in both directions (constriction/relaxation), takes part in platelet aggregation, excites nociceptive pain neurons, and influences CNS neurons. Serotonin also plays a role in the symptoms of GI inflammation, acting through different mechanisms to exert pro- or anti-inflammatory activity [5,10–12]. Common substances have been shown to influence serotonin secretion, which may be responsible for the presence of ambiguous disease symptoms and prevalent digestive diseases. Bisphenol A, a chemical compound in plastic bottles made of PE, was shown in an animal study to enhance the number of 5-HT-positive cells in the mucosal layer of the small intestine [13]. GI tract disorders are closely associated with serotoninergic transmission. We review the current knowledge of peripheral serotonin neurotransmission with special emphasis on the effects essential for GI action and reference to drugs affecting the alimentary system.

2. Serotonin in the GI Tract

A highly organized ENS, also called the "abdominal brain" or "second brain", regulates absorption, secretion, and gut motility. It is the only organ that, although under the control of the CNS, can function in isolation independent of the brain. Serotonin is secreted by EC cells apically to the intestine lumen and baso-laterally in response to mechanical and chemical stimulation [14,15]. Through the mucosal projections of primary afferent neurons, intrinsic and extrinsic nerves conduct information to the CNS. Submucosal projections of intrinsic primary afferent neurons (IPANs) initiate peristaltic and secretory reflexes, whereas myenteric projections are responsible for giant contractions and mediate excitatory neurotransmission regulating GI motility [16]. Mechanical stimulation of the bowel (by food) provides secretion of 5-HT that activates IPANs containing calcitonin gene-related peptide (CGRP) in the mucosa, which synapse with ascending and descending interneurons. Through excitatory motor neurons, ascending interneurons cause contraction of smooth muscle mediated by acetylcholine, substance P, and neurokinin A. Descending interneurons cause smooth muscle relaxation, activating inhibitory motor neurons to release nitric oxide (NO), vasoactive intestinal peptide (VIP), and pituitary adenylate cyclase-activating peptide (PACAP) [17]. Longitudinal smooth muscles contract and relax in reverse fashion to circular muscle under the regulation of the same neurotransmitters [18,19].

2.1. GI Serotonin—Linkage to Metabolism

Investigations on human carcinoid EC cell lines have given information about its response to some nutrients. It was confirmed that EC cells are sensitive to luminal glucose levels through glucose–sensing mechanisms for both an acute increase and chronic reduction in glucose availability. EC cells express a range of G-protein-coupled receptors that are tuned to other nutrients, such as amino acids triggering serotonin release. Similarly, production of secondary bile acids and short-chain fatty acids by gut microbiota activates EC cells for 5-HT secretion. In vitro EC cells respond to neuromodulatory agents, which suggests that these cells may be responsive to neural signals in the CNS and ENS. Luminal 5-HT is required for intestinal nutrients and water absorption and takes part in bicarbonate and electrolyte secretion into the lumen, as well as bile acid turnover, bile acid synthesis, and liver secretion [20].

Serotoninergic intestinal activity depends on local stimulation. 5-HT secreted by EC cells acts as a paracrine messenger because there are no direct connections to the activated nerves. There is also confirmed hormonal signaling with other enteroendocrine cells. Mouse models have shown the role of gut-derived serotonin (GDS) in lipolysis and gluconeogenesis. Sumara et al., identified that 5-HT acts directly on adipocytes through the Htr2b receptor and promotes lipolysis during fasting. As a result, free fatty acids and glycerol are released as a substrate for liver gluconeogenesis. Htr2b is the most highly expressed 5-HT liver receptor. Serotonin has been observed to favor gluconeogenesis by enhancing the activity of two rate-limiting enzymes, FBPase and G6Pase. Through the same receptor, GDS suppresses glucose uptake in hepatocytes, possibly by suppressing glucokinase activity and glucose transporter 2 (Glut2) degradation. In diabetes type 2, there is often lipolysis and liver gluconeogenesis, and these results suggest that decreasing GDS synthesis could ameliorate type 2 diabetes [21]. Some EC cells express specific receptors, including receptors for glucagon-like peptide 1 and 2 (GLP1, GLP2) in diabetes and GI tract motility, respectively. GLP2 is secreted in response to food intake and influences GLP1 secretion from L cells in the ileum in response to an elevated glucose concentration. Thus, serotonin may act as a kind of mediator in inhibiting gastric emptying and stimulating gastric secretion with GLP2, and takes part in the metabolic reaction for glucose intake with GLP1 [20]. The intestinal microbiome performs a range of essential functions on the host metabolism.

Although the gut bacterial system, including that of Corynebacterium spp., Streptococcus spp., and Enterococcus spp., can synthesize and secrete 5-HT, it provides signals through metabolites, such as fatty and biliary acids, to EC cells to maintain the gut content and plasma serotonin levels [22].

Only a small amount of 5-HT is synthesized with bacterial beta-glucuronidase from glucuronide-conjugated serotonin. Some microbial metabolites promote TPH1 expression and 5-HT release. The pathway goes through specific receptors present in the colon, including olfactory receptor 78 (OLF78) for short-chain fatty acids, G-protein-coupled receptor 35 (GPR35) for small aromatic acids, G-protein-coupled bile acid receptor 1 (GPBAR1) for secondary bile acids, free fatty acid receptor 2 (FFAR2), and other G-protein coupled receptors [23,24]. The enteric microbiota is crucial and takes part in regulating a variety of neurotransmitters, including those playing an important role in diseases of the GI tract, such as histamine, serotonin, and glutamate. Non-specific and specific symptoms of GI tract failure seem to be a common problem in health services all over the world. According to the National Centre for Health Statistics (NCHS) in the US, there were 37.2 million visits to physician offices and 7.9 million to the emergency department with diseases of the digestive system as a primary diagnosis in 2018 [25].

2.2. *Serotonin in GI Tract Disorders*

2.2.1. Irritable Bowel Syndrome (IBS)

IBS is a bothersome disease that may occur with several leading symptoms with predominant complaints according to Rome IV criteria of constipation (IBS-C), diarrhea (IBS-D), mixed type (IBS-M), and unclassified (IBS-U) [26]. Symptoms may vary and are dependent on diet and lifestyle, and even may be influenced by psychological factors. There are no reliable, established, standardized tests to assess disease activity. One of the crucial factors that may influence the disease course is intestinal microbiota, and communication between the gut microbiota and CNS was proposed as the brain-gut microbiome (BGM). The microorganism composition is relatively stable, and an imbalance in homeostasis caused by usage of antibiotics or other drugs, diet change, and/or exposure to enteritis may lead to dysbiosis and clinical deterioration [27,28]. Bacterial overgrowth in the small intestine (SIBO) leads to a disturbance in intestinal absorption and release of toxic products, such as methane gas, influencing motor activity and delayed bowel transit [22]. There are several microbial neurotransmitters, including 5-HT, which seems to be an essential molecule that induces IBS symptoms through the activation of immune cells, changes in gut motility, and increased visceral hypersensitivity and epithelial permeability. Excessive serotonin release promotes GI motility and may be responsible for IBS-D symptoms, and bacteria-derived 5-HIAA directly accelerates colonic motility via activation of L-type calcium channels [29]. In contrast, increased SERT function and downregulation of TPH1 in animal models has been shown to reduce GI motility and lead to delayed intestinal transit [30,31]. Through 5-HT as a neurotransmitter, the gut microbiota stimulates mesenteric sensory fibers and vagal and spinal afferent fibers, influencing the presence of chronic pain in IBS patients, and the pro-inflammatory action of serotonin exacerbates abdominal pain intensity [32,33].

2.2.2. Inflammatory Bowel Disease (IBD)

IBD consists of two diseases—ulcerative colitis (UC) and Crohn's disease (CD). CD may affect all of the small and large bowel, whereas UC is limited to the colon. There are different types of immune responses involved in GI inflammation. CD is characterized by type 1 or type 17, with increased production of IL-12, IL-17, IL-23, IFNγ and TGFβ, whereas UC is typified by type 2 with higher levels of IL-5 and IL-13 [34,35]. There is high symptom heterogeneity, and the main factors affecting the course of IBD are genetic predisposition, infectious history, diet, and microbiota, which seems to play an important role in intestinal inflammation [36]. Kwon et al., compared the influence of serotonin on chemically induced colitis in a mouse model and showed that serotonin selected for more colitogenic microbiota by regulating bacterial growth and inhibiting beta-defensin production in colonic epithelial cells. A significantly reduced intestinal concentration of 5-HT decreased the severity of colitis. Microbial transfer between guts with 5-HT reduced and normalized the mediated colitis severity, indicating the protective function of microflora with reduced serotonin levels [37]. In humans, *Escherichia coli*, available as probiotic bacteria, regulates tryptophan hydroxylase 1, enhancing the 5-HT level. It may be beneficial in IBS-C to have a decreased serotonin level, and in IBD, an increased level of serotonin may be associated with exacerbation of the clinical course due to enhanced inflammation [38]. Microbiota-derived short-chain fatty acids, through upregulation of G-protein coupled receptors, strengthen the epithelial barrier integrity and, by inducing regulatory T cells, have anti-inflammatory potential. On the other hand, short-chain fatty acids upregulate TPH transcription, which increases mucosal production of serotonin, supporting inflammation and colitis manifestation [26].

Peripheral serotonin is important for a proper immune response but also impacts various inflammatory conditions, such as IBD. The main source of 5-HT for the immune response is platelets. Platelets cannot produce 5-HT themselves, but they take it from the bloodstream by SERT. In contrast, mast cells, monocytes/macrophages, and T cells partially participate in serotonin production. Serotonin acts as a chemotactic agent, increases pro-inflammatory cytokine secretion (e.g., IL-1, IL-6, IL-8, and NFkB), and enhances phagocytosis. Serotonin can affect both T cells and lymphocytes through their 5-HT receptors [39–42]. 5-HT increases the production of reactive species, enhances cytokine production, and promotes adhesion of monocytes to GI epithelial cells [43].

2.2.3. Carcinoid

Carcinoid is one of the best described neuroendocrine tumors (NETs), and carcinoid syndrome (CS) is the most frequent of the NET ectopic hormonal syndromes. CS occurs when a sufficient amount of tumor-related compounds are secreted into systemic circulation. Despite the fact that numerous potential mediators are reported to be responsible for the clinical symptoms of CS, the most frequently used for laboratory confirmation is 5-HIAA, the product of 5-HT degradation. Overproduction of serotonin is noted in 98–100% of cases, and persevering diarrhea is one of the symptoms of CS [44]. Serotonin stimulates colonic motor functions via 5-HT3 and chloride ion secretion via the 5-HT2A and 5-HT4 receptors [9].

In February 2017, the Food and Drug Administration (FDA) approved telotristat ethyl for the treatment of CS diarrhea in patients inadequately controlled by somatostatin analogue therapy. The European Medicine Agency (EMA) followed suit in September of that year. The drug is a first-in-class, small molecule, peripheral TPH inhibitor [45]. TPH is one of the main causes of the effects of CS, such as frequent bowel movements associated with diarrhea and other symptoms [46]. Telotristat ethyl is given as a tablet three times daily and is generally well tolerated. The proportion of patients reporting at least one adverse event related to the drug is similar to that observed with placebo. The most common adverse events are abdominal pain, nausea, increased gamma-glutamyltransferase, and fatigue [47]. However, the drug was labeled with a black triangle due to EMA regulations for new drugs and biologics approved since January 2011. The symbol displayed in their package leaflet and the summary of product characteristics (SmPC) for healthcare professionals means that the medications are under 'additional monitoring' by regulatory authorities, and is meant to encourage doctors and patients to report any adverse effects [48].

2.3. 5-HT Receptors and Drugs Acting in the GI Tract

Multimodal serotonin GI function and enteric pathologies are a result of the presence of different types of 5-HT receptor families. 5-HT1 includes five subtypes: 5-HT1A, 5-HT1B, 5-HT1D, 5-HT1e, and 5-HT1F. However, for 5-HT1e, a functional response in native cells or tissue has not been identified [9]. What was the 5-HT1C receptor was finally classified as 5-HT2C, so it does not exist in the 5-HT1 family. Representatives of this group of receptors have been confirmed in many tissues. The most extensively distributed is the 5-HT1A receptor, which is present in the CNS, cardiovascular system, and GI tract. Extensive investigations of the distribution of the 5-HT1 receptors and their involvement in a variety of physiological and pathological responses have led to a broad knowledge base on 5-HT1 receptor identification, expression, and pharmacology. Much is known about 5-HT1A receptors, especially in area of targeting for pharmacotherapy in a broad spectrum of neuropsychiatric disorders, such as major depression, anxiety, schizophrenia, pain, attention deficiency hyperactivity disorder, cognitive deficits, Parkinson's disease, and recently sexual dysfunction and respiratory deficits [9]. Its role in the human GI tract seems to be rather limited. The main confirmed role is a contribution to gastric contractility. Application of a selective 5-HT1A receptor agonist, R137696, resulted in fundus relaxation with no effect on distension-induced dyspeptic symptoms [49]. Similar observations concerning the administration of sumatriptan, a 5-HT1D agonist, was reported by Coullie et al., who noted that relaxation of the gastric fundus resulted in a prolonged half-emptying time of liquids and solids [50]. Sumatriptan also increases lower esophageal sphincter (LES) contraction but increases the frequency of reflux. This is probably due to sumatriptan evoking stomach postprandial relaxation and delayed meal retention [51]. The 5-HT1B receptor is present in the CNS and vessels, but 5-HT1B/1D agonists have been observed to have a prokinetic influence on GI tract muscles [52]. Different types of 5-HT receptor antagonists act through different types of intestine musculature. 5-HT1D antagonists decrease contraction of the circular muscle of human small intestine, whereas 5-HT1B antagonists decrease contraction of the longitudinal muscle [53]. A few publications have distinguished the 5-HT1P receptor as a separate subtype [54–56], but it needs to be defined and is suspected to be either the 5-HT7 receptor or a heterodimer consisting of the dopamine D2 receptor with either the 5-HT1B or 5-HT1D receptor with a functional role in the ENS, as it was not detected in the CNS [57]. The 5-HT1P receptor may be critical in the initiation and maintenance of peristaltic and secretory reflexes; it activates submucosal IPANs, and receptor agonists can be expected to enhance diarrhea, whereas antagonists stimulate constipation, or even paralytic ileus [56,57]. Several antidepressant and antimigraine drugs acting via the 5-HT1 receptor have been registered and approved. Sumatriptan prototypical triptane with affinity for different 5-HT1 receptors affects the smooth muscles in the GI tract and, in 1992, was the first triptane approved by the FDA for migraine treatment. Triptanes of mixed affinity to 5-HT1 receptors were available on the market later. Sumatriptan, zolmitriptan, naratriptan, and riazatriptan are full agonists of all 5-HT1 receptors. Frovatriptan is a full agonist to 5-HT1B and 5-HT1D receptors with partial agonism towards 5HT1A and 5-HT1F receptors. Attempts to develop 5-HT1D selective agonists have been unsuccessful, but a new class of drugs was recognized during the research into selective subtypes of 5-HT1 receptor agonists. These are "ditans" that selectively act at the 5-HT1F receptor. Activation of a second messenger for the 5-HT1B receptor, but not the 5-HT1D or 5-HT1F receptors, correspond to the contractile potency of isolated human blood vessels in vitro and in anesthetized canines in vivo [58]. Lasmiditan is considered to be a first-in class "ditan" registered by the FDA in October 2019 [59] and is under evaluation by the EMA. None of the triptanes or lasmiditan have been registered directly for GI tract diseases [60]. However, sumatriptan given to a patient with functional dyspepsia delays gastric emptying, improves gastric accommodation, and reduces the perception of gastric distension and early satiety [61]. Thus, 5-HT1B and 5-HT1D receptors may be involved in the mechanism of vomiting, though this has not been elucidated [62].

The 5-HT2 receptor family consists of three subtypes: 5-HT2A, 5-HT2B, 5-HT2C. This family has excitatory activity, but 5-HT2A also has inhibitory effects. 5-HT2A receptors were first identified in the brain but soon after were found to mediate several effects in the periphery, including platelet aggregation, chloride ion secretion [63], and triggering the contraction of smooth muscles due to its presence in myenteric and submucosal neurons, enterocytes, and both the longitudinal and circular muscles of the GI tract [64]. Many cell types in the periphery express 5-HT2A receptors, including platelets, fibroblasts, lymphocytes, and myocytes [9]. 5-HT2B receptors are present in the longitudinal and circular muscle layers and myenteric neurons. Their activation results in the contraction of smooth muscle in the stomach fundus and longitudinal muscle in the intestine. In preclinical studies, these receptors were postulated to take part in the development of the ENS [5]. 5-HT2C receptors have no known role in GI physiology. There are a number of drugs that act through 5-HT2 receptors. Some are used in migraine, including methysegrid (withdrawn from the market due to cases of retroperitoneal fibrosis), pizotifen, and cyproheptadine. Atypical antipsychotics, such as risperidone, olanzapine, clozapine, and sertindole, block 5-HT2A receptors with high affinity but have limited selectivity versus 5-HT2C and dopamine receptors [8a]. The discovery that 5-HT2A receptor inverse agonists have antipsychotic effects opened an alternative pathway for treating psychosis and drove the development of pimavanserin, a 5HT2A inverse agonist. Pimavanserin lacks dopamine receptor affinity but exhibits antipsychotic activity [65]. In 2016, the FDA and EMA approved pimavanserin for the treatment of psychosis in Parkinson's disease. Considering the GI system, 5-HT2B receptor expression has been found in spontaneous human carcinoid tumors [66] and hepatitis C-type hepatocellular carcinoma [67]. This suggests 5-HT receptors as a therapeutic target.

There is still little evidence on the expression of 5-HT1C receptor outside the CNS. Low levels of the 5-HT2C receptor mRNA has been noted in pancreatic islet cells [68] and been induced in cultured adipocytes [69]. The physiological role of 5-HT2C in the above-mentioned areas still needs to be elucidated.

The 5-HT3 receptor is different in structure and function from the other six families of 5-HT receptors. The 5-HT3 receptors have a pentameric composition of five identical or nonidentical subunits (from A to E). Only 5-HT3A subunits form functional homomeric 5-HT3 receptors. Other subunits have been identified (from B to E), but only 5-HT3B has been investigated to any extent. Co-expression of the 5-HT3B subunit with 5-HT3A creates the 5-HT3AB receptor. The presence of at least one 5-HT3A subunit is necessary for heteromeric forms [9]. The number and arrangement of 5-HT3C, 5-HT3D, and 5-HT3E subunits in functional receptors has not been determined, though their expression at the protein level was not confirmed too long ago [70]. 5-HT3 receptors create the only group that is ion channel gated by ligand and permeable to sodium, potassium, and calcium. They are expressed mostly in the CNS but are also important in the GI tract, as they take part in gut motility and chemotherapy-induced nausea and emesis. Receptor immunoreactivity was confirmed in the myenteric and submucosal plexuses, cells of Cajal, and the circular and longitudinal muscle cells. Receptor genes were present in both the colon and intestine [71,72]. A preclinical study showed that myenteric IPAN excitation occurs through 5-HT3 receptor activation, and the myenteric and submucosal neurons respond to stimulation [73]. 5-HT3 receptors also play a role in GI mucosal secretion, as their activation results in chloride secretion and serotonin release from EC cells [74,75]. Some studies have confirmed that 5-HT3A receptor mRNA, in particular, is present at high levels in the stomach and colon rather than the small intestine. These receptors are expressed in cholinergic nerves and PDGFRα-positive cells in the myenteric plexus, directly influencing motility. Their activation accelerates gastric emptying and colon transit [76]. 5-HT3 receptors play a role in rotavirus –induced diarrhea. Hagbom showed that serotonin is secreted by EC cells in response to rotavirus enterotoxin NSP4, which acts via 5-HT3 receptor and increases bowel motility [77]. The mechanism of chemotherapy-dependent nausea is via excitation by anticancer drugs (e.g., cisplatin) of EC cells to release serotonin, which activates 5-HT3 receptors and vagal sensory afferent neurons conduct signals to the emetic center in the brain stem [17,78]. In patients treated by cisplatin, higher urinary levels of 5-HIAA confirmed the correlation with the development of emesis. What is important about transmission depends on vagal excitation rather than serotonin release; thus, 5-HT3 antagonist (ondansetron) does not affect the increased 5-HIAA urinary levels [79].

Dependent on anticancer drug doses and type, ondansetron combined with dexamethasone gives complete protection from vomiting in up to 70–80% of cases without adverse effects on intestinal activity and stool consistency [17,80,81]. Ondansetron was first approved in the EU in 1990 and in the US in 1991. It is indicated in the EU for the management of nausea and vomiting induced by cytotoxic chemotherapy and radiotherapy (adults and children > 6 months) and for the prevention and treatment of post-operative nausea and vomiting (adults and children > 1 month). The FDA issued a warning about the risk of abnormal heart rhythms from high doses of ondansetron in 2011, followed by the EMA in 2012 [82]. The SmPC was updated in November 2019 with important changes to the section on "Fertility, pregnancy and lactation". The SmPC now states that ondansetron should not be used in the first trimester of pregnancy due to the risk of congenital cardiac malformations and oral cleft [83]. Alosetron and cilansetron were implemented into IBS-D treatment but were suspected in the development of ischemic colitis requiring advanced surgical treatment, despite no serious constipation. Due to such serious adverse events, these drugs were withdrawn from the market in 2000. The FDA approved a supplemental new drug application in 2002, which allows for the remarketing of alosetron, but under conditions of restricted use [17,60]. Several other drugs also act on the GI tract via the 5-HT3 receptor. These are non-selective 5-HT3A antagonists, such as metoclopramide, which acts as an antagonist to both dopamine D2 and 5-HT3A receptors. It was approved by the FDA and EMA in 1979 and is recommended to avoid postoperative and chemotherapy-induced emesis. However, in 2013, some restrictions to the use of metoclopramide were introduced by the EMA [84] that were mainly aimed to minimize the known risks of potentially serious adverse neurological reactions. It was recommended that metoclopramide should be prescribed only for short-term use (up to five days) and not be used in children < 1 year of age, and in children > 1 year of age, it may only be used as a second-choice treatment for the prevention of delayed nausea and vomiting after chemotherapy and for the treatment of post-operative nausea and vomiting. In adults, it is used for the prevention and treatment of nausea and vomiting, such as that associated with chemotherapy, radiotherapy, surgery, and in the management of migraine. Moreover, the maximum allowable doses in adults and children were reduced, and higher strength formulations removed from the market [84]. 5-HT3A selective antagonists consist of palonosetron (approved by FDA in 2003 and EMA in 2009 as antiemetic), alosetron (approved and reapproved in 2002 in IBS treatment), granisetron (approved by FDA in 1993 and EMA in 2012 as antiemetic), tropisetron (approved for chemotherapy-induced emesis), and ondansetron (approved by FDA in 1991 as antiemetic in patients receiving chemotherapy and in postoperative emesis) [60].

The 5-HT4 receptor family represents G protein-coupled metabotropic receptors with seven splice variants associated with adenylyl cyclase activity. These receptors are widely distributed within the CNS and periphery, including the heart, GI tract, adrenal and salivary glands, urinary bladder, and lungs [9]. Stimulation of the receptors by an agonist affects the modulation of GI motility and contraction of the esophagus and potentiates peristaltic reflex by colon relaxation and contraction depending on the method of stimulation. In a preclinical investigation, activation of the 5-HT4 receptors located on circular smooth muscle cells resulted in colon relaxation, whereas activation via receptors located on neurons leads to excitatory and inhibitory neurotransmitter release (calcitonin gene-related peptide, vasoactive inhibitory peptide, substance P) [85]. 5-HT4 receptors are important in the early development of enteric neurons, affecting neurogenesis after injury or surgical wound healing after gut anastomosis in adults. Thus, in an animal model, the receptor agonist mosapride promoted the regeneration of an impaired myenteric plexus and recovered the defecation reflex in the rectum [86,87]. In the ileum and right colon, serotonin increases chloride secretion via the 5-HT4 receptors and, with short-chain fatty acids, HCO_3 luminal secretion [16]. In addition, voltage-controlled ion channel stimulation influences not only intestinal muscles, but also heart atria [88–90], which may be responsible for the cardiac toxicity of pure older agonists, such as cisapride. The arrhythmogenic effect of stimulation of atrial 5-HT4 receptors was proposed long ago [91], and the antiarrhythmic effects of 5-HT4 antagonists were presented in a porcine model of atrial fibrillation [92]. Atrial 5-HT4 expression was increased in human chronic atrial fibrillation [93]. QT prolongation and ventricular tachyarrhythmias are thought to be due to potassium channel dysfunction, and cisapride can trigger tachycardia and supraventricular arrhythmia via 5-HT4 atrial receptors [94]. Later, the mechanism through which cisapride promotes cardiac arrhythmias was found to be unrelated to 5-HT4 receptor agonism. The cardiac risk is thought to be related to its affinity for hERG channels, which results in QT prolongation and is enhanced by the concomitant use of inhibitors of CYP involved in cisapride metabolism [95]. Nevertheless, cisapride was withdrawn from the US market in 2000 [76] and suspended from the European market in 2002 [96] due to serious adverse cardiac events. The affinity of the 5-HT4 receptor for particular ligands has been noted to depend on which COOH-terminal splice variant is expressed by a particular cell. This differentiation may explain why the same agonist facilitates increased GI motility with high intrinsic activity, whereas the intrinsic activity in cardiac muscle is low [97,98]. The only drugs acting as selective 5HT4 agonists that remain on the market are mosapride, which improves gastric emptying and reduces gastro-esophageal reflux symptoms, and prucalopride for the treatment of chronic constipation in adults for whom laxatives do not work well enough [99]. Prucalopride has also been investigated in idiopathic, diabetic, and connective tissue disease-related gastroparesis [100,101]. Partial agonists of 5-HT4 receptors, such as tegaserod, seem to be safer by not resulting in heart toxicity and, therefore, are useful in treating the symptoms of IBS-C. Tegaserod reduces the severity of colitis, increases the proliferation of crypt epithelial cells via receptor stimulation, and reduces oxidative stress-induced apoptosis, which was confirmed in animal models before implementation in IBS treatment [102]. Some data also indicate a beneficial role of tegaserod in gastro-esophageal reflux disease (GERD) and gastroparesis treatment. It improves esophageal acid clearance, reduces lower esophageal sphincter (LES) relaxation, and enhances gastric meal passage. This reduces the low postprandial esophagus exposition for stomach acid and decreases GERD symptoms [100,101]. Only a few of the drugs mentioned above were approved in the US and EU with a mechanism acting via the 5-HT4 receptor, though tegaserod was also withdrawn from the market in 2007 due to adverse cardiovascular effects [58].

The 5-HT5 and 5-HT6 receptors are present mostly in the CNS [103–105]. They are probably involved in psychiatric disorders, but also anxiety and memory processes [106].

The 5-HT7 receptors have five splice variants that are abundantly present in the vessels and extravascular smooth muscles of the GI tract [5]. They are present in the human stomach, small intestine, and colon, and their activity has been confirmed in myenteric and submucosal IPANs [107]. The activation of these receptors in IPANs produces slow excitatory postsynaptic potentials, resulting in muscle relaxation. In animal models, selective 5-HT7 antagonists have been shown to inhibit the excitatory potential and reduce the accommodation of the circular muscles during the relaxation phase of peristalsis. Overstimulation of the receptors has been postulated to be responsible for abdominal bloating and the exaggerated relaxation of circular muscles, resulting in the symptoms of functional bowel diseases. 5-HT7 agonists may improve after-feeding symptoms, such as postprandial satiety [108]. A similar effect has been investigated for other fundus-relaxing drugs, including sumatriptan and buspirone, which are not classical 5-HT7 agonists. The 5-HT7 receptor is expressed in enteric neurons and CD11c/CD86 cells of the colon in animal models suffering from induced CD. Receptor stimulation has shown an anti-inflammatory effect, likely by the regulation of cytokine production by activated immune cells. The 5-HT7 receptor takes part in cytokine production by antigen-presenting dendritic cells and LPS-stimulated macrophages, except that dendritic cells are able to modulate T-cell function through the 5-HT7 receptor. Thus, the 5-HT7 receptor blockade results in severe inflammation severity, whereas its stimulation results in the clinical remission of symptoms [109]. In contrast to these results, in 2,4,6 trinitrobenzene sulfonic acid-induced colitis, blockade of the receptor does not have such an effect on the severity of inflammation. Thus, this activity may be model-dependent and require further studies [110]. There have been solely antidepressant and antipsychotic drugs approved in the US and EU that have a mechanism of action involving the 5-HT7 receptor [61].

The peripheral effects of acting on serotonin receptors and therapeutic outcomes are presented in Figure 2.

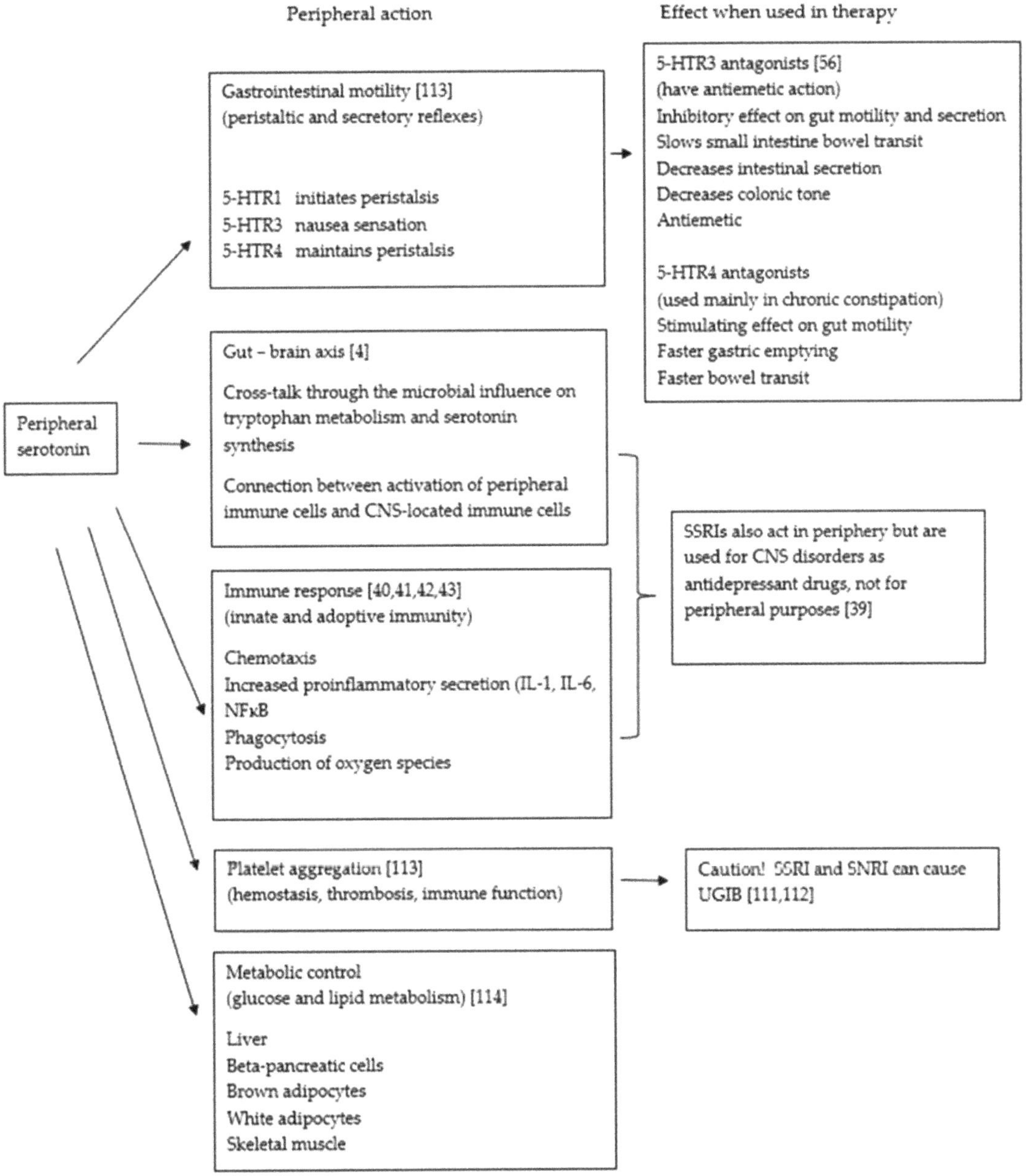

Legend: CNS—central nervous system, SSRI—selective serotonin reuptake inhibitor, SNRI—serotonin noradrenalin reuptake inhibitor, UGIB—upper gastrointestinal bleeding

Figure 2. Peripheral effects of acting on serotonin receptors and therapeutic outcomes [111–114].

3. Conclusions

In summarizing the multimodal role of serotonin, it is worth underlining that the effects of its activity differ according to the receptors on which it acts. Serotonin takes part in both the physiology and pathophysiology of the GI tract. In general, it increases intestinal motility but, depending on the receptors, may play opposite roles in the upper and lower part of the GI tract. In IBS with diarrhea, the plasma level of serotonin is increased, whereas in patients with constipation it is decreased. Thus, the proposed pharmacological treatment involves 5-HT3 receptor antagonism to slow the passage or 5-HT4 receptor agonism as a prokinetic agent. Models of IBD have confirmed that serotonin plays a role in enhancing inflammation, whereas a decreased level of 5-HT is accompanied by a decreased severity of disease signs and symptoms. An anti-inflammatory reaction goes through activation of 5-HT4 and 5-HT7 receptors. Immunology of the response of the 5-HT receptor involves immune cells, including dendritic cells, macrophages, neutrophils, and lymphocytes, and is altered by the pro-inflammatory cytokines TNFα, IL-1β, IL-6, and IFNγ and the anti-inflammatory IL-10. Although some drugs acting on 5-HT receptors are registered in GI tract diseases, there is still much to be elucidated in terms of their mechanism of action, efficacy, and safety.

Author Contributions: T.G.—investigation, writing—original draft preparation, D.M.-G.—writing—review and editing, project administration. All authors have read and agreed to the published version of the manuscript.

Funding: This research was founded by Medical University of Warsaw, statutory grant 1M9/N/2022.

Institutional Review Board Statement: Not applicable.

Informed Consent Statement: Not applicable.

Data Availability Statement: Not applicable.

Acknowledgments: This research subject was supported by the CePT infrastructure, fianced by the European Union—the European Regional Development Fund within the Operational Program "Innovative economy"for 2007–2013. Authors thank Hanna Guzel for her technical support.

Conflicts of Interest: The authors declare that they have no conflict of interest.

References

1. Liu, N.; Sun, S.; Wang, P.; Sun, Y.; Hu, Q.; Wang, X. The mechanism of secretion and metabolism of gut-derived 5-hydrixytryptamine. *Int. J. Mol. Sci.* **2021**, *22*, 7931. [CrossRef] [PubMed]
2. Montesinos, M.S.; Machado, J.D.; Camacho, M.; Diaz, J.; Morales, Y.G.; Alvarezde la Rosa, D.; Carmona, E.; Castaneyra, A.; Viveros, O.H.; O'Connor, D.T.; et al. The crucial role of chromogranins in storage and exocytosis revealed using chromaffin cells from chromogranin A null mouse. *J. Neurosci.* **2008**, *28*, 3350–3358. [CrossRef] [PubMed]
3. Martin, A.M.; Young, R.L.; Leong, L.; Rogers, G.B.; Spencer, N.J.; Jessup, C.F.; Keating, D.J. The diverse metabolic roles of peripheral serotonin. *Endocrinology* **2016**, *158*, 1049–1063. [CrossRef] [PubMed]
4. Jones, L.A.; Sun, E.W.; Martin, A.M.; Keating, D.J. The ever-changing roles of serotonin. *Int. J. Biochem. Cell Biol.* **2020**, *125*, 105776. [CrossRef]
5. Pytliak, M.; Vargova, V.; Mechirova, V.; Felsoci, M. Serotonin receptors—From molecular biology to clinical applications. *Physiol. Res.* **2011**, *60*, 15–25. [CrossRef]
6. Yabut, J.M.; Crane, J.D.; Green, A.E.; Keating, D.J.; Khan, W.I.; Steinberg, G.R. Emerging roles for serotonin in regulating metabolism: New implications for an ancient molecule. *Endocr. Rev.* **2019**, *40*, 1092–1107. [CrossRef]
7. Gershon, D.M. 5-hydroxytryptamine (serotonin) in the gastrointestinal tract. *Curr. Opin. Endocrinol. Diabetes Obes.* **2013**, *10*, 14–21. [CrossRef]
8. Rapport, M.M.; Green, A.A.; Page, I.H. Serum vasoconstrictor (serotonin); isolation and characterization. *J. Biol. Chem.* **1948**, *176*, 1243–1251. [CrossRef]
9. Barnes, N.M.; Ahern, G.P.; Becamel, C.; Bockaert, J.; Camilleri, M.; Chaumont-Dubel, S.; Claeysen, S.; Cunningham, K.A.; Fone, K.C.; Gershon, M.; et al. International Union of Basic and Clinical Pharmacology. CX. Classification of Receptors for 5-hydroxytryptamine; Pharmacology and Function. *Pharm. Rev.* **2021**, *73*, 310–520. [CrossRef]
10. Ghia, J.E.; Li, N.; Wang, H.; Collins, M.; Deng, Y.; El-Sharkawy, R.T.; Cote, F.; Mallet, J.; Khan, W.I. Serotonin has a key role in pathogenesis of experimental colitis. *Gastroenterology* **2009**, *137*, 1649–1660. [CrossRef]

molecules

MDPI

Review

Antibiotics and the Nervous System—Which Face of Antibiotic Therapy Is Real, Dr. Jekyll (Neurotoxicity) or Mr. Hyde (Neuroprotection)?

Magdalena Hurkacz [1,2], Lukasz Dobrek [1] and Anna Wiela-Hojeńska [1,*]

[1] Department of Clinical Pharmacology, Wroclaw Medical University, 50-556 Wroclaw, Poland; magdalena.hurkacz@umw.edu.pl (M.H.); lukasz.dobrek@umw.edu.pl (L.D.)
[2] Clinical Pharmacy Service, Jan Mikulicz-Radecki University Clinical Hospital, 50-556 Wroclaw, Poland
* Correspondence: anna.wiela-hojenska@umw.edu.pl

Abstract: Antibiotics as antibacterial drugs have saved many lives, but have also become a victim of their own success. Their widespread abuse reduces their anti-infective effectiveness and causes the development of bacterial resistance. Moreover, irrational antibiotic therapy contributes to gastrointestinal dysbiosis, that increases the risk of the development of many diseases, including neurological and psychiatric. One of the potential options for restoring homeostasis is the use of oral antibiotics that are poorly absorbed from the gastrointestinal tract (e.g., rifaximin alfa). Thus, antibiotic therapy may exert neurological or psychiatric adverse drug reactions which are often considered to be overlooked and undervalued issues. Drug-induced neurotoxicity is mostly observed after beta-lactams and quinolones. Penicillin may produce a wide range of neurological dysfunctions, including encephalopathy, behavioral changes, myoclonus or seizures. Their pathomechanism results from the disturbances of gamma-aminobutyric acid-GABA transmission (due to the molecular similarities between the structure of the β-lactam ring and GABA molecule) and impairment of the functioning of benzodiazepine receptors (BZD). However, on the other hand, antibiotics have also been studied for their neuroprotective properties in the treatment of neurodegenerative and neuroinflammatory processes (e.g., Alzheimer's or Parkinson's diseases). Antibiotics may, therefore, become promising elements of multi-targeted therapy for these entities.

Keywords: antibiotics; neurotoxicity; adverse drug reaction; neurotransmission

Citation: Hurkacz, M.; Dobrek, L.; Wiela-Hojeńska, A. Antibiotics and the Nervous System—Which Face of Antibiotic Therapy Is Real, Dr. Jekyll (Neurotoxicity) or Mr. Hyde (Neuroprotection)? *Molecules* **2021**, *26*, 7456. https://doi.org/10.3390/molecules26247456

Academic Editor: Alicja Nowaczyk

Received: 9 November 2021
Accepted: 7 December 2021
Published: 9 December 2021

1. Introduction. Antibiotics and Antibiotic-Induced Adverse Drug Reactions

Antibiotics are one of the most widely used classes of drug that have revolutionized the treatment of infectious diseases, enabling the causal treatment of these conditions. The discovery of antibiotic agents and their introduction into clinical practice is considered to be one of the greatest medical breakthrough of the 20th century [1]. Mankind has used antibacterial agents of natural origin since the dawn of its history, based on empirical knowledge and centuries-old tradition in various healing systems (e.g., traditional Chinese medicine and others). Traces of tetracyclines, incorporated into the hydroxyapatite mineral portion of bones, have been found in skeletal remains of ancient people (e.g., of the Roman period or even in Sudanese Nubian human remains dated back to 350–550 CE) [2]. The beginning of the modern "antibiotic era" and antibiotic therapy used to treat human infections is usually associated with names of Paul Ehrlich, Gerhard Domagk and Alexander Fleming. These researchers became famous in the history of medicine with the introduction of the first modern, arsenic-based antimicrobial agent named Salvarsan, effective in the treatment of syphilis (Ehrlich; 1909), the discovery of the sulfa drug, sulfonamidochrysoidine (Protonsil), endogenously releasing active sulfanilamide (Domagk; 1935; Nobel Prize laureate in Medicine or Physiology in 1939 for the development of antibacterial effect of Protonsil) and the discovery of penicillin (Fleming; 1929; Nobel Prize laureate in Medicine or Physiology in 1945 for the discovery of penicillin and its curative effect in various infectious diseases) [2,3]. Obviously, these "milestones" of antibiotic therapy would not have been possible without the prior work of other researchers, such as Antonie van Leeuwenhoek, Robert Hooke, Robert Koch and Louis Pasteur who laid the basics for modern microbiology [3]. Then, "the golden age of antibiotic discovery" began, which lasted for about 20 years and resulted in the introduction of most of the currently used antibiotics in clinical practice. The twilight of this period, which also includes the present times, is the aftermath and one of the fundamental problems of antibiotic therapy, i.e., the development of bacterial strains resistant to various antibiotics, which results in the loss of the anti-infective effectiveness of many of the preparations used so far. Uncontrolled infectious diseases are again becoming an emerging problem in modern medicine. Estimates indicate that mortality rates due to multidrug-resistant bacterial infections have become increasingly higher—each year, about 25,000 of patients treated in the EU die from multidrug-resistant bacterial induced infections and in the USA about 63,000 deaths are caused by hospital-acquired infections [2]. Currently, bacterial resistance is not limited to primary inpatients, but is especially true for outpatients. The ongoing antibiotic resistance crisis is determined by various factors, the most important of which include the excessive and unreasonable antibiotic consumption (due to the fact that in many countries antibiotics use is unregulated and available over the counter without a rational medical recommendation), inappropriate prescribing and extensive agricultural use (primarily to promote growth of housed animals and to prevent infections) [4]. Complex genetic mechanisms, including plasmids, bacteriophages, naked DNA or transposons, are the background for the development of bacterial resistance to antibiotics. Spontaneous mutations are also an important cause, allowing the acquisition of bacterial resistance to antibiotics without the exchange of genetic material between various strains [5]. The problem of widespread bacterial resistance to many, if not most, antibiotics still used in the current therapy is a major threat and disadvantage. New solutions are expected (including the discovery of new structures with antimicrobial activity) that would allow us to be "one step" ahead of bacteria in the fight to control infection. To sum up, despite the undisputed benefits of antibiotics, which have saved millions of lives from the consequences of infectious diseases, the current treatment of these diseases is becoming more and more challenging.

Additionally, a significant problem of antibiotic therapy is the occurrence of many possible antibiotic-related adverse drug reactions (ADR). An adverse drug reaction is regarded as an expected, unwanted, harmful or unpleasant effect attributed to the use of a medication that occurs during its usual clinical use. According to the commonly accepted definition given by Edward and Aronson, "an adverse drug reaction is an appreciably harmful or unpleasant reaction, resulting from an intervention related to the use of the medicinal product, which predicts hazard from future administration and warrants prevention or specific treatment, or alternation of the dosage regimen, or withdrawal of the product". ADRs appear in both outpatients and hospitalized patients and manifest a wide spectrum of clinical entities, ranging from mild symptoms to life-threatening disorders. Estimates indicate that ADRs occur in 5–10% of cases of hospital admissions and, in as many as 0.1–0.3% ADRs, may be serious and cause death [6–8].

Antibiotics, along with antiplatelets, anticoagulants, cytotoxics, immunosuppressants, diuretics or antidiabetics, have been particularly implicated in ADR inducement. Perhaps the most characteristic for antibiotic-related ADRs are the symptoms caused by hypersensitivity and allergic reactions, which most often take the form of skin reactions (rash, hives, itching), but these can also be severe disorders such as angioedema or anaphylactic shock. Other characteristic antibiotic-induced ADRs are complex symptoms originating from the gastrointestinal tract (e.g., nausea, vomiting, bloating, diarrhea/constipation) determined by the altered secretion, absorption and motility due to dysbiosis. There are also reported class-specific (or even compound-specific) antibiotic-related ADRs, for example: the possibility of developing pseudomembranous colitis induced by *Clostridium difficile* colonization after application of antibiotics with broad antibacterial activity, aminoglycoside-associated

11. Manocha, M.; Khan, W.I. Serotonin and GI disorders: An update of clinical and experimental studies. *Clin. Transl. Gastroenterol.* **2012**, *3*, e13. [CrossRef]
12. Gershon, M.D.; Liu, M.T. Serotonin and neuroprotection in functional bowel disorders. *Neurogastroenterol. Motil.* **2007**, *19*, 19–24. [CrossRef]
13. Gonkowski, S. Bisphenol A (BPA)-induced changes in the number of serotonin-positive cells in the mucosal layer of porcine small intestine-the preliminary studies. *Int. J. Mol. Sci.* **2020**, *21*, 1079. [CrossRef] [PubMed]
14. Gershon, M. Roles played by 5-hydroxytryptamine in the physiology of the bowel. *Aliment. Pharmacol.* **1999**, *13*, 15–30. [CrossRef]
15. Racke, K.; Reimann, A.; Schworer, H.; Kilbinger, H. Regulation of 5-HT release from enterochromaffin cells. *Behav. Brain Res.* **1995**, *73*, 83–87. [CrossRef]
16. Gershon, M.D.; Tack, J. The serotonin signalling system: From basic understanding to drug development for functional GI disorders. *Gastroenterology* **2007**, *132*, 397–414. [CrossRef] [PubMed]
17. Nowaczyk, A.; Kowalska, M.; Nowaczyk, J.; Grześk, G. Carbon monoxide and nitric oxide as examples of the youngest class of transmitters. *Int. J. Mol. Sci.* **2021**, *22*, 6029. [CrossRef] [PubMed]
18. Beattie, D.T.; Smith, J.A.M. Serotonin pharmacology in the gastrointestinal tract: A review. *Naunyn-Schmiedeberg's Arch Pharmacol.* **2008**, *377*, 181–203. [CrossRef]
19. Grider, J.R. Neurotransmitters mediating the intestinal peristaltic reflex in the mouse. *J. Pharm. Exp.* **2003**, *307*, 460–467. [CrossRef]
20. Martin, A.M.; Lumsden, A.L.; Young, R.L.; Jessup, C.F.; Spencer, N.J.; Keating, D.J. Regional differences in nutrient-induced secretion of gut serotonin. *Physiol. Rep.* **2017**, *5*, e13199. [CrossRef]
21. Sumara, G.; Sumara, O.; Kim, J.K.; Karsenty, G. Gut-derived serotonin is a multifunctional determinant to fasting adaptation. *Cell Met.* **2012**, *16*, 588–600. [CrossRef]
22. Mishima, Y.; Ishihara, S. Molecular Mechanisms of microbiota-mediated pathology in irritable bowel syndrome. *Int. J. Mol. Sci.* **2020**, *21*, 8664. [CrossRef] [PubMed]
23. Bellono, N.W.; Bayrer, J.R.; Leitch, D.B.; Castro, J.; Zhang, C.; O'Donnel, T.A.; Brierley, S.M.; Ingraham, H.A.; Julius, D. Enterochromaffin cells are gut chemosensors that couple to sensory neural pathways. *Cell* **2017**, *170*, 185–198.e16. [CrossRef] [PubMed]
24. Lund, M.L.; Egerod, K.L.; Engelstoft, M.S.; Dmytriyeva, O.; Theodorsson, E.; Patel, B.A.; Schwartz, T.W. Enterochromaffin 5-HT cells—A major target for GLP-1 and gut microbial metabolites. *Mol. Metab.* **2018**, *11*, 70–83. [CrossRef]
25. Digestive diseases. National Center of Health Statistics. Centers for Disease Control and Prevention. Available online: https://www.cdc.gov/nchs/fastats/digestive-diseases.htm (accessed on 18 December 2021).
26. Mishima, Y.; Ishihara, S. Enteric microbiota –mediated serotoninergic signalling in pathogenesis of irritable bowel syndrome. *Int. J. Mol. Sci.* **2021**, *22*, 10235. [CrossRef]
27. Sartor, R.B.; Wu, G.D. Roles for intestinal bacteria, viruses, and fungi in pathogenesis of inflammatory bowel diseases and therapeutic approaches. *Gastroenterology* **2017**, *152*, 327–339.e4. [CrossRef] [PubMed]
28. Richard, M.L.; Sokol, H. The gut mycobiota: Insights into analysis, environmental interactions and role in gastrointestinal diseases. *Nat. Rev. Gastroenterol. Hepatol.* **2019**, *16*, 3310345. [CrossRef] [PubMed]
29. Waclawikova, B.; Bullock, A.; Schwalbe, M.; Aranzamendi, C.; Nelemans, S.A.; van Dijk, G.; El Aidy, S. Gut bacteria-derived 5-hydroxyidole is a potent stimulant of intestinal motility via its action on L-type calcium channels. *PLoS Biol.* **2021**, *19*, e3001070. [CrossRef]
30. Golubeva, A.V.; Joyce, S.A.; Moloney, G.; Burokas, A.; Sherwin, E.; Arboleya, S.; Flynn, I.; Khochanskiy, D.; Moya-Perez, A.; Peterson, V.; et al. Microbiota-Related changes in bile acid & tryptophan metabolism are associated with gastrointestinal dysfunction in a mouse model of autism. *EBioMedicine* **2017**, *24*, 166–178. [CrossRef] [PubMed]
31. Margolis, K.G.; Li, Z.; Stevanovic, K.; Saurman, V.; Israelyan, N.; Anderson, G.M.; Snyder, I.; Veenstra-VanderWeele, J.; Blakley, R.D.; Gershon, M.D. Serotonin transporter variant drives preventable gastrointestinal abnormalities in development and function. *J. Clin. Investig.* **2016**, *126*, 2221–2235. [CrossRef] [PubMed]
32. Kato, S. Role of serotonin 5-HT3 receptors in intestinal inflammation. *Biol. Pharm. Bull.* **2013**, *36*, 1406–1409. [CrossRef]
33. Mawe, G.M.; Hoffman, J.M. Serotonin signalling in the gut-functions, dysfunctions and therapeutic targets. *Nat. Rev. Gastroenterol. Hepatol.* **2013**, *10*, 473–486. [CrossRef]
34. Strober, W.; Fuss, I.J. Proinflammatory cytokines in the pathogenesis of inflammatory bowel diseases. *Gastroenterology* **2011**, *140*, 1756–1767. [CrossRef] [PubMed]
35. Abraham, C.; Cho, J.H. Inflammatory bowel disease. *N. Engl. J. Med.* **2009**, *361*, 2066–2078. [CrossRef]
36. Wang, H.; Foong, J.P.P.; Harris, N.L.; Bornstein, J.C. Enteric neuroimmune interactions coordinate intestinal responses in health and disease. *Mucosal Immunol.* **2021**, *15*, 27–39. [CrossRef] [PubMed]
37. Kwon, Y.H.; Wang, H.; Denou, E.; Ghia, J.E.; Rossi, L.; Fointes, M.E.; Bernier, S.P.; Shajib, M.S.; Banskota, S.; Collins, S.M.; et al. Modulation of gut microbiota composition n by serotonin signalling influences intestinal immune response and susceptibility to colitis. *Cell. Mol. Gastroenterol. Hepatol.* **2019**, *7*, 709–728. [CrossRef] [PubMed]
38. Nzakaizwanayo, J.; Dedi, C.; Standen, G.; Mac Farlane, W.M.; Patel, B.A.; Jones, B.V. Escherihia coli Nissle 1917 enhances bioavailability of serotonin in gut tissues through modulation of synthesis and clearance. *Sci. Rep.* **2015**, *5*, 17324. [CrossRef] [PubMed]

39. Wu, D.; Denna, T.H.; Storkersen, J.N.; Gerriets, V.A. Beyond a neurotransmitter: The role of serotonin in inflammation and immunity. *Pharm. Res.* **2019**, *140*, 100–114. [CrossRef]
40. Herr, N.; Bode, C.; Duerschmied, D. The effects of serotonin in immune cells. *Front Cardiovasc Med* **2017**, *4*, 48. [CrossRef]
41. Shaijb, M.S.; Khan, I. The role of serotonin and its receptors in activation of immune responses and inflammation. *Acta Physiol.* **2015**, *2113*, 561–574. [CrossRef]
42. Deuerschmied, D.; Siudan, G.L.; Demers, M.; Herr, N.; Carb, C.; Brill, C.H.; Cifuni, S.M.; Mauler, M.; Cicko, S.; Bader, M.; et al. Platelet serotonin promotes the recruitment of neutrophils to sites of acute inflammation in mice. *Blood* **2013**, *121*, 1008–1015. [CrossRef]
43. Regmi, S.C.; Park, S.; Ku, S.K.; Kim, J. Serotonin regulates innate immune responses of colonic epithelial cells through Nox-2-dervied reactive oxygen species. *Free Radic. Biol. Med.* **2014**, *69*, 377–389. [CrossRef] [PubMed]
44. Ito, T.; Lee, L.; Jensen, R.T. Carcinoid-syndrome: Recent advances, current status and controversies. *Curr. Opin. Endocrinol. Diabetes Obes.* **2018**, *25*, 22–35. [CrossRef] [PubMed]
45. Lyseng-Williamson, K.A. Telotristat ethyl: A review in carcinoid syndrome diarrhoea. *Drugs* **2018**, *78*, 941–950. [CrossRef]
46. Chan, D.L.; Singh, S. Developments in the treatment of carcinoid syndrome: Impact of telotristat. *Clin. Risk Manag.* **2018**, *14*, 323–329. [CrossRef] [PubMed]
47. Xermelo. Summary of Product Characteristics. Available online: https://www.ema.europa.eu/en/documents/product-information/xermelo-epar-product-information_en.pdf (accessed on 18 December 2021).
48. Medicines under Additional Monitoring. European Medicines Agency. Available online: https://www.ema.europa.eu/en/human-regulatory/post-authorisation/pharmacovigilance/medicines-under-additional-monitoring (accessed on 18 December 2021).
49. Boeckxstaens, G.E.; Tytgant, G.M.N.; Wajs, E.; Van Nueten, L.; De Ridder, F.; Meulemans, A.; Tack, J. The influence of the novel 5-HT1A agonist R137696 on the proximal stomach function in healthy volunteers. *Neurogastroenterol. Motil.* **2006**, *18*, 919–926. [CrossRef]
50. Coulie, B.; Tack, J.; Maes, B.; Geypens, B.; De Roo, M.; Jenssens, J. Sumatriptan, a selective 5-HT1 receptor agonist, induces a lag phase for gastric emptying of liquids in humans. *Am. J. Physiol.* **1997**, *272*, G902–G908. [CrossRef] [PubMed]
51. Sifrim, D.; Holloway, R.H.; Tack, J.; Zelter, A.; Misotten, T.; Coulie, B.; Janssens, J. Effect on sumatriptan, a 5-HT1 agonist, on the frequency of transient lower oesophageal sphincter relaxations and gastroesophageal reflux in healthy subjects. *Am. J. Gastroenterol.* **1999**, *94*, 3158–3164. [CrossRef] [PubMed]
52. Morelli, N.; Gori, S.; Choub, A.; Maluccio, M.R.; Orlandi, G.; Guazelli, M.; Murri, L. Do 5HT1B/1D receptor agonists have an effect on mood and anxiety disorders? *Cephalagia* **2007**, *27*, 471–472. [CrossRef] [PubMed]
53. Borman, R.A.; Burleigh, D.E. 5-HT1D and 5-HT2B receptors mediate contraction of smooth muscle in human small intestine. *Ann. N. Y. Acad. Sci.* **1997**, *812*, 222–223. [CrossRef]
54. Kirchgessner, A.L.; Liu, M.T.; Tamir, H.; Gershon, M.D. Identyfication and localization of 5-HT1P receptors in the guinea pig pancreas. *Am. J. Physiol.* **1992**, *262*, 553–566. [CrossRef]
55. Kirchgessner, A.L.; Liu, M.T.; Howard, M.J.; Gershon, M.D. Detection of the 5-HT1A receptor and 5-HT1A receptor mRNA in the rat bowel and pancreas: Comparison with 5-HT1P receptors. *J. Comp. Neurol.* **1993**, *327*, 33–250. [CrossRef] [PubMed]
56. Gershon, M.D. Review article: Serotonin receptors and transporters—Roles in normal and abnormal gastrointestinal motility. *Aliment. Pharm.* **2004**, *20*, 3–14. [CrossRef]
57. Branchek, T.A.; Mawe, G.M.; Gershon, M.D. Characterization and localization of a peripheral neural 5-hydroksytryptamine receptor subtype (5-HT1P) with a selective agonist, 3H-5-hydroxyindalpine. *J. Neurosci.* **1998**, *8*, 2582–2595. [CrossRef]
58. Rubio-Beltran, E.; Labastida-Ramirez, A.; Haanes, K.A.; van den Bogaerdt, A.; Bogers, A.; Zanelli, E.; Meeus, L.; Danser, A.H.J.; Gralinski, M.R.; Senese, P.B.; et al. Characterization of binding, functional activity, and contractile responses of the selective 5-HT_{1F} receptor agonist Lasmiditan. *Br. J. Pharm.* **2019**, *176*, 4681–4695. [CrossRef]
59. Clemow, D.B.; Johnson, K.W.; Hochstetler, H.M.; Ossipov, M.H.; Hake, A.M.; Blumenfeld, A.M. Lasmiditan mechanism of action—Review of a selective 5-HT1F agonist. *J. Headache Pain* **2020**, *21*, 71. [CrossRef]
60. International Union of Basic and Clinical Pharmacology IUPHAR. Available online: https://www.guidetopharmacology.org/GRAC/FamilyDisplayForward?familyId=1 (accessed on 18 October 2021).
61. Tack, J.; Caenepeel, P.; Corsetti, M.; Janssens, J. Role of tension receptors in dyspeptic patients with hypersensitivity to gastric distension. *Gastroenterology* **2004**, *127*, 1058–1066. [CrossRef] [PubMed]
62. Johnston, K.D.; Lu, Z.; Rudd, J.A. Looking beyond 5-HT(3) receptors: A review of the wider role of serotonin in the pharmacology of nausea and vomiting. *Eur. J. Pharm.* **2014**, *722*, 13–25. [CrossRef]
63. De Clerck, F.; David, J.L.; Janssen, P.A.J. Inhibition of 5-hydrxytryptamine-induced and -amplified human platelet aggregation by ketanserin (R 41 468) a selective 5-HT2-receptor antagonist. *Agents Actions* **1982**, *12*, 388–397. [CrossRef]
64. Engel, G.; Hoyer, D.; Kalkman, H.; Wick, M.B. Pharmacological similarity between 5-HT-D receptor on the guinea pig ileum and the 5-HT2 binding site. *Br. J. Pharm.* **1985**, *84*, 106.
65. Muneta-Arrate, I.; Diez-Alarcia, R.; Horrillo, I.; Meana, J.J. Pimavanserin exhibits serotonin 5-HT2A receptor inverse agonism for Gαi1- and neutral antagonism for Gαq/11- proteins in human brain cortex. *Eur. Neuropsychopharmacol.* **2020**, *36*, 83–89. [CrossRef] [PubMed]

66. Launay, J.M.; Birraux, G.; Bondoux, D.; Callebert, J.; Choi, D.S.; Loric, S.; Maroteaux, L. Ras involvement in signal transduction by the serotonin 5-HT2B receptor. *J. Biol. Chem.* **1996**, *271*, 3141–3147. [CrossRef] [PubMed]
67. Iizuka, N.; Oka, M.; Yamada-Okabe, H.; Hamada, K.; Nakayama, H.; Mori, N.; Tamesa, T.; Okada, T.; Takemoto, N.; Matoba, K.; et al. Molecular signature in three types of hepatocellular carcinoma with different viral origin by oligonucleotide microarray. *Int. J. Oncol.* **2004**, *24*, 565–574. [CrossRef] [PubMed]
68. Zhang, Q.; Zhu, Y.; Zhou, W.; Gao, L.; Yuan, L.; Han, X. Serotonin receptor 2C and insulin secretion. *PLoS ONE* **2013**, *8*, e54250. [CrossRef]
69. Stunes, A.K.; Reseland, J.E.; Hauso, O.; Kidd, M.; Tommeras, K.; Waldum, H.L.; Syversen, U.; Gustafsson, B.I. Adipocytes express a functional system for serotonin synthesis, reuptake and receptor activation. *Diabetes Obes. Metab.* **2011**, *13*, 551–558. [CrossRef]
70. Kappeler, J.; Möller, D.; Lasitschka, F.; Autschbach, F.; Hovius, R.; Rappold, D.; Brüss, M.; Gershon, M.D.; Niesler, B. Serotonin receptor diversity in the human colon: Expression of serotonin type 3 receptor subunits 5-HT3C, 5-HT3D, and 5-HT3E. *J. Comp. Neurol.* **2011**, *519*, 420–432. [CrossRef]
71. Niesler, B.; Frank, B.; Kapeller, J.; Rappold, G.A. Cloning, physical mapping and expression analysis of the human 5-HT3 serotonin receptor-like genes HTR3C, HTR3D and HTR3E. *Gene* **2003**, *310*, 101–111. [CrossRef]
72. Glatzle, J.; Sternini, C.; Robin, C.; Zittel, T.T.; Wong, H.; Reeve, J.R.; Raybould, H.E. Expression of 5-HT 3 receptors in the rat gastrointestinal tract. *Gastroenterology* **2002**, *123*, 217–226. [CrossRef]
73. Bertrand, P.P.; Kunze, W.A.; Furness, J.B.; Bornstein, J.C. The terminals of myenteric intrinsic primary afferent neurons of the guinea-pig ileum are excited by 5-hydrokxytryptamine acting at 5-hydroxytryptamine-3 receptors. *Neuroscience* **2000**, *101*, 459–469. [CrossRef]
74. Hansen, M.B.; Skadhauge, E. Signal transduction pathways for serotonin as an intestinal secretagogue. *Comp. Biochem. Physil. A Physiol.* **1997**, *118*, 283–290. [CrossRef]
75. Shworer, H.; Ramadori, G. Autoreceptors can modulate 5-hydroxytryptamine release from porcine and human small intestine in vitro. *Naunyn-Schmiedeberg's Arch. Pharmacol.* **1998**, *357*, 548–552. [CrossRef]
76. Aikiyo, S.; Kishi, K.; Kaji, N.; Mikawa, S.; Kondo, M.; Shimada, S.; Hori, M. Contribution of serotonin 3A receptor to motor function and its expression in the gastrointestinal tract. *Digest* **2021**, *102*, 516–526. [CrossRef]
77. Hagbom, M.; Hellysaz, A.; Istrate, C.; Nordgren, J.; Sharma, S.; de-Faria, F.M.; Magnusson, K.E.; Svensson, L. The 5-HT3 receptor affects rotavirus-induced motility. *J. Virol.* **2021**, *95*, e0075121. [CrossRef] [PubMed]
78. Hesketh, P.J. Understanding the pathobiology of chemotherapy induced nausea and vomiting. Providing a basis for therapeutic progress. *Oncology* **2004**, *18*, 9–14.
79. Cubeddu, L.X.; Hoffman, I.S.; FuenMayor, N.T.; Finn, A.L. Efficacy of ondansetron (GR 38032F) and the role of serotonin in cisplatin-induced nausea and vomiting. *N. Eng. J. Med.* **1990**, *322*, 810–816. [CrossRef]
80. Roiola, F.; Fatigoni, S. New antiemetic drugs. *Ann. Oncol.* **2006**, *17*, 96–100. [CrossRef]
81. Clemens, C.H.M.; Samson, M.; Van Berge Henegouwen, G.P.; Fabri, M.; Smout, A.J.P.M. Effect on allosteron on left colonic motility in non-constipated patients with irritable bowel syndrome and healthy volunteers. *Aliment. Pharm.* **2002**, *16*, 993–1002. [CrossRef]
82. U.S. Food and Drug Administration. FDA Drug Safety Communication: New Information Regarding QT Prolongation with Ondansetron (Zofran). Available online: https://www.fda.gov/Drugs/DrugSafety/ucm310190.html (accessed on 17 October 2021).
83. Damkier, P.; Caplan, Y.C.; Shechtman, S.; Diav-Citrin, O.; Cassina, M.; Weber-Schoendorfer, C. Ondansetron in pregnancy revisited: Assessment and pregnancy labelling by the European Medicines Agency (EMA) & Pharmacovigilance Risk Assessment Committee (PRAC). *Basic Clin. Toxicol. Pharm.* **2021**, *128*, 579–582. [CrossRef]
84. European Medicines Agency Recommends Changes to the Use of Metoclopramide Changes Aim Mainly to Reduce the Risk of Neurological Side Effects. Available online: https://www.ema.europa.eu/en/documents/press-release/european-medicines-agency-recommends-changes-use-metoclopramide_en.pdf (accessed on 17 October 2021).
85. Tanyiama, K.; Makimoto, N.; Furuichi, A.; Sakurai-Yamashita, Y.; Nagase, Y.; Kaibara, M.; Kanematsu, T. Functions of peripheral 5-hydroxytryptamine receptors, especially 5-hydroksytryptamie 4 receptor, in gastrointestinal motility. *J. Gastroenterol.* **2000**, *35*, 575–582. [CrossRef] [PubMed]
86. Matsuyoshi, H.; Kuniyasu, H.; Okumura, M.; Misawa, H.; Katsui, R.; Zhang, G.X.; Obata, K.; Takaki, M. A 5-HT(4)-receptor activation-induced neural plasticity enhances in vivo reconstructs of enteric nerve circuit insult. *Neurogastroenterol. Motil.* **2010**, *22*, 806–813.e226. [CrossRef] [PubMed]
87. Kawahara, I.; Kuniyasu, H.; Matsuyoshi, H.; Goto, K.; Obata, K.; Misawa, H.; Fujii, H.; Takaki, M. Comparison of effects of a selective 5-HT reuptake inhibitor versus a 5-HT4 receptor agonist on in vivo neurogenesis at the rectal anastomosis in rats. *Am. J. Physiol. Gastrointest Liver Physiol.* **2012**, *302*, G588–G597. [CrossRef]
88. Kaumann, A.J.; Levy, F.O. 5-hydroksytryptamine receptors in the human cardiovascular system. *Pharmacol. Ther.* **2006**, *111*, 674–706. [CrossRef]
89. Brattelid, T.; Kvingedal, A.M.; Krobert, K.A.; Andressen, K.W.; Bach, T.; Hystad, M.E.; Kaumann, A.J.; Levy, F.O. Cloning, pharmacological characterisation and tissue distribution of a novel 5-HT4 receptor splice variant, 5-HT4(i). *Naunyn-Schmiedeberg's Arch. Pharmacol.* **2004**, *369*, 616–628. [CrossRef] [PubMed]

90. Brattelid, T.; Qvigstad, E.; Lynham, J.A.; Molenaaa, T.; Aasschgeiran, O.; Skomedal, T.; Osnes, J.B.; Levy, F.O.; Kaumann, A.J. Functional serotonin 5-HT4 receptors in porcine and human ventricular myocardium with increased 5-HT4 mRNA in heart failure. *Naunyn-Schmiedeberg's Arch. Pharmacol.* **2004**, *370*, 157–166. [CrossRef] [PubMed]
91. Kaumann, A.J. Do human atrial 5-HT4 receptors mediate arrhythmias? *Trends Pharm. Sci* **1994**, *15*, 451–455. [CrossRef]
92. Rahme, M.M.; Cotter, B.; Leistad, E.; Wadhwa, M.K.; Mohabir, R.; Ford, A.P.; Eglen, R.M.; Feld, G.K. Electrophysiological and antiarrhythmic effects of the atrial selective 5-HT(4) receptor antagonist RS-100302 in experimental atrial flutter and fibrillation. *Circulation* **1999**, *100*, 2010–2017. [CrossRef]
93. Lezoualc'h, F.; Steplewski, K.; Sartiani, L.; Mugelli, A.; Fischmeister, R.; Bril, A. Quantitative mRNA analysis of serotonin 5-HT4 receptor isoforms, calcium handling proteins and ion channels in human atrial fibrillation. *Biochem. Biophys. Res. Commun.* **2007**, *357*, 218–224. [CrossRef] [PubMed]
94. De Ponti, F.; Crema, F. Treatment functional GI disease: The complex pharmacology of serotonergic drugs. *Br. J. Clin.* **2002**, *54*, 680–681. [CrossRef]
95. Tack, J.; Camilleri, M.; Chang, L.; Chey, W.D.; Galligan, J.J.; Lacy, B.E.; Müller-Lissner, S.; Quigley, E.M.M.; Schuurkes, J.; De Maeyer, J.H.; et al. Systematic review: Cardiovascular safety profile of 5-HT4 agonists developed for gastrointestinal disorders. *Aliment. Pharm.* **2012**, *35*, 745–767. [CrossRef]
96. CisaprideWithdrawal Requires Alternative Therapy. Clevland Clinic Center for Continuing Education. Available online: https://www.clevelandclinicmeded.com/medicalpubs/pharmacy/mayjune2000/cisapride.htm (accessed on 15 October 2021).
97. Cisapride. European Medicine Agency. Available online: https://www.ema.europa.eu/en/medicines/human/referrals/cisapride (accessed on 15 October 2021).
98. Sanger, G.J. Translating 5-HT receptor pharmacology. *Neurogastroenterol. Motil.* **2009**, *21*, 1235–1238. [CrossRef]
99. Resolor. Summary of Product Characteristics. Available online: https://www.ema.europa.eu/en/documents/product-information/resolor-epar-product-information_en.pdf (accessed on 2 February 2022).
100. Carbone, F.; Van den Houte, K.; Clevers, E.; Andrews, C.N.; Papathanasopoulos, A.; Holvoet, L.; Van Oudenhove, L.V.; Caenepeel, P.; Arts, J.; Vanuytsel, T.; et al. Prucalopride in Gastroparesis: A Randomized Placebo-Controlled Crossover Study. *Am. J. Gastroenterol.* **2019**, *114*, 1265–1274. [CrossRef]
101. Tack, J.; Rotondo, A.; Meulemans, A.; Thielemans, L.; Cools, M. Randomized clinical trial: A controlled pilot trial of the 5-HT4 receptor agonist revexepride in patients with symptoms suggestive of gastroparesis. *Neurogastroenterol. Motil.* **2016**, *28*, 487–497. [CrossRef] [PubMed]
102. Spohn, S.N.; Bianco, F.; Scott, R.B.; Keenan, C.M.; Linton, A.A.; O'Neill, C.H.; Bonora, E.; Dicay, M.; Lavoie, B.; Eilcox, R.L.; et al. Protective actions of epithelial 5-hydrokxytryptamine 4 receptors in normal and inflamed colon. *Gastroenterology* **2016**, *151*, 933–944. [CrossRef] [PubMed]
103. Rodriguesz-Stanley, S.; Zubaidi, S.; Proskin, H.M.; Klarstein, J.R.; Shetzline, M.A.; Miner, P.B.; Philip, B. Effect of tegaserod on esophageal pain threshold, regurgitation, and symptom relief in patients with functional heartburn and mechanical sensitivity. *Clin. Gastroenterol. Hepatol.* **2006**, *4*, 442–450. [CrossRef] [PubMed]
104. Kahrilas, P.J.; Quigley, E.M.M.; Castell, D.O.; Specjhler, S.J. The effects of tegaserod (HTF919) on esophageal acid exposure in gastroesophageal reflux disease. *Aliment. Pharm.* **2000**, *14*, 1503–1509. [CrossRef]
105. Grailhe, R.; Grabtree, G.W.; Hen, R. Human 5-HT(5) receptors: The 5-HT(5A) receptor is functional but 5-HT(5B) receptor was lost during mammalian evolution. *Eur. J. Pharmacol.* **2001**, *418*, 157–167. [CrossRef]
106. Thomas, D.R. 5-HT5A receptor as a therapeutic targets. *Pharmacol. Ther.* **2006**, *111*, 707–714. [CrossRef] [PubMed]
107. Kohen, R.; Metcalf, M.A.; Khan, M.; Druck, T.; Huebner, K.; Lachowicz, J.E.; Meltzer, H.Y.; Sibley, D.R.; Roth, B.L.; Hamblin, M.W. Cloning, characterization, and chromosomal localization of a human 5-HT6 serotonin receptor. *J. Neurochem.* **1996**, *66*, 613–618. [CrossRef] [PubMed]
108. Johnson, C.N.; Ahmed, M.; Miller, M.D. 5-HT6 receptor antagonists: Prospects for the treatment of cognitive disorders including dementia. *Curr. Opin. Drug Discov. Devel* **2008**, *11*, 642–654.
109. Monro, R.L.; Bornstein, J.C.; Bertarnd, P.P. Slow excitatory postsynaptic potentials in myenteric AH neurons of the guinea pig ileum are reduced by the 5-hydroxytryptamine (7) receptor antagonist SB 269970. *Neuroscience* **2005**, *134*, 975–986. [CrossRef]
110. Tonini, M. 5-hydroxytryptamine effects in the gut: The 3, 4, and 7 receptors. *Neurogastroenterol. Motil.* **2005**, *17*, 637642. [CrossRef] [PubMed]
111. Zeiss, R.; Connemann, B.J.; Schönfeldt-Lecuona, C.; Gahr, M. Risk of Bleeding Associated With Antidepressants: Impact of Causality Assessment and Competition Bias on Signal Detection. *Front. Psychiatry* **2021**, *12*, 727687. [CrossRef] [PubMed]
112. Zeiss, R.; Hiemke, C.; Schönfeldt-Lecuona, C.; Connemann, B.J.; Gahr, M. Risk of bleeding associated with antidepressant drugs: The competitive impact of antithrombotics in quantative signal detection. *Drugs-Real World Outcomes* **2021**, *8*, 547–554. [CrossRef] [PubMed]
113. Kanova, M.; Kohout, P. Serotonin—Its synthesis and roles in the healthy and the critically ill. *Int. J. Mol. Sci.* **2021**, *22*, 4837. [CrossRef] [PubMed]
114. Choi, W.; Moon, J.H.; Kim, H. Serotoninergic regulation of Energy metabolism in peripheral tissues. *J. Endocrinol.* **2020**, *245*, R1–R10. [CrossRef]

renal toxicity, fluoroquinolone-related tendonitis and Achilles tendon rupture, myelosuppression after linezolid, cardiac arrythmias induced by macrolides or diffuse interstitial pneumonitis, and pulmonary fibrosis that might be the consequence of nitrofurantoin administration [9,10]. However, many antibiotics are considered to exert hepato- and nephrotoxicity, peripheral blood disorders (anemia, leukopenia, thrombocytopenia) or electrolyte abnormalities. Among other potential ADRs induced during antibiotic therapy, uncommon, but possible, neurotoxicity should also be mentioned, mostly associated with the use of beta-lactams or quinolones. Post-antibiotic neurological disorders are manifested by hearing loss or labyrinthine dysfunction (characteristic for erythromycin and azithromycin), and by ototoxicity and vestibular dysfunction (pathognomonic for aminoglycosides) or by other forms of neurotoxicity, affecting either peripheral or the central nervous system [11]. Generally, drug-induced neurological disorders (DIND) are manifested by a very broad spectrum of disorders, e.g., cerebrovascular disease, delirium, headache, nerve and muscle disorders, movement disturbances, seizure attacks, sleep abnormalities and others [12,13]. They are listed in Table 1 below. Among the potential drugs responsible for the development of DIND, antibiotics should also be mentioned. Most commonly, the above-mentioned aminoglycosides and macrolides are characterized by harmful potential toward the nervous system, but this also applies to quinolones, sulfonamides, penicillin, carbapenems, tetracyclines, oxazolidinones, polymyxins' and metronidazole. These are listed in the next chapter. The toxic effects of antibiotics on the central nervous system are not as well understood as their other side effects and may be confused with symptoms of various neurological or psychiatric diseases.

Table 1. Examples of drug-induced neurological disorders (DIND).

Disorder/Syndrome	Symptoms	Drugs
Cerebrovascular disorders	Stroke due to deep venous thrombosis or pulmonary embolism Cerebellar syndrome	estrogens/progestins (oral contraceptives) antiepileptic drugs (phenytoin, carbamazepine), lithium, selected antibiotics
Cognitive impairment and delirium	Dementia Fluctuations in cognition, mood, attention and arousal	1-st generation antihistamines, antiparkinsonian agents, skeletal muscle relaxants, tricyclic antidepressants, antipsychotics, benzodiazepines
Neuroleptic malignant syndrome	Muscular rigidity, tremor, possible muscle tissue breakdown, autonomic instability, high fever, changes in cognition	antipsychotics (neuroleptics)
Nerve and muscle disorders	Muscular weakness, loss of coordination, possible paralysis	benzodiazepines selected antibiotics
Movement disorders	Akathisia, dystonia, pseudo-parkinsonism	dopamine receptor blockers: 1-st generation neuroleptics and antiemetics (metoclopramide), anticholinergic agents (benztropine, diphenhydramine), benzodiazepines
Epilepsy	Seizures or impairment of consciousness and/or movements	benzodiazepines (when suddenly withdrawn), diuretics (due to electrolyte imbalance), antiarrhythmics, bupropion, antipsychotics (chlorpromazine, clozapine), lithium, opiate analgesics (fentanyl, meperidine, tramadol), selected antibiotics
Serotonin syndrome	Cognitive and behavioral changes, autonomic instability, high blood pressure, sweating, agitation, tremor, fever, nausea and vomiting	serotonin reuptake inhibitors serotonin-norepinephrine reuptake inhibitors, tricyclic antidepressants, opiate analgesics (meperidine, dextromethorphan), anti-migraine drugs-triptans, selected antibiotics
Sleep disorders	Insomnia or excessive daytime sleepiness with decreased ability to concentrate, think and reason	stimulants: adrenergic agents, antidepressants, corticosteroids, antiparkinsonian agents, sleep-inducing agents (when overused or suddenly discontinued)
Disorders of the sense organs	Hearing and vision impairment	selected antibiotics

The pathogenesis underlying DIND is complex. To damage nervous system structures, a drug or its metabolites must either cross the blood–brain barrier (BBB) or become incorporated into the neuron by peripheral axonal uptake and retrograde axonal transport. The first mechanism is mainly used by lipophilic drugs, and their potential neurotoxicity is obviously exacerbated by already existing damage to the BBB. The direct mechanisms by which drugs may produce neurotoxic effects include impairment of neuronal energy production with subsequent disturbances of ion channels' functioning, disturbances in synthesis and release of neurotransmitters from neuronal terminals, or noxious effects of cellular structures of neurons exerted by drug metabolites. Neuronal ATP synthesis may be affected not only by hypoxia, ischemia or hypoglycemia but also by drugs that disrupt the metabolism by hindering energy production or enhancing energy consumption, contributing to uncoupling of electron flow and oxidative phosphorylation, oxidative stress or inhibition of adenosine enzymatic breakdown. These disturbances lead to the subsequent intracellular ion entry (Ca^{2+}, Na^{+}) and release of excitatory glutamate which in the "vicious circle" mechanism intensify already existing damage and activity of Ca^{2+}-dependent cellular phenomena. Finally, the release of neurotransmitters (serotonin, noradrenaline, dopamine, acetylcholine) is disturbed and the calcium-dependent apoptotic processes of nerve cells occur. The triggering factors facilitating the DIND involve drug related factors (e.g., polydrug abuse, formation of neurotoxic metabolites during endogenous drug metabolism) and individual related factors (age, gender, gestational drug exposure, antioxidant status, diet) or influence of environmental conditions (chronic stress, temperature, exposure to environmental toxins and pollutions) [14,15].

2. Antibiotic-Related Neurotoxicity—A General Outline and Pathogenesis

Antibiotics may be causative agents of peripheral or central nervous system dysfunction. The neurogenic ADRs of antibiotics are more common in elderly patients with kidney and/or liver insufficiency and in patients with preexisting neurological abnormalities. As with other ADRs, antibiotic-induced neurological disorders are potentially reversible as long as they are quickly recognized and corrected.

The risk of post-antibiotic peripheral neuropathy occurs with prolonged administration of some antibiotics, e.g., metronidazole. Seizures, twitching and hallucinations are possible neurological ADRs caused mostly by penicillin, imipenem-cilastin, cephalosporins or ciprofloxacin [11]. However, central nervous system toxicities were also demonstrated for sulfonamides, tetracyclines, chloramphenicol, colistin, aminoglycosides, metronidazole, isoniazid, rifampin, ethionamide, cyclo-serine, and dapsone. Cranial nerve toxicities, manifested by myopia, optic neuritis, deafness, vertigo, and tinnitus, were associated with the use of erythromycin, sulfonamides, tetracyclines, chloramphenicol, colistin, aminoglycosides, vancomycin, isoniazid, and ethambutol. Symptoms of paresthesias, motor weakness or sensory impairment, which are considered to be a clinical manifestation of peripheral neuropathy, were associated with the use of penicillin, sulfonamides, chloramphenicol, colistin, metronidazole, isoniazid, ethionamide, and dapsone. Neuromuscular blockade and weakening of the neuromuscular strength were related to the use of tetracyclines, polymyxins, lincomycin, clindamycin, and aminoglycosides. Antibiotic-related neurotoxicity depends on the dosing schedule and the functional status of the liver and kidneys. There are reports that penicillin G intravenous administration may lead to harmful effect in the central nervous system when given more than 50 million units per day in adults [16]. The maximum recommended dose of imipenem-cilastin in adults with preserved renal function that does not cause neurological disorders is 4 g per day and estimates indicate that seizures occurring in patients using this antibiotic occur in 2% of cases [17]. Similarly, fluoroquinolone use was found to be associated with seizures and headaches in 1–2% of recipients. The other, unusual effects observed in patients treated with fluoroquinolones (ofloxacin, sparfloxacin) included orofacial dyskinesia and a Tourette-like syndrome [18]. Neuromuscular blockade and the possibility of intensification of the action of intraoperative muscle relaxants is the most commonly known neurological ADR of aminoglycosides, but the symptoms were also demonstrated for tetracyclines, polymyxins, lincomycin, clindamycin, although to a much lesser extent. Thus, aminoglycosides should be avoided in patients with inherited neuromuscular disturbances, e.g., myasthenia gravis [16]. Ototoxicity or vestibular dysfunction are also well-known neurological ADRs of aminoglycosides. These disturbances are usually dose- and frequency-dependent and correlated with other risk factors for cranial nerve VIII damage, such as advanced age, fever, anemia, baseline creatinine level and concomitant use of other ototoxic agents (e.g., furosemide, salicylate) [19–21]. Macrolides-erythromycin and azithromycin administration may cause the bilateral hearing loss or labyrinthine dysfunction and vertigo, and patients with hepatic insufficiency are especially predestined to develop these disturbances. In most cases, these complications were described as dose-dependent and usually reversible within 2 weeks after discontinuation of the treatment, although there have also been reports of irreversible hearing loss [22–25].

A summary of the neurotoxic effects related to the use of different classes of antibiotics is given in Table 2 below [26,27].

Table 2. Possible and most common adverse drug reactions in the form of neurotoxicity of different classes of antibiotics.

Class of Antibiotic	Neurotoxicity
penicillin	confusion, disorientation, tardive seizure, encephalopathy, tremors
cephalosporins	lethargy, tardive seizures, myoclonus, encephalopathy, chorea, athetosis,
carbapenems	headache, seizures, encephalopathy, myoclonus, peripheral neuropathy
glycopeptides	ototoxicity
macrolides	ototoxicity, seizures, confusion, agitation, insomnia, delirium, exacerbation of myasthenia gravis
aminoglycosides	ototoxicity-class effect, peripheral neuropathy, neuromuscular blockade class-effect, autonomic dysfunction
oxazolidinones	encephalopathy, peripheral neuropathy, optic neuropathy
polymyxins	Encephalopathy, paresthesias, ataxia, diplopia, potosís and nystagmus, vertigo, confusion, ataxia, seizures
tetracyclines	cranial nerve toxicity, neuromuscular blockade, intracranial hypertension
lincosamides	movement disturbances
chloramphenicol	optic neuropathy
sulfonamides /trimethoprim	tremor, transient psychosis, encephalopathy, aseptic meningitis
quinolones	headache, seizures, confusion, insomnia, encephalopathy, myoclonus, orofacial dyskinesias, ataxia, chorea, extra-pyramidal disturbances
metronidazole	headache, dizziness, confusion, encephalopathy, optic neuropathy, peripheral neuropathy
nitrofurantoin	intracranial hypertension, peripheral neuropathy
isoniazid, ethambutol, cyclo-serine	peripheral neuropathy, seizures, optic neuropathy

3. Antibiotics and the Dysbiosis of the Gastrointestinal Tract and Its Relation to Neurotoxicity

The human digestive tract is inhabited by many microorganisms that form a specific ecosystem, which includes, among others, bacteria, fungi, yeasts and viruses. All these living microorganisms are collectively named "the microbiota" (this term has replaced the previously used term "microflora"), while the collection of genes of the microorganisms constituting the microbiota is called "the microbiome" (containing about 3 million genes). More broadly, the microbiota is also considered to be a collection of all microorganisms found in the various compartments of the human body, including the above-mentioned gut microbiota and organisms inhabiting the skin, distal urogenital or respiratory systems [28–30]. The term "microbiota" was introduced by the Nobel Laureate Joshua Lederberg in 2001 to define the whole system of commensal, syn-biotic and pathogenic microorganisms that share a living space with the human host [31,32].

The microorganisms inhabiting the gut are an integral part of its host's well-being and the composition of the microbiota is individual and unique for every human being. It is formed during childbirth, but modified after birth by many factors: age, genetic conditions of the host, diet, infections and use of antibacterial drugs or probiotics/prebiotics/symbiotics. Under physiological conditions, the intestine is colonized by approximately 10^{13}–10^{14} bacteria represented primarily by *Firmicutes, Bacteroidetes, Actinobacteria, Proteobacteria, Fusobacteria* and *Verrucomicrobia*. In health, all intestinal microorganisms are in a state of dynamic equilibrium known as eubiosis. This state has protective, trophic and metabolic functions in the gastrointestinal tract, but also plays a role in controlling the brain activity and behavior. The phenomenon is widely known as the gut–brain axis (GBA) [33]. This axis is functionally based on communication between the central and the enteric nervous system (mostly via vagus nerve fibers), linking centers of the brain with peripheral intestinal functions. GBA appears to be bidirectional, namely through signaling from gut-microbiota to the brain ("bottom-up") and from the brain to gut-microbiota by means of neural, endocrine, immune, and humoral pathways. The background for signaling from the gut to the brain are several microbiologically derived metabolites (short-chain fatty acids (SCFAs) butyrate, propionate, and acetate, secondary bile acids, tryptophan metabolites). These agents act primarily through interactions with enteroendocrine cells, enterochromaffin cells and the musical immune system, also resulting in an increased release of cytokines (Il-1β, Il-6, TNF-α). There are two barriers to GBA signaling: the intestinal barrier and the blood–brain barrier (BBB). In conditions of dysbiosis (pathological change of eubiosis) there is an increase in the permeability of the intestinal wall ("leaky gut") and the transfer of bacterial mediators to the blood and inflammation takes place. Dysbiosis is also associated with disruptive BBB changes since abnormal gut microbiota may affect proper traffic between the circulatory system and the cerebrospinal fluid of the central nervous system. The descending modulation of GBA activity takes place indirectly through changes in the activity of the autonomic nervous system and directly through luminal release of neurotransmitters (catecholamines, serotonin, dynorphins). Autonomic fibers (both sympathetic and parasympathetic, the most important being the vagus nerve) control gut functions including motility, secretion, epithelial fluid maintenance, intestinal permeability and mucosal immune response and these phenomena affect the microbial habitat, thus influencing the composition and activity of microbiota [34–37].

Abnormalities in gut microbiome and GBA interactions have been implicated in the pathogenesis of functional gastrointestinal disorders (e.g., irritable bowel syndrome; IBS) but also in neurologic and psychiatric entities [33,34]. There is also evidence that the dysbiosis-induced stimulation of the vagal nerve, that conveys information between the gut and the central nervous system, intensifies the expression of neurotrophic elements determining the development of new neurons and synaptic connections, which has been shown to be associated with mood disorders [34,38]. Moreover, it has been demonstrated that bacterial strains residing in the intestines may be implicated in affecting the brain by impacting the production or response to neurotransmitters (GABA, serotonin) [34,39,40]. Abnormal gut microbiota may produce a large number of amyloids and other toxins and act as a source of systemic inflammation, thus contributing to increased risk of Alzheimer's disease development [34,41]. The intestinal dysbiosis also predisposes to Parkinson's disease development due to the fact that gut inflammatory pathomechanisms play a significant role in alpha-synuclein misfolding [34,42]. It was also found that higher concentrations of *Enterobacteriaceae* were directly proportional to gait and postural instability [34,43]. Studies also revealed the role of the gut microbiome in amyotrophic lateral sclerosis (ALS). In an experimental ALS mouse model, a tight junction structure, greater intestinal permeability, and an abnormal microbiota profile with lower butyrate-producing bacteria were observed compared to controls. Butyrate, a bacterial metabolic by-product, has been proposed to normalize the gut microbiota, as well as to enhance the lifespan of ALS [34,44]. Abnormalities of the gut microbiota and the "leaky gut" syndrome development that allows bacterial metabolites to cross the intestinal barrier is also considered to be implicated in the pathogenesis of some psychiatric entities. The results of some studies demonstrated that persistent, low-grade inflammation as a result of a "leaky gut" predisposes the host to the development of anorexia nervosa, depression and anxiety conditions [34,45,46].

To sum up, the gut microbiota significantly influences the interaction between the gut and the brain through complex neuroendocrine and immune processes. It has long been known that dysbiosis of the intestinal microbiota is associated with various disorders of the nervous system. It is worth mentioning that the use of antibiotics leads to the rebuilding of microbiota composition and activity. Therefore, the administration of antibiotics, in the context of their effect on GBA, can be viewed dichotomously. On the one hand, by increasing the risk of dysbiosis development when used irrationally, these antibacterial agents may promote neurotoxicity. On the other hand, if properly applied, by eliminating pathogenic bacterial strains, antibiotics can significantly reduce the risk of neurological disorders resulting from GBA abnormalities [47].

4. Short Description of the Detailed Neurotoxicity of Particular Classes of Antibiotics

4.1. Metronidazole

Metronidazole has been used for decades as a broad-spectrum antimicrobial agent effective in the treatment of anaerobic bacterial and protozoal infections and in Helicobacter pylori eradication [48]. Metronidazole-induced encephalopathy (MIE) was first described in 1977 [49]. The most common reported neurologic disturbances are mild and involve dizziness, headache, confusion, vertigo and insomnia [48]. However, an inappropriate, excessive use of the drug may lead to neurological complications, the severity of which reflects total drug exposure. Therefore, it is recommended to reduce rationally both the duration of treatment and adopted doses while maintaining its effectiveness [50,51]. Neurological complications become more common when the drug is used in a dose exceeding 2 g/day for prolonged time [52]. Severe neuropsychiatric disturbances have been observed in patients treated with metronidazole in a total dose of 42 g for 4 weeks of continuous therapy. However, the symptoms are observed to resolve after the discontinuation of the therapy in most patients [53]. The encephalopathy symptoms may be still present within 1–12 weeks following high-dose metronidazole treatment and the imaging abnormalities resolve between 3 to up to 16 weeks after stopping metronidazole administration [52]. In rare cases, persistent MRI abnormalities of the brain and clinical symptoms of encephalopathy have been reported despite discontinuation of the treatment [54]. Metronidazole use is associated with the risk of both central and peripheral neurotoxicity [48,50,55]. Usually, the metronidazole-induced neurotoxicity is characterized by a gradual onset and mostly affects patients with concomitant renal and/or liver dysfunctions [56,57]. The peripheral neuropathy induced by higher doses of metronidazole manifests by sensi-motor neuropathy and in some patients it may be accompanied by autonomic neuropathy in the form of vasomotor and temperature dysregulations. The reason for sequential involvement of peripheral sensory, motor and finally autonomic fibers evoked by the drug is unknown [52,58]. Moreover, the induction of cerebellar and vestibular system damage with subsequent ataxia after metronidazole, often demonstrated in experimental studies, remains unclear [52]. The proposed pathomechanism of metronidazole-induced neurotoxicity is related to the basic antimicrobial action of metronidazole and is associated with the drug's ability to generate free radicals. These intermediate molecules may cause oxidation of catecholamines and other neurotransmitters and contribute to production of semiquinone and nitro-anion secondary neurotoxic radicals [52,58]. Moreover, inhibition of neuronal protein synthesis and radical injury to nerve tissue may result in peripheral nerve injury ("axonal swelling" and localized neuronal ischemia with perineural edema) leading to mixed neuropathy symptoms development. The proposed, complementary mechanism of metronidazole neurotoxicity is also the inhibition of GABAergic neurotransmission and modulation of the GABA receptor [50,52,55,58]. The hypothesis is in line with the experimental observations that central metronidazole-associated neurotoxicity is ameliorated by diazepam [59].

4.2. *Sulfonamides/Trimethoprim*

Sulfonamides as antagonists of para-aminobenzoic acid (PABA; folate precursor), were the first antimicrobial agents used in the treatment of infections evoked by many Gram-positive cocci and Gram-negative bacilli. Currently, sulfonamides have diminished importance due to resistance, but are still used in the treatment of certain infections (dysentery, plague, tetanus, typhoid and paradour), and as second-line drugs in the treatment of infections of the urinary tract and the respiratory system. They are also externally used on the skin for the prevention of post-burn infections and topically to treat bacterial conjunctivitis. Moreover, these drugs are still important in the prophylaxis and treatment of some opportunistic infections associated with immunodeficiency in the course of AIDS. At present the most clinically relevant is sulfomethoxazole (SMX) administered with trimethoprim (TMP; a dihydrofolate reductase inhibitor) [60]. SMX/TMP administration produces various ADRs, including gastrointestinal, dermatological disturbances, hematological and hypersensitivity reactions. Some neurological disruptions in the form of tremor and transient psychosis with agitation and visual and auditory hallucinations were also reported [26,27,60]. The first reports of psychiatric disorders related to the use of sulfa drugs appeared as early as 1942 [61]. More recently, Walker et al. [62] confirmed the development of temporary psychosis in 20% of immunosuppressed HIV-negative, renal transplantation patients, with *Pneumocystis jirovecii* infection, treated with SMX/TMP. The symptoms appeared between 3–10 days after initiation of the SMX/TMP administration and resolved within 24 h after discontinuation of the treatment. In another study Lee et al. [63] demonstrated that almost 12% of HIV-infected patients with *P. jirovecii*-induced pneumonia treated intravenously with SMX/TMP presented acute psychosis symptoms after an average of 5 days of the drug administration. The symptoms resolved after discontinuation of treatment or, in some cases, after SMX/TMP dose reduction or change of the route of administration from i.v. to oral while maintaining the applied dose. Moreover, SMX/TMP administration was also reported to be, rarely, associated with the aseptic meningitis development or transient-occurring tremor in immunocompromised patients [64,65].

The mechanisms contributing to sulfonamide-induced acute behavioral changes remain unknown. However, it is postulated that the psychiatric disturbances may be related to the SMX/TMP-dependent deficiency of the tetrahydrobiopterin synthesis. This factor is also utilized in the formations of essential central neurotransmitters, e.g., serotonin or dopamine, thus the resulting disturbances in central neurotransmission may be co-responsible for the generation of symptoms of transient psychosis [66]. Some reports also indicate a relationship between a powerful antioxidant level-glutathione and SMX/TMP neurotoxicity. It is also likely that the decrease of preventive glutathione enables the formation of unstable, neurotoxic sulfonamide by-products. This hypothesis would be in line with the observations that sulfonamide neurological ADRs are often noticed in HIV-infected or geriatric patients with depleted endogenous reserves of glutathione [67,68].

Of note, the SMX/TMP neurotoxicity is less commonly reported in children, probably due to the lower doses used in the therapy, the lack of significant concurrent diseases and drug interactions resulting from polypharmacotherapy [69].

4.3. Beta-Lactams

The beta-lactam antibiotics include penicillin, cephalosporins, carbapenems and monobactams. Except for monobactams, this group of antibiotics, together with quinolones, have been reported to account mostly for neurological ADRs development. The risk factors of beta-lactam induced neurotoxicity include: renal dysfunction (both acute and chronic) that decreases drug clearance, a blood level decrease in albumin binding of the antibiotics (e.g., hypoalbuminemia), liver insufficiency with downregulation of the hepatic metabolism by cytochromes P450 system, advanced age, high dosing, previous, concomitant diseases of the nervous system, low birth weight in newborns and all pathological conditions predisposing to increased permeability of BBB [26,27,49,60,70]. The most common potential neurological disturbances attributed to penicillin were abnormalities found in electroencephalograms (with epileptiform discharges), myoclonia, seizures and the presence of disorientation, confusion, delusions or hallucinations [26,27,60,70–72]. The convulsant effect of penicillin was first observed in 1945 by Walker and Johnson [27,49]. These antibiotics also stimulate T-cells and are responsible for the occurrence of drug-induced aseptic meningitis (DIAM) [49,72]. Hoigne's syndrome is a specific neuropsychiatric entity associated with the intramuscular use of procaine penicillin. The incidence of the condition is estimated at about 0.8–16.8/1000 injections [71]. The symptoms include panic attacks, depersonalization, auditory, visual, gustatory and somatosensory hallucinations, which are accompanied by adrenergic overstimulation (tachycardia, high blood pressure, shortness of breath) and possible generalized seizures. The attack usually lasts a few minutes and is preceded by residual asthenia and anxiety [73,74]. The potential underlying mechanism of the phenomena is that of embolic events in brain vessels, secondary to accidental penetration of procaine penicillin in the vascular system during injection or the direct toxic effect exerted by procaine with presumed limbic excitation [75]. Penicillin neurotoxicity is manifested primarily upon intravenous or intrathecal administration [27]. Among the penicillin agents, piperacillin and tazobactam appear to be most potent to produce neurotoxicity symptoms [60,76,77], although ampicillin or benzylpenicillin-induced epileptogenic potential has also been reported in the literature [78,79]. It has been shown that symptoms of encephalopathy can occur 1.5 to 7 days after piperacillin or piperacillin/tazobactam administration [72].

Cephalosporin-induced neurological ADRs are similar to those observed after penicillin administration and include, abnormal electroencephalogram, non-convulsive status epilepticus, myoclonus, chorea-athetosis, seizures and psychotic symptoms [26,27,60,70,71]. The variety of clinical presentation, ranging from simple EEG abnormalities to mental status changes, myoclonus, seizures or even coma have been reported within all four generations of cephalosporins, with the most frequent findings related to cefepime, cefoperazone, ceftazidine, cefuroxime and cefazolin [60,80]. The time to develop encephalopathy ranges from 1 to 10 days after medication initiation, and resolves in 2 to 7 days following discontinuation. Renal failure may be responsible for drug accumulation, which promotes the occurrence of neurotoxic effects. These manifest themselves at serum trough concentrations ranging from 15 to 20 mg/L. Other risk factors for encephalopathy are preexisting brain injury, increased serum concentration and overdose of the drug. Analogous to penicillin, they may mediate DIAM through specific drug-IgG binding in cerebrospinal fluid [49]. Cefazolin, ceftazidime, and cefepime-cephalosporins, with higher $GABA_A$ receptor affinity and increased BBB penetration, are thought to be more predisposed to cause neurotoxic symptoms [72]. It should be noted that sepsis and systematic inflammation compromise the integrity of BBB and may make it easier for drugs to overcome it [49]. The probability of neurotoxicity of cefotaxime or ceftriaxone is lower than in the above-mentioned group [27], although the study of Lacroix et al. reported the incidence of serious CNS complications associated with ceftriaxone therapy to be seven times higher than that published in the literature. Reported CNS ADRs between 1995 and 2017 identified ceftriaxone as both the leading cause of hospitalization and life-threatening situations, or even death [81].

Carbapenems including imipenem, meropenem, panipenem, ertapenem, and doripenem are also antibiotics that were demonstrated to share common symptoms of neurotoxicity with other beta lactams. Treatment with carbapenems may induce headache, seizures and encephalopathy [26,27,60,70,71]. Seizure incidence of imipenem was estimated in up to 1.5–2% and this decreases with the newer carbapenems, with a value found for doripenem of 1.1% [82,83]. The pro-convulsive effects may be related to its action on the a-amino-3-hydroxy-5-methyl-isoxazolepropionate (AMPA) and NMDA receptor complexes [49].

There is no unambiguously convincing evidence supporting the significant neurotoxicity of monobactams. The leaflet dedicated to these preparations mentions the possibility of seizures, confusion, dizziness, vertigo, paresthesia or insomnia, but they are reported very rarely [70,71].

The mechanisms responsible for beta lactam neurotoxicity are related to the ability of these drugs to exert inhibitory effects on GABA neurotransmission. This effect is thought to be due to the structural resemblance of the beta lactam ring and its affinity to GABA receptor binding since the degradation of the beta-lactam structure prevents the occurrence of seizures [49,84]. Thus, GABA complex receptor inhibition via competitive (for cephalosporins) or non-competitive affecting of the $GABA_A$ subunits is the basic hypothesis for beta lactam neurotoxicity [26,84,85]. The complementary hypotheses raise issues of the release of various cytokines with potential for neurotoxicity and an ability to increase the excitatory action of N-methyl-D-aspartate (NMDA) and alpha-amino-3-hydroxy-5-methylisoxazolepropionate receptors with overactivity of the glutamatergic system and accumulation of neurotoxic metabolites [26,49,80,84–88].

4.4. Glycopeptides

It would be difficult to imagine the practice of infectious diseases treatment over the past 20 years without glycopeptide antibiotics. Their safety profile is favorable, although vancomycin (with intravenous use) and teicoplanin can induce sensorineural hearing loss, with possible association to tinnitus, dizziness and vertigo [89–92]. Penetration of vancomycin into cerebrospinal fluid is poor, but has increased in patients with meningitis. Encephalopathy and mononeuritis multiplex are rarely observed during the use of this drug [93]. The mechanism of vancomycin ototoxicity involves direct damage by the drug to the auditory branch of the eighth cranial nerve [91]. Moreover, an explanation for this toxicity may be oxidative stress, which leads to loss of sensory cochlear cells [94]. Transient or permanent hearing loss has been reported during vancomycin use, especially in patients treated with high doses, those receiving concomitant other drugs with ototoxic effects (e.g., aminoglycosides), with renal dysfunction or those with pre-existing hearing impairment. The risk of hearing loss is greater in elderly patients [91,92]. Ototoxicity with teicoplanin has been observed, but it does not occur often [92]. Currently available data suggests that the second generation lipoglycopeptides, dalbavancin and oritavancin, have no effect on hearing loss or dysfunction [95,96].

4.5. Macrolides

Macrolides show a similar spectrum of antimicrobial activity as benzylpenicillin making them useful alternatives for people with a history of penicillin and cephalosporin allergy. Erythromycin, the prototype macrolide, has been used since 1952, and clarithromycin or azithromycin are popular in treating upper respiratory infections but their administration may be accompanied by confusion, obtundation, agitation, insomnia, delirium, disorientation, psychosis and exacerbation of myasthenia gravis. The timing of these dose-dependent symptoms can range from 3 to 10 days after drug ingestion. Some may be permanent. Risk factors include psychiatric illness, renal insufficiency or excess dosage of medication [27,60,72]. Steinmam and Steinman were the first to point out visual hallucinations induced by clarithromycin taken 500 mg twice daily for acute bronchitis. This complication developed within 24 h of taking the drug. The 56-year-old patient described them as "constantly evolving landscape of sharks, priests, red lines and other technicolor" [97]. The mechanisms of CNS toxicity of macrolides are unclear. Several hypotheses include drug interactions (metabolism through isoenzyme CYP3A4), adverse effects of the lipid-soluble active metabolite of clarithromycin (14-hydroxyclarithromycin) on the CNS, alterations of cortisol and prostaglandin metabolism, as well as interactions with glutaminergic and GABA pathways [27,60,97–99]. Macrolides also induce ototoxicity. It has been suggested that patients may recover from transient hearing loss associated with macrolide therapy, but develop tinnitus, which may be generated in the auditory centers of the brain by deviant neuronal activity caused by macrolide use [100].

4.6. *Aminoglycosides*

Aminoglycosides are used in patients with serious gram-negative infections. They have been known to cause ototoxicity, peripheral neuropathy, encephalopathy and neuromuscular blockade [26,27,60]. Hearing loss may occur in 20–63% of patients using aminoglycosides for many days. Acute ototoxicity is related to ion channel blockade and calcium antagonism and chronic ototoxicity is based on drug access to perilymph and endolymph, and penetration of the hair cells [101]. The cause of the toxic effect on the hearing organ is the excitotoxic activation of NMDA receptors within the cochlea as a result, with subsequent oxygen radicals formulation, which is postulated to contribute to cell death [26]. The mechanism responsible for neuromuscular blockade is inhibition of quantal release of acetylcholine in the neuromuscular junction pre-synaptically and a postjunctional binding of aminoglycosides to the acetylcholine receptor complex [26,27]. Inflammation and fever increase the risk of aminoglycoside-induced hearing loss. Another cause of hearing loss may be coexisting renal insufficiency, which decreases excretion of aminoglycosides from the blood [102].

4.7. *Oxazolidinones*

This class of antibiotics is used to treat serious skin and bacterial infections, often after other antibiotics have been ineffective. They are active against a large spectrum of gram-positive bacteria, including methicillin- and vancomycin-resistant staphylococci, vancomycin-resistant enterococci, penicillin-resistant pneumococci, and anaerobes. Manifestations of oxazolidinone neurotoxicity, especially linezolid, include peripheral and optic neuropathy, serotonin syndrome, encephalopathy, and delirium. Peripheral neuropathy appears to be most commonly reported. It is more likely to occur during prolonged courses of treatment (>28 days, median 5 months). Optic neuropathies in patients treated for *Staphylococcus aureus* infections may be asymptomatic or lead to decreased visual acuity, blurred vision, central scotomas, and dyschromatopsia, The mechanism of linezolid neuropathies is unclear. It may be associated with mitochondrial injury. In addition, the drug has the ability to penetrate the central nervous and ocular system. Risk factors for developing neuropathy include pre-existing neurologic diseases, alcohol abuse, diabetes, chemotherapy and antiviral therapy. It generally improves or completely resolves after discontinuation of the medicine, although occasionally can be permanent. Linezolid is a nonselective inhibitor of monoamine oxidase. Inhibition of monoamine oxidase A increases levels of serotonin, and monoamine oxidase B elevates catecholamines. Epinephrine, norepinephrine, and dopamine are reported to be involved in serotonin syndrome, delirium or encephalopathy associated with the administration of this drug. When it is used with, e.g., selective serotonin and norepinephrine reuptake inhibitors, it can increase the risk of serotonin syndrome. Linezolid, which has dopaminergic properties, may cause serotonin syndrome if used with a monoamine oxidase inhibitor. Its administration with an anticholinergic substances increases encephalopathy risk [27,60,103,104].

4.8. Polymyxins

Polymyxins are peptide antibiotics of natural origin, first obtained in 1947 by fermentation in *Bacillus polymyxa* subspecies colistinus. In the early 1980s, data on the safety risks of their use related to severe episodes of renal failure, as well as incompletely understood neurotoxicity, and the availability of antibiotics with fewer potential side effects reduced their use in therapy. The incidence of neurological complications with these antibiotics ranges from 7–27%, including dizziness, generalized or muscle weakness, confusion, hallucinations, seizures, paresthesias, ataxia and, less commonly, diplopia, nystagmus and ptosis [60]. Paresthesias are more common with intravenous administration than intramuscular use. Ventilation-dependent respiratory disturbances were observed after intramuscular administration of polymyxins. They lasted from 10 to 48 h. This was probably a myasthenia-like syndrome. The polymyxin chemical structure contains a fatty acid, which may interact with the lipophilic content of neurons. Neuromuscular blockade may be related to inhibition of acetylcholine release in the synaptic cleft. Risk factors of neurotoxicity include renal dysfunction, hypoxia and concomitant use of such medication as nephrotoxic agents, sedatives, muscle relaxants, anesthetic drugs or corticosteroids [60]. Colistin neurotoxicity, especially observed in patients with renal failure or receiving high doses, includes facial paresthesias (pricking, tingling, numbness), dizziness, speech impairment, visual disturbances, confusion, and psychosis. Neuromuscular blockade manifested by myasthenia-like syndrome or as respiratory muscle paralysis producing apnea has also been observed. Colistin neurotoxicity primarily involving paresthesias, and in only sporadic cases apnea, especially in patients with intramuscular administration of the drug, with acute or chronic renal failure and receiving medications, induces respiratory muscle weakness [99,105]. Two mechanisms account for colistin neurotoxicity and neuromuscular blockade. One involves presynaptic action of the drug, preventing the release of acetylcholine into the synaptic gap. The other is biphasic, involving a short phase of competitive blockade between acetylcholine and colistin, followed by a prolonged depolarization phase, leading to loss of calcium from neurons, resulting in altered mitochondrial permeability. This results in mitochondrial dysfunction in neuronal cells and accumulation of reactive oxygen species. This in turn is the cause of oxidative stress and further nerve damage [26,106].

4.9. Tetracyclines

Tetracyclines are a class of broad-spectrum bacteriostatic antibiotics discovered in the 1940s, including tetracycline, minocycline, and doxycycline, which have shown to be effective against aerobic and anaerobic bacteria, as well as Gram-positive and Gram-negative bacteria (with the exceptions of *Proteus* species and *Pseudomonas aeruginosa*). They are largely prescribed in dermatology and infectious diseases, both for the anti-bacterial and anti-inflammatory actions. Neurotoxicity associated with this class of antibiotics include cranial nerve toxicity, neuromuscular blockage and intracranial hypertension [26,27,60]. During therapy with tera-cyclines, symptoms such as blurred vision, loss of balance, light-headedness, dizziness, vertigo or tinnitus were observed [60].

4.10. Quinolones

Quinolones are a family of antibiotics with a wide range of antimicrobial activity, which are active against both Gram-positive and Gram-negative bacteria, including mycobacteria, and anaerobes. Since their discovery in the early 1960s, they have become increasingly important in the treatment of both community and serious hospital-acquired infections. In the 1970s and 1980s, the scope of the quinolone class was greatly expanded by the groundbreaking development of fluoroquinolones, which exhibit a much broader spectrum of action and improved pharmacokinetics compared with first-generation quinolones [107]. Unfortunately, several European Medicines Agency (EMA) recommendations have recently been made to healthcare providers regarding risk factors for musculoskeletal, neurological and psychiatric adverse reactions observed among quinolone users [108].

Many members of this group of antibiotics (norfloxacin > ciprofloxacin > ofloxacin, levofloxacin) are known for their neurotoxic effects. These may manifest as headache, confusion, decline of attention, tremors, psychosis, seizures, myoclonic jerks, insomnia, encephalopathy, delirium, sleep disturbances, toxic psychosis or Tourette-like syndrome, and moreover as extrapyramidal manifestations such as gait disturbance, dysarthria and choreiform movements. Scavone et al. observed that third-generation quinolones were always associated with higher reporting probability of neurological and psychiatric adverse drug effects compared to second generation. These effects were presented 1 to 2 days after antibiotic therapy and were dose-dependent. Their etiology is likely to be multifactorial and include inhibition of $GABA_A$ receptor, stimulation of NMDA receptor and ligand-gated glutamate receptors which reduce seizure threshold. It has also been suggested that oxidative stress is increased by these drugs. No less important is the relationship between their chemical structure and the symptoms observed, e.g., ciprofloxacin, norfloxacin as a quinolone with 7-piperazine and clinafloxacin, and tosufloxacin as a quinolone with 7-pyrrolidine have been observed to be highly associated with epilepsy. The epileptogenic potential of fluoroquinolones is increased by simultaneously used non-steroidal anti-inflammatory drugs (NSAIDs). Moreover, these antibiotics penetrate through the BBB and induce eosinophilic meningitis. Risk factors for neurotoxicity include older age, hypoxemia, pre-existing central nervous system diseases, electrolyte disturbance, thyrotoxicosis, renal and hepatic dysfunction. Hemodialysis may be a useful treatment for encephalopathy associated with quinolone treatment in patients with impaired renal function [27,49,72,99,108–110].

4.11. Other Antibacterial Agents (Chloramphenicol, Nitrofurantoin, Isoniazid, Ethambutol, Cycloserine)

Chloramphenicol is a broad spectrum antibiotic, which was first isolated from *Streptomyces venezuelae* in 1947. It is currently of limited use due to adverse effects and frequently observed antimicrobial resistance. It must be used only in those serious infections for which less potentially dangerous drugs are ineffective or contraindicated. Headache, mild depression, mental confusion, and delirium have been described in patients receiving this medicine. Optic and peripheral neuritis have been reported, usually following long-term therapy. If this occurs, the drug should be promptly withdrawn [26].

Nitrofurantoin, a synthetic nitrofuran derivative, has been available for the treatment of uncomplicated lower urinary tract infection since 1952. It is effective against *E. coli* and many gram-negative organisms. Nitrofurantoin treatment has been associated with neurotoxicity effects including peripheral neuropathy, dizziness, vertigo, diplopia, cerebellar dysfunction and intracranial hypertension. These are observed particularly in women and elderly patients. The etiology is attributed to axon loss [111].

Isoniazid, cyclo-serine and ethambutol-medications used for treating tuberculosis, may cause both central and peripheral neuropathy. Isoniazid administration may be accompanied by peripheral neuropathy, psychosis and seizures. The importance of isoniazid interference with GABA synthesis is emphasized in the etiology of seizures, through inhibition of pyridoxal-5 phosphate. This compound is a cofactor for the enzymatic activity of glutamic acid decarboxylase, thus reducing the concentration of GABA and enhanced seizure susceptibility. Status epilepticus was also observed after therapeutic doses of the medicine. Cyclo-serine may be the cause of neuropsychiatric adverse events including anxiety, agitation, depression, psychosis, and, rarely, seizures. The frequencies of psychiatric and central nervous system adverse events are 5.7 and 1.1%, respectively. They may be associated with elevated plasma concentrations of the drug. Cyclo-serine crosses the blood–brain barrier and decreases GABA production. It binds to N-methyl-d-aspartate receptors, which in part explains the commonly associated neurotoxicity. At the recommended dosage for cyclo-serine (250 to 500 mg once daily), the neurotoxicity can range from mild to severe and has resulted in psychosis and treatment discontinuation in some cases. Concurrent use of alcohol increases the risk of developing psychosis and seizures. Another complication of ethambutol therapy can be optic nerve neuropathy. This is dose-dependent, with the lowest risk at total daily doses < 15 mg/kg. Its risk factors include older age, hypertension, renal insufficiency, and duration of treatment. Symptoms are manifested by gradual onset of reduced visual acuity, dyschromatopsia and central or mid-central visual field losses observed several months after the drug was started. They are probably related to mitochondrially induced papillary bundle dysfunction [27,99,112].

To sum up, the mechanisms contributing to the neurotoxic adverse effects of antibiotics are multiple and specific to a given class of those drugs. They are summarized in Table 3 below.

Table 3. Summary of the mechanisms of neurotoxicity of particular classes of antibiotics.

Class of Antibiotic	Mechanisms of Neurotoxicity
penicillin cephalosporins	GABA complex receptor inhibition via competitive or non-competitive affecting the $GABA_A$ subunits; an increase of the N-methyl-D-aspartate (NMDA) and alpha-amino-3-hydroxy-5-methylisoxazolepropionate receptors stimulation resulting in the overactivity of glutamatergic system
glycopeptides	direct damage of the auditory branch of the eighth cranial nerve; an increase of the oxidative stress leading to loss of sensory cochlear cells
macrolides	drug interactions (metabolism through isoenzyme CYP3A4); direct neurotoxic effect produced by the lipid-soluble active metabolites; alterations of cortisol and prostaglandin metabolism; interactions with glutaminergic and GABA pathways
aminoglycosides	Ototoxicity-determined by the overactivation of NMDA receptors within the cochlea with subsequent oxygen radicals formulation; neuromuscular blockade-due to the presynaptic inhibition of quantal release of acetylcholine in the neuromuscular junction and a postjunctional blockade of the acetylcholine receptor complex
oxazolidinones	mitochondrial injury; nonselective inhibition of monoamine oxidase leading to increased serotonin and catecholamines levels
polymyxins	neuromuscular blockade-due to the presynaptic decrease of acetylcholine release into the synaptic gap; induction of prolonged depolarization following the transient postsynaptic blockade, with loss of calcium from neurons and altered mitochondrial permeability; accumulation of reactive oxygen species
quinolones	inhibition of $GABA_A$ receptor; stimulation of NMDA receptor and ligand-gated glutamate receptors; an increase of the oxidative stress
sulfonamides /trimethoprim	deficiency in the tetrahydrobiopterin synthesis resulting in disturbances in synthesis of central neurotransmitters
metronidazole	an increase of oxidative stress; oxidation of catecholamines and other neurotransmitters; inhibition of GABA-ergic neurotransmission
other anti-infective agents: nitrofurantoin, isoniazid, ethambutol	loss of axons; decrease of GABA synthesis, NMDA receptors activation

5. Methods of Reducing the Frequency and Severity of Antibiotic-Induced Neurologic and Psychiatric Entities

Modern optimal antibiotic therapy requires extensive knowledge of the mechanisms of drug action, their pharmacokinetic properties, adverse effects, identification of their risk factors, especially underestimated neurotoxicity, toxicity thresholds limiting dosing, infection site and antibiotic penetration, and careful monitoring of the consequences of their action. It is necessary to control the clinical condition of patients, to examine the efficiency of organs responsible for elimination of drugs from the body. Early recognition of renal failure may reduce the frequency or severity of neurologic and psychiatric symptoms associated with antibiotic administration. EEG may be helpful in differentiating between drug complications in the form of non-convulsive status epilepticus (NCSE) and encephalopathy. Sometimes temporary use of anti-convulsant medication may be needed. Myasthenic syndrome accompanying treatment with polymyxins may require ventilatory support depending on the degree of respiratory impairment. Hemodialysis or hemofiltration may be needed in patients with impaired renal function if antibiotic-induced neurotoxicity is observed [26,113].

In recent years, much attention has been given to increasing the optimization of antibiotic therapy based on pharmacokinetic and pharmacodynamic (PK/PD) modelling [114–117]. To evaluate the efficacy and safety of antimicrobial therapy, three basic ratios were developed: Cmax/MIC (minimal inhibitory concentration), T > MIC, AUC_{24}/MIC. Concentration-dependent antibiotics include aminoglycosides and metronidazole. Their efficacy best correlates with peak concentration (Cmax) to MIC. Clinical PK/PD target for amikacin/gentamicin efficacy is Cmax/MIC $\geq$ 8–10, clinical PK/PD threshold for amikacin toxicity is Cmin > 5 mg/L, for gentamicin > 1 mg/L. The group of antibiotics whose effectiveness is determined by the time the concentration remains above the MIC of the bacterial pathogen include penicillin, cephalosporins, carbapenems, monobactams, macrolides (erythromycin, clarithromycin), linezolid. Clinical PK/PD target for carbapenems/penicillin efficacy is 50–100% fT>MIC, for cephalosporins 45–100%, clinical PK/PD threshold for meropenem nephro- or neurotoxicity is Cmin > 44.5–64 mg/L, for neurotoxicity of cefepime Cmin $\geq$ 20–22 mg/L, for piperacillin Cmin > 64–361 mg/L. Concentration-dependent antibiotics with a time-dependent component for which the best predictor of efficacy is the area under the concentration-time curve during a 24 h time period (AUC_{24}) to the MIC ratio include: glycopeptides, oxazolidinones, fluoroquinolones, polymixins, daptomycin, azithromycin and tigecycline. Clinical PK/PD target for vancomycin efficacy is $AUC_{0\text{–}24}$/MIC $\geq$ 400, threshold for its toxicity $AUC_{0\text{–}24}$ > 700 mg·h/L, Cmin > 20 mg/L [118]. This individualized approach has allowed two directions for optimizing antibiotic therapy, especially in intensive care patients: dose adjustment based on therapeutic drug monitoring (TDM) or modification of drug dosing by using higher initial and maintenance doses or by using prolonged or continuous infusions [119–121].

TDM, the measurement of drug concentrations in biological fluid (typically plasma) is particularly important with respect to drugs with a narrow therapeutic index, with a defined relationship between their concentration and pharmacological effect, significant intra-and/or inter-individual pharmacokinetic variability, established target concentration range, which are the cause of numerous drug complications and interactions with other drugs, long duration of therapy, absence of pharmacodynamic markers of therapeutic response and/or toxicity, and availability of cost-effective drug assay (precise, accurate, highly selective bioanalytical assay methods for drug measurement). It is widely used for aminoglycosides, and vancomycin, for beta-lactam antibiotics, particularly for piperacillin and meropenem, is becoming increasingly common [113,122,123]. It is important to remember that the drug concentration is only complementary but not a substitute for clinical judgement, and we treat the individual patient, not the laboratory value.

Imami et al. retrospectively reviewed a series of cases of people treated with potentially neurotoxic antibiotics hospitalized at St Vincent Hospital in Sydney between 2013 and 2015. Adverse events of neurotoxicity, nephrotoxicity, hepatotoxicity and *Clostridium difficile* infections were assessed. Based on the measurements of drug concentrations (piperacillin, meropenem, fluo-cloxacillin), their direct relationship with the complication was demonstrated. The breakpoint for which the risk of neurotoxicity is 50% for piperacillin was found to be Cmin > 361.4 mg/L, for meropenem > 64.2 mg/L, and for flucloxacillin > 125.1 mg/L. Therefore, measuring the concentrations of these antibiotics, especially in patients with an increased risk of neurological complications, is a method of optimizing their use [124].

Oda et al. reported a case of using Bayesian estimation calculations in conjunction with the measurement of cefepime concentration to reduce the dose in people with pneumonia to prevent neurological complications. After receiving a dose of 1.0 g every 8 h, the patient developed aphasia on the fifth day. Measurement of the drug concentration in the serum showed 71.3 mg/l, which was 2–3 times higher than the recommended value (22–35 mg/L).

Bayesian pharmacokinetic calculations indicated the need to reduce the dose to 0.5 g every 12 h. After 3 days, the neurological symptoms improved and the treatment was continued successfully [125].

Another case was described by Smith et al. and concerned an 82-year-old patient admitted to the intensive care unit with a diagnosis of severe community-acquired pneumonia, septic shock and multiple organ failure. After administration of cefepime, the patient developed convulsions. Blood and cerebrospinal fluid drug concentrations were measured and increased values were found. After dose adjustments and a decrease in cefepime levels, the seizures subsided [126].

In 2020, a summary of an expert discussion panel on the use of TDM in relation to antibiotics, antifungal and antiviral drugs in intensive care units was published. It was emphasized that from a clinical practice point of view dosing drugs under TDM control is beneficial for the aminoglycosides, voriconazole and ribavirin. Therapeutic ranges have been defined for some of the antibiotics. Routine use of TDM has been recommended for therapy with aminoglycosides, beta-lactam antibiotics, linezolid, teicoplain, vancomycin and voriconazole in critically ill patients. The authors pointed out that, although drug concentration monitored therapy was first used in the 1940s, it still requires the development of globally uniform standards of care, especially with regard to the treatment of patients with comorbidities and multi-organ disorders [118].

According to a systematic review by Barreto et al., clinical observations have shown that, in critically ill patients, beta-lactam antibiotic levels must be monitored, and the recommended minimum concentrations should be greater than the MIC for at least half the time between doses. The free drug fraction is recommended to be measured during the first 48 h of therapy, and should be above the MIC breakpoint of the most likely pathogen before blood culture results are available. This concentration should be maintained for the entire period between doses, and after this time the minimum concentration should reach a value of 1–2x of the observed MIC of the pathogen obtained in microbiological cultures. Neurotoxicity has also been shown to be the most dose-dependent adverse event, although direct evidence is not yet available to indicate the concentration above which this complication is likely to occur [127].

A retrospective cohort study published in 2017, which included 53 patients admitted to the intensive care unit with no neurological abnormalities prior to commencing continuous infusion of piperacillin at the standard dose and subjected to serum piperacillin determination, showed that 23 patients developed a neurological disorder, in which piperacillin causation was consistent chronologically and semiologically. The minimum concentration value of 157.2 mg/L, regardless of other variables, was the factor of the occurrence of neurotoxicity with 96.7% specificity and 52.2% sensitivity. This is a phenomenon that may be a limitation in antibiotic therapy if the patient has pathogens less sensitive to this antibiotic [128].

Optimization of antibiotic therapy also requires the use of guidelines adapted to local needs and adherence to these by medical staff. Unfortunately, a multi-center study has shown that 37.8% of antibiotic use in European hospitals does not comply with this restriction. Antimicrobial stewardship programs are a promising strategy. One of the methods is a pharmacokinetic dosing nomogram. This describes the influence of a covariate (e.g., weight) on a drug exposure target (e.g., concentration). It can be combined with TDM. Clinical pharmacological advice, which is delivered by the clinical pharmacologist who interprets the therapeutic drug monitoring results of antimicrobials in relation to the site of infection, the pathophysiological characteristics of the patient, and potential drug–drug interactions are very important in personalized treatment [129,130]. The interprofessional team should include a clinical pharmacist, who can play an important role by monitoring antimicrobial prescriptions and providing advice or educating medical and nursing staff, because approximately 50% of hospitalized patients receive at least one antibiotic, and 20-30% cases of antibiotic therapy are unnecessary. Clinical pharmacist intervention has been shown to be effective in enhancing appropriate use of antibiotics and reducing their toxicity, which may improve patient care. Moreover these had a positive impact not only on the clinical, but on financial outcomes [131–135].

6. Neuroprotective Action of Antibiotics

In recent years, old, well-known drugs have been increasingly used in new indications. Such a strategy is referred to as "repositioning drugs", "redirecting drugs" or "finding new uses for old drugs". It is an efficient and cost-effective pathway to new drug development. Antibiotics are also being studied for their anti-amyloidogenic and anti-inflammatory properties. Results of ongoing observations suggest the possible use of antibiotics in Alzheimer's disease, Parkinson's disease or multiple sclerosis. Tetracyclines, and especially doxycycline, are promising in this area. Interest in their use in Alzheimer's disease dates back to the early 2000s when it was discovered that tetracyclines could inhibit the aggregation of the β-amyloid peptide (Aβ). Moreover they have anti-oxidative and anti-apoptotic activities [136–138]. Many studies have confirmed the neurotrophic, anti-inflammatory, antioxidant and anti-apoptotic effects of minocycline, a long-acting, semi-synthetic tetracycline. This antibiotic is characterized by high lipophilicity and can easily penetrate the blood–brain barrier, has long half-life time and excellent tissue penetration. It alters the reactivity of microglia cells, counteracts inflammatory processes, and reduces neurodegenerative processes within the central nervous system. Its effectiveness has been proven in experimental models for the treatment of Alzheimer's disease, Parkinson's disease, Huntington's disease, multiple sclerosis, neuropathic pain, stroke, hypoxic-ischemic encephalopathy and hypomyelination. It has been shown to reduce white matter and hippocampal lesions and improve cerebral blood flow. The drug reduces the expression of pro-inflammatory markers responsible for increasing the activity of chemokine CCL2, IL-1β, IL-6, TNF-α and iNOS. Minocycline has antioxidant and antiapoptotic properties, manifested by caspase inhibition. In turn, ceftriaxone was found to increase the expression of astrocytic glutamate transporter 1 (GLT-1), decreasing excitotoxicity and neuroinflammation by detoxifying the brain from glutamate. It should be emphasized that persistently elevated amounts of this compound in the synaptic space may contribute to neurodegenerative diseases and ischemic stroke [139]. It affects the markers of oxidative status and neuroinflammation [138]. Rifampicin is also a broad-spectrum antibiotic whose protective effect on the brain has been demonstrated in many experimental studies. Its mechanism of action includes inhibitory effect on free oxygen radicals, tau and Aβ protein accumulation, microglial activation, apoptotic cascades [140]. Use of antibiotics in neuroprotection is promising, creates new potential treatment options for neurodegenerative diseases, but requires many more studies using not only laboratory models but also human subjects.

7. Conclusions

The study of neuroprotective drugs that lead to rescue, recovery or regeneration of the nervous system, its cells, structure and function, has been ongoing for many years. These are based on three main strategies, i.e., the synthesis of new drugs, the use of natural products with as yet unidentified properties, and attempts to develop therapies based on existing drugs, so-called "drug repositioning" or "drug reprofiling". The latter area seems worthy of attention, as the pharmacokinetic and pharmacodynamic profile of such drugs is already known, and the effort put into such a strategy requires incomparably less time and cost than developing new drugs. Unfortunately, this is not an easy task, as there are many neurochemical modulators of nervous system damage. Clinical trials often fail to demonstrate their efficacy, and the doses used prove toxic [141]. Patients with nervous system dysfunctions are also a very heterogeneous group in terms of both their etiology and their age, etc., and they are additionally burdened with various risk factors. Experimental models also differ significantly from clinical conditions. The development of such drugs requires a better understanding of the etiology and pathogenesis of nervous system diseases. It is believed that neuroinflammatory mechanisms may account for many of the processes responsible for the neuronal degeneration observed in Alzheimer's disease,

Parkinson's disease, stroke, and other neurodegenerative diseases. They undoubtedly represent a significant health problem and challenge for 21st century medicine. Antibiotics are also being investigated in this aspect and promising observational results provide new potential avenues for their use as neuroprotective rather than just anti-infective drugs. Rifaximin is currently in phase II clinical trials based on the association between changes in the gut microbiota and neuropsychiatric diseases. It is hypothesized that it may improve memory and daily functioning in people with Alzheimer's disease by reducing blood levels of ammonia and/or levels of pro-inflammatory cytokines secreted by gut bacteria [142]. On the other hand, it is very important to pay attention to the possibility of neurotoxicity during antibiotic therapy. Multidirectional monitoring of patients at high risk of neurotoxicity is necessary to prevent or reduce its severity. As described above, its causes are not fully understood. It is also necessary to conduct multidirectional research dedicated to the elucidation of mechanisms responsible for nervous system dysfunction under the influence of antimicrobial drugs. To achieve an effective antimicrobial effect, and at the same time not to induce drug-related complications, the choice of antibiotic and therapy depend on clinical diagnosis, pathogens isolated from patient or those most frequently causing a specific infection in a population and their sensitivity to antibiotics, concomitant diseases present in the patient (taking into account past diseases, chronic diseases, impaired renal or hepatic function, age, allergies, etc.), and properties of the antibiotic itself (pharmacodynamics, pharmacokinetics, possible side effects, toxicity).

Author Contributions: Conceptualization, M.H. and A.W.-H.; methodology, M.H. and A.W.-H.; resources, M.H., L.D. and A.W.-H.; writing—original draft preparation, M.H., L.D. and A.W.-H.; writing—review and editing, M.H., L.D., A.W.-H.; supervision, L.D. and A.W.-H.; project administration, M.H., L.D.; funding acquisition, A.W.-H. All authors have read and agreed to the published version of the manuscript.

Funding: This research received no external funding.

Conflicts of Interest: The authors declare no conflict of interest.

References

1. Hutchings, M.I.; Truman, A.W.; Wilkinson, B. Antibiotics: Past, present and future. *Curr. Opin. Microbiol.* **2019**, *51*, 72–80. [CrossRef] [PubMed]
2. Aminov, R.I. A brief history of the antibiotic era: Lessons learned and challenge for the future. *Front. Microbiol.* **2010**, *1*, 134. [CrossRef]
3. Gould, K. Antibiotics: From prehistory to the present day. *J. Antimicrob. Chemother.* **2016**, *71*, 572–575. [CrossRef] [PubMed]
4. Ventola, C.L. The antibiotic resistance crisis. Part 1: Causes and threats. *Pharm. Ther.* **2015**, *40*, 277–283.
5. Levy, S.B.; Marshall, B. Antibacterial resistance worldwide: Causes, challenges and responses. *Nat. Med.* **2004**, *10*, S122–S129. [CrossRef]
6. Schatz, S.N.; Weber, R.J. Adverse Drug Reactions. In *PSAP 2015 Book 2 CNS/Pharmacy Practice: Pharmacotherapy Self-Assessment Program*; Murphy, J.E., Lee, M.W.-L., Eds.; American College of Clinical Pharmacy: Lenexa, KS, USA, 2015; pp. 5–22.
7. Coleman, J.J.; Pontefract, S.K. Adverse drug reactions. *Clin. Med.* **2016**, *16*, 481–485. [CrossRef]
8. Edwards, I.R.; Aronson, J.K. Adverse drug reactions: Definitions, diagnosis, and management. *Lancet* **2000**, *356*, 1255–1259. [CrossRef]
9. Zagaria, M.A.E. Antibiotic therapy: Adverse effects and dosing considerations. *US Pharm* **2013**, *38*, 18–20.
10. Mohsen, S.; Dickinson, J.A.; Somayaji, R. Update on the adverse effects of antimicrobial therapies in community practice. *Can. Fam. Phys.* **2020**, *66*, 651–659.
11. Granowitz, E.V.; Brown, R.B. Antibiotic adverse reactions and drug interactions. *Crit. Care Clin.* **2008**, *24*, 421–442. [CrossRef] [PubMed]
12. Demler, T.L. Drug-induced neurologic conditions. *US Pharm* **2014**, *39*, 47–51.
13. Jain, K.K. Chapter 1: Epidemiology and Clinical Significance. In *Drug-Induced Neurological Disorders*, 3rd revised and expanded ed.; Hogrefe Publishing: Gottingen, Germany, 2012; pp. 1–5.
14. Jain, K.K. Chapter 2: Pathomechanisms of Drug-Induced Neurological Disorders. In *Drug-Induced Neurological Disorders*, 3rd revised and expanded ed.; Hogrefe Publishing: Gottingen, Germany, 2012; pp. 7–12.
15. Soleimani, S.M.A.; Ekhtiari, H.; Cadet, J.L. Drug-induced neurotoxicity in addiction medicine: From prevention to harm reduction. *Prog. Brain Res.* **2016**, *223*, 19–41.
16. Snavely, S.R.; Hodges, G.R. The neurotoxicity of antibacterial agents. *Ann. Intern. Med.* **1984**, *101*, 92–104. [CrossRef] [PubMed]

17. File, T.M.; Tan, J.S. Recommendations for using imipenem-cilastatindthe most broad spectrum antibiotic. *Hosp. Formul.* **1987**, *22*, 534–542.
18. Ruiz, M.E.; Wortmann, G.W. Unusual effects of common antibiotics. *Clevel. Clin. J. Med.* **2019**, *86*, 277–281. [CrossRef] [PubMed]
19. Moore, R.D.; Smith, C.R.; Leitman, P.S. Risk factors for the development of auditory toxicity in patients receiving aminoglycosides. *J. Infect. Dis.* **1984**, *149*, 23–30. [CrossRef]
20. Gatell, J.M.; Ferran, F.; Araujo, V.; Bonet, M.; Soriano, E.; Traserra, J.; SanMiguel, J.G. Univariate and multivariate analyses of risk factors predisposing to auditory toxicity in patients receiving aminoglycosides. *Antimicrob. Agents Chemother.* **1987**, *31*, 1383–1387. [CrossRef] [PubMed]
21. Selimoglu, E. Aminoglycoside-induced ototoxicity. *Curr. Pharm. Des.* **2007**, *13*, 119–126. [CrossRef] [PubMed]
22. Swanson, D.J.; Sung, R.J.; Fine, M.J.; Orloff, J.J.; Chu, S.Y.; Yu, V.L. Erythromycin ototoxicity: Prospective assessment with serum concentrations and audiograms in a study of patients with pneumonia. *Am. J. Med.* **1992**, *92*, 61–68. [CrossRef]
23. Wallace, M.R.; Miller, L.K.; Nguyen, M.T.; Shields, A.R. Ototoxicity with azithromycin. *Lancet* **1994**, *343*, 241. [CrossRef]
24. Umstead, G.S.; Neumann, K.H. Erythromycin ototoxicity and acute psychotic reaction in cancer patients with hepatic dysfunction. *Arch. Intern. Med.* **1986**, *146*, 897–899. [CrossRef]
25. Ress, B.D.; Gross, E.M. Irreversible sensorineural hearing loss as a result of azithromycin ototoxicity. A case report. *Ann. Otol. Rhinol. Laryngol.* **2000**, *109*, 435–437. [CrossRef]
26. Grill, M.F.; Maganti, R.K. Neurotoxic effects associated with antibiotic use: Management considerations. *Br. J. Clin. Pharmacol.* **2011**, *72*, 381–393. [CrossRef]
27. Rezaei, N.J.; Bazzazi, A.M.; Alavi, S.A.N. Neurotoxicity of the antibiotics: A comprehensive study. *Neurol. India* **2018**, *66*, 1732–1740. [PubMed]
28. Wang, B.; Yao, M.; Lv, L.; Ling, Z.; Li, L. The human microbiota in health and disease. *Engineering* **2017**, *3*, 71–82. [CrossRef]
29. Cani, P.D. Human gut microbiome: Hopes, threats and promises. *Gut* **2018**, *67*, 1716–1725. [CrossRef]
30. Fan, Y.; Pedersen, O. Gut microbiota in human metabolic health and disease. *Nat. Rev. Microbiol.* **2021**, *19*, 55–71. [CrossRef] [PubMed]
31. Liu, X. Microbiome. *Yale J. Biol. Med.* **2016**, *89*, 275–276.
32. Lederberg, J. Ome Sweet'Omics—A Genealogical Treasury of Words. *Scientist* **2001**, *15*, 8.
33. Shaik, L.; Kashyap, R.; Thotamgari, S.R.; Singh, R.; Khanna, S. Gut-Brain Axis and its Neuro-Psychiatric Effects: A Narrative Review. *Cureus* **2020**, *12*, e11131. [CrossRef] [PubMed]
34. Martin, C.R.; Osadchiy, V.; Kalani, A.; Mayer, E.A. The Brain-Gut-Microbiome Axis. *Cell. Mol. Gastroenterol. Hepatol.* **2018**, *6*, 133–148. [CrossRef] [PubMed]
35. Carabotti, M.; Scirocco, A.; Maselli, M.A.; Severi, C. The gut-brain axis: Interactions between enteric microbiota, central and enteric nervous systems. *Ann. Gastroenterol.* **2015**, *28*, 203–209. [PubMed]
36. Cryan, J.F.; O'Riordan, K.J.; Cowan, C.S.M.; Sandhu, K.V.; Bastiaanssen, T.F.S.; Boehme, M.; Codagnone, M.G.; Cussotto, S.; Fulling, C.; Golubeva, A.V.; et al. The Microbiota-Gut-Brain Axis. *Physiol. Rev.* **2019**, *99*, 1877–2013. [CrossRef] [PubMed]
37. Rutsch, A.; Kantsjo, J.B. Ronchi, F. The Gut-Brain Axis: How microbiota and host inflammasome influence brain physiology and pathology. *Front. Immunol.* **2020**, *11*, 604179. [CrossRef]
38. Follesa, P.; Biggio, F.; Gorini, G.; Caria, S.; Talani, G.; Dazzi, L.; Puligheddu, M.; Marrosu, F.; Biggio, G. Vagus nerve stimulation increases norepinephrine concentration and the gene expression of BDNF and bFGF in the rat brain. *Brain Res.* **2007**, *1179*, 28–34. [CrossRef]
39. Ozogul, F.; Ozogul, Y. The ability of biogenic amines and ammonia production by single bacterial cultures. *Eur. Food Res. Technol.* **2007**, *225*, 385–394. [CrossRef]
40. Pokusaeva, K.; Johnson, C.; Luk, B.; Uribe, G.; Fu, Y.; Oezguen, N.; Matsunami, R.K.; Lugo, M.; Major, A.; Mori-Akiyama, Y.; et al. GABA-producing Bifidobacterium dentium modulates visceral sensitivity in the intestine. *Neurogastroenterol. Motil.* **2017**, *29*, e12904. [CrossRef] [PubMed]
41. Cattaneo, A.; Cattane, N.; Galluzzi, S.; Provasi, S.; Lopizzo, N.; Festari, C.; Ferrari, C.; Guerra, U.P.; Paghera, B.; Muscio, C.; et al. Association of brain amyloidosis with pro-inflammatory gut bacterial taxa and peripheral inflammation markers in cognitively impaired elderly. *Neurobiol. Aging* **2017**, *49*, 60–68. [CrossRef] [PubMed]
42. Devos, D.; Lebouvier, T.; Lardeux, B.; Biraud, M.; Rouaud, T.; Pouclet, H.; Coron, E.; des Varannes, S.B.; Naveilhan, P.; Nguyen, J.M.; et al. Colonic inflammation in Parkinson's disease. *Neurobiol. Dis.* **2013**, *50*, 42–48. [CrossRef] [PubMed]
43. Scheperjans, F.; Aho, V.; Pereira, P.A.; Koskinen, K.; Paulin, L.; Pekkonen, E.; Haapaniemi, E.; Kaakkola, S.; Eerola-Rautio, J.; Pohja, M.; et al. Gut microbiota are related to Parkinson's disease and clinical phenotype. *Mov. Disord.* **2015**, *30*, 350–358. [CrossRef] [PubMed]
44. Wu, S.; Yi, J.; Zhang, Y.G.; Zhou, J.; Sun, J. Leaky intestine and impaired microbiome in an amyotrophic lateral sclerosis mouse model. *Physiol. Rep.* **2015**, *3*, e12356. [CrossRef]
45. Morita, H.; Obata, K.; Abe, C.; Shiba, D.; Shirakawa, M.; Kudo, T.; Takahashi, S. Feasibility of a Short-Arm Centrifuge for Mouse Hypergravity Experiments. *PLoS ONE* **2015**, *10*, e0133981. [CrossRef] [PubMed]
46. Borgo, F.; Riva, A.; Benetti, A.; Casiraghi, M.C.; Bertelli, S.; Garbossa, S.; Anselmetti, S.; Scarone, S.; Pontiroli, A.E.; Morace, G.; et al. Microbiota in anorexia nervosa: The triangle between bacterial species, metabolites and psychological tests. *PLoS ONE* **2017**, *12*, e0179739. [CrossRef]

47. Obrenovich, M.; Jaworski, H.; Tadimalla, T.; Mistry, A.; Sykes, L.; Perry, G.; Bonomo, R.A. The Role of the Microbiota-Gut-Brain Axis and Antibiotics in ALS and Neurodegenerative Diseases. *Microorganisms* **2020**, *8*, 784. [CrossRef]
48. Guglielmo, B.J. Metronidazole neurotoxicity: Suspicions confirmed. *Clin. Infect. Dis.* **2021**, *72*, 2101–2102. [CrossRef]
49. Xioa, M.; Huang, X. Unmasking antibiotic-associated neurological disorders: The underminer in Intensive Care Unit. *J. Clin. Neurosci.* **2021**, *91*, 131–135. [CrossRef]
50. Zareifopoulos, N.; Panayiotakopoulos, G. Neuropsychiatric Effects of Antimicrobial Agents. *Clin. Drug Investig.* **2017**, *37*, 423–437. [CrossRef]
51. Tango, R.C. Psychiatric side effects of medications prescribed in internal medicine. *Dialogues Clin. Neurosci.* **2003**, *5*, 155–165.
52. Puri, V. Metronidazole neurotoxicity. *Neurol. India* **2011**, *59*, 4–5. [CrossRef]
53. Goolsby, T.A.; Jakeman, B.; Gaynes, R.P. Clinical relevance of metronidazole and peripheral neuropathy: A systematic review of the literature. *Int. J. Antimicrob. Agents* **2018**, *51*, 319–325. [CrossRef]
54. Hobbs, K.; Stern-Nezer, S.; Buckwalter, M.S.; Fischbein, N.; Caulfield, A.F. Metronidazole-induced encephalopathy: Not always a reversible situation. *Neurocrit. Care* **2015**, *22*, 429–436. [CrossRef]
55. Park, K.I.; Chung, J.M.; Kim, J.Y. Metronidazole neurotoxicity: Sequential neuroaxis involvement. *Neurol. India* **2011**, *59*, 104–107. [CrossRef]
56. Knorr, J.P.; Javed, I.; Sahni, N.; Cankurtaran, C.Z.; Ortiz, J.A. Metronidazole-induced encephalopathy in a patient with end-stage liver disease. *Case Rep. Hepatol.* **2012**, *2012*, 209258. [CrossRef]
57. Yamamoto, T.; Abe, K.; Anjiki, H.; Ishii, T.; Kuyama, Y. Metronidazole-induced neurotoxicity developed in liver cirrhosis. *J. Clin. Med. Res.* **2012**, *4*, 295–298. [CrossRef]
58. Roy, U.; Panwar, A.; Pandit, A.; Das, S.K.; Joshi, B. Clinical and Neuroradiological Spectrum of Metronidazole Induced Encephalopathy: Our Experience and the Review of Literature. *J. Clin. Diagn. Res.* **2016**, *10*, OE01–OE09. [CrossRef]
59. Evans, J.; Levesque, D.; Knowles, K.; Longshore, R.; Plummer, S. Diazepam as a treatment for metronidazole toxicosis in dogs: A retrospective study of 21 cases. *J. Vet. Intern. Med.* **2003**, *17*, 304–310. [CrossRef]
60. Mattappalil, A.; Mergenhagen, K.A. Neurotoxicity with antimicrobials in the elderly: A review. *Clin. Ther.* **2014**, *11*, 1489–1511. [CrossRef] [PubMed]
61. Little, S. Nervous and mental effects of the sulphonamides. *JAMA* **1942**, *119*, 467–474. [CrossRef]
62. Walker, L.E.; Thomas, S.; McBride, C.; Howse, M.; Turtle, L.C.W.; Vivancos, R.; Beeching, N.J.; Beadsworth, M.B.J. 'Septrin psychosis' among renal transplant patients with *Pneumocystis jirovecii* pneumonia. *J. Antimicrob. Chemother.* **2011**, *66*, 1117–1119. [CrossRef]
63. Lee, K.Y.; Huang, C.H.; Tang, H.J.; Yang, C.J.; Ko, W.C.; Chen, Y.H.; Lee, Y.C.; Hung, C.C. Acute psychosis related to use of trimethoprim/sulfamethoxazole in the treatment of HIV-infected patients with Pneumocystis jirovecii pneumonia: A multicentre, retrospective study. *J. Antimicrob. Chemother.* **2012**, *67*, 2749–2754. [CrossRef]
64. Patey, O.; Lacheheb, A.; Dellion, S.; Zanditenas, D.; Jungfer-Bouvier, F.; Lafaix, C. A rare case of cotrimoxazole-induced eosinophilic aseptic meningitis in an HIV-infected patient. *Scand. J. Infect. Dis.* **1998**, *30*, 530–531.
65. Patterson, R.G.; Couchenour, R.L. Trimethoprim-sulfamethoxazole-induced tremor in an immunocompetent patients. *Pharmacotherapy* **1999**, *19*, 1456–1458. [CrossRef]
66. Haruki, H.; Hovius, R.; Pedersen, M.G.; Johnsson, K. Tetrahydrobiopterin Biosynthesis as a Potential Target of the Kynurenine Pathway Metabolite Xanthurenic Acid. *J. Biol. Chem.* **2016**, *291*, 652–657. [CrossRef]
67. Sekhar, R.V.; Patel, S.G.; Guthikonda, A.P.; Reid, M.; Balasubramanyam, A.; Taffet, G.E.; Jahoor, F. Deficient synthesis of glutathione underlies oxidative stress in aging and can be corrected by dietary cysteine and glycine supplementation. *Am. J. Clin. Nutr.* **2011**, *94*, 847–853. [CrossRef]
68. Stuhec, M. Trimethoprim-sulfamethoxazole-related hallucinations. *Gen. Hosp. Psychiatry* **2014**, *36*, 230.e7–230.e8. [CrossRef]
69. Karpman, E.; Kurzrock, E.A. Adverse reactions of nitrofurantoin, trimethoprim and sulfamethoxazole in children. *J. Urol.* **2004**, *172*, 448–453. [CrossRef]
70. Kathait, J.; Rawat, A.S. Beta-lactam antibiotics induced neurotoxicity. *IOSR J. Pharm.* **2020**, *10*, 1–7.
71. Deshayes, S.; Coquerel, A.; Verdon, R. Neurological Adverse Effects Attributable to β-Lactam Antibiotics: A Literature Review. *Drug Saf.* **2017**, *40*, 1171–1198. [CrossRef]
72. Warstler, A.; Bean, J. Antimicrobial-induced cognitive side effects. *Ment. Health Clin.* **2016**, *6*, 207–214. [CrossRef]
73. Ilechukwu, S.T. Acute psychotic reactions and stress response syndromes following intramuscular aqueous procaine penicillin. *Br. J. Psychiatry* **1990**, *156*, 554–559. [CrossRef]
74. Cummings, J.L.; Barritt, C.F.; Horan, M. Delusions induced by procaine penicillin: Case report and review of the syndrome. *Int. J. Psychiatry Med.* **1987**, *16*, 163–168. [CrossRef] [PubMed]
75. Araskiewicz, A.; Rybakowski, J.K. Hoigné's syndrome: A procaine-induced limbic kindling. *Med. Hypotheses* **1994**, *42*, 261–264. [CrossRef]
76. Lin, C.S.; Cheng, C.J.; Chou, C.H.; Lin, S.H. Piperacillin/tazobactam-induced seizure rapidly reversed by high flux hemodialysis in a patient on peritoneal dialysis. *Am. J. Med. Sci.* **2007**, *333*, 181–184. [CrossRef]
77. Huang, W.T.; Hsu, Y.J.; Chu, P.L.; Lin, S.H. Neurotoxicity associated with standard doses of piperacillin in an elderly patient with renal failure. *Infection* **2009**, *37*, 374–376. [CrossRef]

78. Shaffer, C.L.; Davey, A.M.; Ransom, J.L.; Brown, Y.L.; Gal, P. Ampicillin-induced neurotoxicity in very-low-birth-weight neonates. *Ann. Pharmacother.* **1998**, *32*, 482–484. [CrossRef]
79. Schliamser, S.E.; Cars, O.; Norrby, S.R. Neurotoxicity of beta-lactam antibiotics: Predisposing factors and pathogenesis. *J. Antimicrob. Chemother.* **1991**, *27*, 405–425. [CrossRef] [PubMed]
80. Grill, M.F.; Maganti, R. Cephalosporin-induced neurotoxicity: Clinical manifestations, potential pathogenic mechanisms, and the role of electroencephalographic monitoring. *Ann. Pharmacother.* **2008**, *42*, 1843–1850. [CrossRef]
81. Lacroix, C.; Bera-Jonville, A.P. Serious neurological adverse events of ceftriaxone. *Antibiotics* **2021**, *10*, 540. [CrossRef]
82. Zhanel, G.G.; Wiebe, R.; Dilay, L.; Thomson, K.; Rubinstein, E.; Hoban, D.J.; Noreddin, A.M.; Karlowsky, J.A. Comparative review of the carbapenems. *Drugs* **2007**, *67*, 1027–1052. [CrossRef]
83. Chastre, J.; Wunderink, R.; Prokocimer, P.; Lee, M.; Kaniga, K.; Friedland, I. Efficacy and safety of intravenous infusion of doripenem versus imipenem in ventilator-associated pneumonia: A multicenter, randomized study. *Crit. Care Med.* **2008**, *36*, 1089–1096. [CrossRef] [PubMed]
84. Chow, K.M.; Hui, A.C.; Szeto, C.C. Neurotoxicity induced by beta-lactam antibiotics: From bench to bedside. *Eur. J. Clin. Microbiol. Infect. Dis.* **2005**, *24*, 649–653. [CrossRef] [PubMed]
85. Wallace, K.L. Antibiotic-induced convulsions. *Crit. Care Clin.* **1997**, *13*, 741–762. [CrossRef]
86. Miller, A.D.; Ball, A.M.; Bookstaver, P.B.; Dornblaser, E.K.; Bennett, C.L. Epileptogenic potential of carbapenem agents: Mechanism of action, seizure rates, and clinical considerations. *Pharmacotherapy* **2011**, *31*, 408–423. [CrossRef] [PubMed]
87. Alkharfy, K.M.; Kellum, J.A.; Frye, R.F.; Matzke, G.R. Effect of ceftazidime on systemic cytokine concentrations in rats. *Antimicrob. Agents Chemother.* **2000**, *44*, 3217–3319. [CrossRef]
88. Koppel, B.S.; Hauser, W.A.; Politis, C.; Van Duin, D.; Daras, M. Seizures in the Critically Ill: The Role of Imipenem. *Epilepsia* **2001**, *42*, 1590–1593. [CrossRef] [PubMed]
89. Altissimi, G.; Colizza, A.; Cianfrone, G.; De Vincentiis, M.; Greco, A.; Taurone, S.; Musacchio, A.; Ciofalo, A.; Turchetta, R.; Angeletti, D.; et al. Drugs inducing hearing loss, tinnitus, dizziness and vertigo: An updated guide. *Eur. Rev. Med. Pharmacol. Sci.* **2020**, *24*, 7946–7952.
90. Huang, V.; Clayton, N.A.; Welker, H. Glycopeptide hypersensitivity and adverse reactions. *Pharmacy* **2020**, *8*, 70. [CrossRef]
91. Bruniera, F.R.; Ferreira, F.M.; Saviolli, L.R.M.; Bacci, M.R.; Feder, D.; Da Luz Goncalves Pedreira, M.; Peterlini, M.A.S.; Azzalis, L.A.; Junqueira, V.B.C.; Fonseca, F.L.A. The use of vancomycin with its therapeutic and adverse effects: A review. *Eur. Rev. Med. Pharmacol. Sci.* **2015**, *19*, 694–700.
92. Finch, R.G.; Eliopoulos, G.M. Safety and efficacy of glycopeptide antibiotics. *J. Antimicrob. Chemother.* **2005**, *55* (Suppl. S2), ii5–ii13. [CrossRef] [PubMed]
93. Ye, Q.-F.; Wang, G.-F.; Wang, Y.-X.; Lu, G.-P.; Li, Z.-P. Vancomycin-related convulsion in a pediatric patient with neuroblastoma: A case report and review of the literature. *World J. Clin. Cases* **2021**, *6*, 3070–3078. [CrossRef] [PubMed]
94. Marissen, J.; Fortmann, I.; Humberg, A.; Rausch, T.K.; Simon, A.; Stein, A.; Schaible, T.; Eichorn, J.; Wintgens, J.; Roll, C.; et al. Vancomycin-induced ototoxicity in very-low-birthweight infants. *J. Antimicrob. Chemother.* **2020**, *75*, 2291–2298. [CrossRef]
95. Simonetti, O.; Rizzetto, G.; Molinelli, E.; Cirioni, O.; Offidani, A. Review: A safety profile of dalbavancin for on- and off-label utilization. *Ther. Clin. Risk Manag.* **2021**, *17*, 223–232. [CrossRef] [PubMed]
96. Townsend, M.L.; Wilson, D.; Pound, M.; Drew, R. Emerging treatment options for complicated skin and skin structure infections: Oritavancin. *Clin. Med. Insight Ther.* **2010**, *2*, 25–35. [CrossRef]
97. Ma, T.K.-W.; Chow, K.-M.; Choy, A.S.M.; Kwan, B.C.-H.; Szeto, C.-C.; Li, P.K.-T. Clinical manifestation of macrolide antibiotic toxicity in CKD and dialysis patients. *Clin. Kidney J.* **2014**, *7*, 507–512. [CrossRef] [PubMed]
98. Essali, N.; Miller, B.J. Psychosis as an adverse effect of antibiotics. *Brain Behav. Immun.-Health* **2020**, *9*, 100148. [CrossRef]
99. Wanleenuwat, P.; Suntharamppillai, N.; Iwanowski, P. Antibiotic-induced epileptic seizures: Mechanisms of action and clinical considerations. *Europ. J. Epilep.* **2020**, *81*, 167–174. [CrossRef]
100. Vanoverschelde, A.; Oosterloo, B.C.; Ly, N.F.; Ikram, M.A.; Goedegebure, A.; Stricker, B.H.; Lahousse, L. Macrolide-associated ototoxicity: A cross-sectional and longitudinal study to assess the association of macrolide use with tinnitus and hearing loss. *J. Antimicrob. Chemother.* **2021**, *76*, 2708–2716. [CrossRef]
101. Chow, K.M.; Szeto, C.C.; Hui, A.C.-F.; Li, P.K.-T. Mechanisms of antibiotic neurotoxicity in renal failure. *Intern. J. Antimicrob. Agents* **2004**, *23*, 213–217. [CrossRef]
102. Steyger, P.S. Mechanisms of aminoglycoside- and cisplatin-induced ototoxicity. *Am. J. Audiol.* **2021**, *30*, 887–900. [CrossRef] [PubMed]
103. Jaspard, M.; Butel, N.; Helali, N.E.; Marigot-Outtandy, D.; Guillot, H.; Peytavin, G.; Veziris, N.; Bodaghi, B.; Flandre, P.; Petitjean, G.; et al. Linezolid-ass0ciated neurologic adverse events in patients with multidrug-resistant tuberculosis, France. *Emerg. Infect. Dis.* **2020**, *26*, 1792–1800. [CrossRef]
104. Bhattacharyya, S.; Darby, R.; Berkowitz, A.L. Antibiotic-induced neurotoxicity. *Curr. Infect. Dis. Rep.* **2014**, *16*, 448. [CrossRef]
105. Spapen, H.; Jacobs, R.; Van Gorp, V.; Troubleyn, J.; Honore, P.M. Renal and neurological side effects of colistin in critically ill patients. *Ann. Intensive Care.* **2011**, *1*, 14. [CrossRef] [PubMed]
106. Camargo, C.; Narula, T.; Jackson, D.A.; Padro, T.; Freeman, W.D. Colistin neurotoxicity mimicking Guillan-Barre syndrome in a patient with cystic fibrosis: Case report and review. *Oxf. Med. Case Rep.* **2021**, *9*, 340–344.
107. Thu, D.M.; Ziora, Z.M.; Blaskovich, M.A.T. Quinolone antibiotics. *Med. Chem. Commun.* **2019**, *10*, 1719–1739.

108. Scavone, C.; Mascolo, A.; Ruggiero, R.; Sportiello, L.; Rafaniello, C.; Berrino, L.; Capuano, A. Quinolones-induced mesculoskeletal, neurological, and psychiatric ADRs: A pharmacovigilance study based on data from the Italian Spontaneous Reporting System. *Front. Pharmacol.* **2020**, *11*, 428. [CrossRef]
109. Al-Ghamdi, S.M.G. Reversible encephalopathy and delirium in patients with chronic renal failure who had received ciprofloxacin. *Saudi J. Kidney Dis. Transplant.* **2002**, *13*, 164–170.
110. Nishikubo, M.; Kanamori, M.; Nishioka, H. Levofloxacin-associated neurotoxicity in a patient with a high concentration of levofloxacin in the blood and cerebrospinal fluid. *Antibiotics* **2019**, *8*, 78. [CrossRef] [PubMed]
111. Novelli, A.; Rosi, E. Pharmacological properties of oral antibiotics for the treatment of uncomplicated urinary tract infections. *J. Chem.* **2017**, *29*, 10–18. [CrossRef] [PubMed]
112. Lu, P.G.; Kung, N.H.; Van Stavern, G.P. Ethambutol optic neuropathy associated with enhancement at the optic chiasm. *Can. J. Ophthalmol.* **2017**, *52*, e178–e181. [CrossRef]
113. Heffernan, A.J.; Sime, F.B.; Taccone, F.S.; Roberts, J.A. How to optimize antibiotic pharmacokinetic/pharmacodynamics for Gram-negative infectionsin critically ill patients. *Curr. Opin. Infect. Dis.* **2018**, *31*, 555–565. [CrossRef]
114. Duszynska, W.; Taccone, F.S.; Hurkacz, M.; Kowalska-Krochmal, B.; Wiela-Hojeńska, A.; Kübler, A. Therapeutic drug monitoring of amikacin in septic patients. *Crit. Care* **2013**, *25*, 17. [CrossRef]
115. Matusik, E.; Lambiotte, F.; Tone, A.; Lemitir, R. Pharmacokinetic modifications and pharmacokinetic/pharmacodynamic optimization of beta-lactams in ICU. *Ann. Pharm. Fr.* **2021**, *1*, 346–360. [CrossRef]
116. Duszynska, W.; Taccone, F.S.; Hurkacz, M.; Wiela-Hojenska, A.; Kübler, A. Continous vs. intermittent vancomycin therapy for Gram-positive infections not caused by methicillin-resistant Staphylococcus aureus. *Minerva Anestesiol.* **2016**, *82*, 284–293.
117. Duszynska, W.; Taccone, F.S.; Switala, M.; Hurkacz, M.; Kowalska-Krochmal, B.; Kübler, A. Continous infusion of piperacillin/tazobactam in ventilator-associated pneumonia: A pilot study on efficacy and costs. *Int. J. Antimicrob. Agents* **2012**, *39*, 153–158. [CrossRef]
118. Abdul-Aziz, M.H.; Alffenaar, J.W.C.; Bassetti, M.; Bracht, H.; Dimopoulos, G.; Marriott, D.; Neely, M.N.; Paiva, J.A.; Pea, F.; Sjovall, F.; et al. Antimicrobial therapeutic drug monitoring in critically ill adult patient: A position paper. *Intensive Care Med.* **2020**, *46*, 1127–1153. [CrossRef] [PubMed]
119. De Velde, F.; Mouton, J.W.; de Winter, B.C.M.; van Gelder, T.; Koch, B.C.P. Clinical applications of population pharmacokinetic models of antibiotics: Challenges and perspectives. *Pharmacol. Res.* **2018**, *134*, 280–288. [CrossRef] [PubMed]
120. Eyler, R.F.; Shvets, K. Clinical pharmacology of antibiotics. *Clin. Pharmacol. Anibiot.* **2019**, *14*, 1080–1090. [CrossRef]
121. Cotta, M.O.; Roberts, J.A.; Lipman, J. Antibiotic dose optimization in critically ill patients. *Med. Intensiva* **2015**, *39*, 563–572. [CrossRef] [PubMed]
122. Buclin, T.; Thoma, Y.; Widmer, N.; Andre, P.; Guidi, M.; Csajka, C.; Decosterd, L.A. The steps to therapeutic drug monitoring: A structured approach illustrated with imatinib. *Front. Pharmacol.* **2020**, *11*, 177. [CrossRef]
123. Ates, H.C.; Roberts, J.A.; Lipman, J.; Cass, A.E.G.; Urban, G.A.; Dincer, C. On-site therapeutic drug monitoring. *Trends Biotechnol.* **2020**, *38*, 1262–1277. [CrossRef] [PubMed]
124. Imani, S.; Buschler, H.; Marriott, D.; Gentili, S.; Sandaradura, I. Too much of a good thing: A retrospective study of β-lactam concentration=toxicity relationships. *J. Antimicrob. Chemother.* **2017**, *1*, 2891–2897. [CrossRef]
125. Oda, K.; Miyakawa, T.; Katanoda, T.; Hishiguchi, Y.; Iwamura, K.; Nosaka, K.; Yamaguchi, A.; Jono, H.; Saito, H. A case of recovery from aphasia following dose reduction of cefepime by Bayesian prediction-based therapeutic drug monitoring. *J. Infect. Chemother.* **2020**, *26*, 498–501. [CrossRef]
126. Smith, N.L.; Freebairn, R.C.; Park, M.A.; Wallis, S.C.; Roberts, J.A.; Lipman, J. Therapeutic drug monitoring when using cefepime in continuous renal replacement therapy: Seizures associated with cefepime. *Crit. Care Resusc.* **2012**, *14*, 312–315. [PubMed]
127. Barreto, E.F.; Webb, A.J.; Pais, G.M.; Rule, A.D.; Jannetto, P.J.; Scheetz, M.H. Setting the beta-lactam therapeutic range for critically ill patients: Is there a floor or even a ceiling? *Crit. Care Explor.* **2021**, *11*, e04466. [CrossRef] [PubMed]
128. Quinton, M.C.; Bodeau, S.; Kontar, L.; Zerbib, Y.; Maizel, J.; Slama, M.; Masmoudi, K.; Lamaire-Hurtel, A.S.; Bebnnis, Y. Neurotoxix concentration of piperacillin during continuous infusion in critically ill patients. *Antimicrob. Agents Chemother.* **2017**, *24*, e.00654-17.
129. Gatti, M.; Cojutti, P.G.; Campoli, C.; Caramelli, F.; Corvaglia, L.T.; Lanari, M.; Pession, A.; Ramirez, S.; Viale, P.; Pea, F. A proof of concept of the role of TDM-based clinical pharmacological advices in optimizing antimicrobial therapy on real-time in different paediatric settings. *Front. Pharmacol.* **2021**, *12*, 755075. [CrossRef] [PubMed]
130. Rawson, T.M.; Wilson, R.C.; O'Hare, D.; Herrero, P.; Kambugu, A.; Lamorde, M.; Ellington, M.; Georgiou, P.; Cass, A.; Hope, W.H.; et al. Optimizing antimicrobial use: Challenges, advances and opportunities. *Nat. Rev. Microbiol.* **2021**, *19*, 747–758. [CrossRef]
131. As-Morey, P.; Ballesteros-Fernandez, A.; Sanmartin-Mestre, E.; Valle, M. Impact of clinical pharmacist intervention on antimicrobial use in a small 164-bed hospital. *Eur. J. Hosp. Pharm.* **2018**, *25*, e46–e51. [CrossRef]
132. Weller, T.M.A.; Jamieson, C.E. The expanding role of the antibiotic pharmacist. *J. Antimicrob. Chemother.* **2004**, *54*, 295–298. [CrossRef]
133. Salman, B.; Al-Hashar, A.; Al-Khirbash, A.; Al-zakwani, I. Clinical and cost implications of clinical pharmacist interventions on antimicrobial use at Sultan Qabooos University Hospital in Oman. *Int. J. Infect. Dis.* **2021**, *109*, 137–141. [CrossRef]

134. Zhang, J.; Li, X.; He, R.; Zheng, W.; Kwong, J.S.; Lu, L.; Lv, T.; Huang, R.; He, M.; Li, X.; et al. The effectiveness of clinical pharmacist-led consultation in the treatment of infectious diseases: A prospective, multicenter, cohort study. *Front. Pharmacol.* **2020**, *11*, 575022. [CrossRef] [PubMed]
135. Hamada, Y.; Ebihara, F.; Kikuchi, K. A strategy for hospital pharmacists to control antimicrobial resistance (AMR) In Japan. *Antibiotics* **2021**, *10*, 1284. [CrossRef] [PubMed]
136. Balducci, C.; Forioni, G. Doxycline for Alzheimer's disease: Fighting β-amyloid oligomers and neuroinflammation. *Front. Pharmacol.* **2019**, *10*, 738. [CrossRef] [PubMed]
137. Yimer, E.M.; Hishe, H.Z.; Tuem, K.B. Repurposing of the β-lactam antibiotic, ceftriaxone for neurological disorders: A review. *Front. Neurosci.* **2019**, *13*, 236. [CrossRef]
138. Danielewski, M.; Ksiądzyna, D.; Szeląg, A. Non-antibiotic use of antibiotics. *Post Mikrobiol.* **2018**, *57*, 301–312. [CrossRef]
139. Cankaya, S.; Cankaya, B.; Kilic, U.; Kilic, E.; Yulug, B. The therapeutic role of minocycline in Parkinson's disease. *Drugs Context* **2019**, *8*, 212553. [CrossRef] [PubMed]
140. Yulug, B.; Hanoglu, L.; Ozansoy, M.; Isik, D.; Kilic, U.; Kilic, E.; Schabitz, W.R. Therapeutic role of rifampicin in Alzheimer's disease. *Psychiatry Clin. Neurosci.* **2018**, *72*, 152–159. [CrossRef]
141. Fogel, D.B. Factors associated with clinical trials that fail and opportunities for improving the likelihood of success: A review. *Contemp. Clin. Trials Commun.* **2018**, *11*, 156–164. [CrossRef]
142. Nowak, D.; Słupski, W.; Rutkowska, M. New therapeutic strategies for Alzheimer's disease. *Adv. Hyg. Exp. Med.* **2021**, *75*, 474–490. [CrossRef]

molecules

MDPI

Review

Neuroprotective Effect of SGLT2 Inhibitors

Agnieszka Pawlos, Marlena Broncel *, Ewelina Woźniak and Paulina Gorzelak-Pabiś

Laboratory of Tissue Immunopharmacology, Department of Internal Diseases and Clinical Pharmacology, Medical University of Lodz, Kniaziewicza 1/5, 91-347 Lodz, Poland; agnieszka.sanetra@stud.umed.lodz.pl (A.P.); ewelina.wozniak@umed.lodz.pl (E.W.); paulina.gorzelak-pabis@umed.lodz.pl (P.G.-P.)

* Correspondence: marlena.broncel@umed.lodz.pl; Tel.: +48-42251-60-03

Abstract: Patients with diabetes are at higher risk of cardiovascular diseases and cognitive impairment. SGLT2 inhibitors (Empagliflozin, Canagliflozin, Dapagliflozin, Ertugliflozin, Sotagliflozin) are newer hypoglycemic agents with many pleiotropic effects. In this review, we discuss their neuroprotective potential. SGLT2 inhibitors (SGLT2i) are lipid-soluble and reach the brain/serum ratio from 0.3 to 0.5. SGLT receptors are present in the central nervous system (CNS). Flozins are not fully SGLT2-selective and have an affinity for the SGLT1 receptor, which is associated with protection against ischemia/reperfusion brain damage. SGLT2i show an anti-inflammatory and anti-atherosclerotic effect, including reduction of proinflammatory cytokines, M2 macrophage polarization, JAK2/STAT1 and NLRP3 inflammasome inhibition, as well as cIMT regression. They also mitigate oxidative stress. SGLT2i improve endothelial function, prevent remodeling and exert a protective effect on the neurovascular unit, blood-brain barrier, pericytes, astrocytes, microglia, and oligodendrocytes. Flozins are also able to inhibit AChE, which contributes to cognitive improvement. Empagliflozin significantly increases the level of cerebral BDNF, which modulates neurotransmission and ensures growth, survival, and plasticity of neurons. Moreover, they may be able to restore the circadian rhythm of mTOR activation, which is quite a novel finding in the field of research on metabolic diseases and cognitive impairment. SGLT2i have a great potential to protect against atherosclerosis and cognitive impairment in patients with type 2 diabetes mellitus.

Keywords: SGLT2i; sodium-glucose cotransporter 2 inhibitors; neuroprotection; atheroprotection; mTOR; type 2 diabetes mellitus; cognitive impairment; inflammation; oxidative stress

Citation: Pawlos, A.; Broncel, M.; Woźniak, E.; Gorzelak-Pabiś, P. Neuroprotective Effect of SGLT2 Inhibitors. *Molecules* **2021**, *26*, 7213. https://doi.org/10.3390/molecules26237213

Academic Editors: Alicja Nowaczyk and Grzegorz Grześk

Received: 3 November 2021
Accepted: 26 November 2021
Published: 28 November 2021

1. Introduction

Type 2 diabetes mellitus (T2DM) is a chronic metabolic disease causing a variety of complications, including atherosclerosis which is associated with increased cardiovascular risk contributing to reduced life expectancy [1]. Additionally, atherosclerosis is an important factor leading to cognitive impairment in the elderly via several mechanisms such as ischemia and a direct molecular link [2,3]. Diabetes mellitus type 2 accelerates the development of atherosclerosis, and patients with T2DM are at a two to four times higher risk of developing vascular diseases than non-diabetics [4]. There is a lot of evidence that proves that diabetic patients are at an increased risk of developing cognitive impairment. Glucose metabolism is also impaired in Alzheimer's disease, as it is sometimes called 'Type 3 diabetes' or 'diabetes of the brain' [5]. According to a meta-analysis performed by Zhang J. et al., patients with diabetes mellitus type 2 have a 53% higher relative risk of Alzheimer's disease than non-diabetic individuals (RR 1.53, 95% CI: 1.42–1.63) [6]. Among diabetics, the presence of micro- and macrovascular complications increases the risk of cognitive decline even further, suggesting that vascular mechanisms, including atherosclerosis, are important players [7]. As diabetic patients with atherosclerosis are especially vulnerable to cognitive impairment, it is necessary to search for drugs that could ensure T2DM control, reduce cardiovascular risk and improve cognitive functions.

SGLT2 inhibitors are newer hypoglycemic drugs that have revolutionized the clinical approach to T2DM management. Their main mechanism of action is inhibiting SGLT2 receptors in the proximal tubules of the kidneys and thus lowering blood glucose levels by blocking its reabsorption from the urine [8]. As it has been proved by large double-blind clinical trials, Empagliflozin not only decreases HbA1c in diabetic patients but also improves their life expectancy by reducing cardiovascular mortality [9]. Canagliflozin, Dapagliflozin, Sotagliflozin significantly decrease the composed primary end-point, including cardiovascular mortality and other cardiovascular outcomes [10–12]. Ertugliflozin showed non-inferiority vs. placebo in reducing cardiovascular mortality and other cardiovascular outcomes [13]. The exact mechanism has not been fully established yet, and SGLT2 inhibitors show many additional beneficial effects which contribute to their wider use, even in non-diabetic patients [14]. There is growing evidence that SGLT2 inhibitors have a neuroprotective potential, as in a murine mixed model of diabetes mellitus and Alzheimer's disease, empagliflozin improved both cerebral microvascular and cognitive impairment [15]. There is no available data on the adverse effects flozins may exert on the Central Nervous System. The most commonly known side effects are genitourinary infections; however, rare but more serious effects also may occur, like euglycemic ketoacidosis [16]. In this review, we are focusing on SGLT2 inhibitors' potential to improve the impaired cognitive functions of diabetic patients with atherosclerosis.

2. Neurological Potential of SGLT2 Inhibitors

SGLT2 inhibitors are lipid-soluble and cross the blood-brain barrier reaching the brain-to-serum ratio of the areas under the curves from 0.3 (Canagliflozin and Dapagliflozin) up to 0.5 (Empagliflozin) [17]. They have the ability to directly affect their target, since SGLT1 and SGLT2 co-receptors are expressed in the human central nervous system and play an important role in maintaining glucose homeostasis. SGLTs are responsible for the transport of glucose, galactose and sodium ions against the concentration gradients [18]. SGLT1 transports two Na+ ions with one D-glucose molecule and SGLT2 one sodium ion with one D-glucose [19]. They may be found in many areas of the central nervous system in several isoforms. SGLT1 inhibitors are present in the pyramidal cells of the brain cortex, Purkinje cerebellum cells, hippocampus pyramidal, and granular cells [20]. They were also detectable in glial cells in the ventromedial hypothalamus [21]. Brain expression of SGLT2 is lower than SGLT1, and it occurs mainly in the microvessels of the blood-brain barrier, but also in the amygdala, hypothalamus, periaqueductal gray (PAG), and in the dorsomedial medulla – the nucleus of the solitary tract (NTS) [22,23]. The presence of SGLT1/SGLT2 was also described in the abluminal membrane of the capillary endothelium [21]. Interestingly, the brain locations where SGLTs are present have been proven to be responsible for learning processes, food intake, energy and glucose homeostasis, and central cardiovascular and autonomic regulation [23,24]. The location of SGLT1 and SGLT2 receptors in the CNS is presented in Figure 1. It is possible that SGLT2 receptors also exert a cardioprotective effect through central mechanisms by directly influencing cardiovascular regulation and autonomic pathways, including the paraventricular nucleus of the hypothalamus, the nucleus of the solitary tract, and the periaqueductal gray [23]. An immunoblotting study of post-mortem human brain tissue showed a significant increase in SGLT1 and SGLT2 expression following brain injury [25]. Results of a study performed in a murine model suggest that, after a brain injury, SGLT1 blockage may bring beneficial effects with regard to the area of the brain lesions, the volume of damaged tissue, edema, and motoric disability [26].

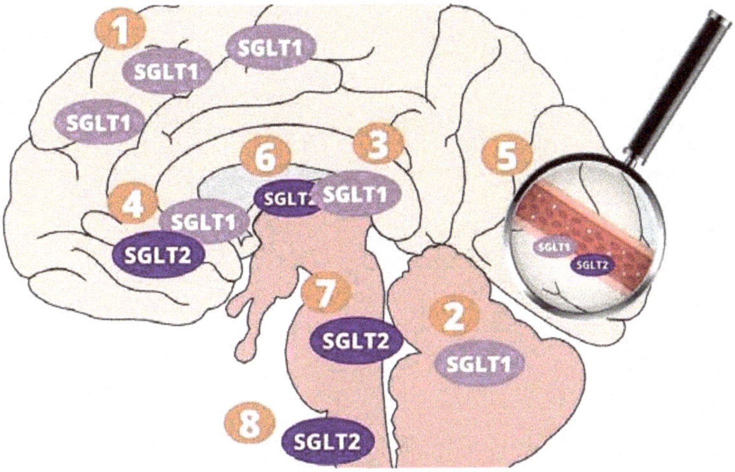

Figure 1. Distribution of SGLT1 and SGLT2 receptors in the Central Nervous System: 1. Pyramidal cells of brain cortex; 2. Purkinje cerebellum cells; 3. Hippocampus pyramidal and granular cells; 4. Hypothalamus; 5. Microvessels; 6. Amygdala; 7. Periaqueductal grey; 8. Dorsomedial medulla—nucleus of the solitary tract (NTS).

SGLT2 inhibitors are not fully selective for SGLT2 co-receptors, and they also affect SGLT1 to various extents (Table 1). Sotagliflozin has the most affinity to SGLT1 receptors. It is even called a "dual SGLT1/SGLT2 inhibitor", however, it is the newest Flozin, and it is not yet used in diabetic patients on a large scale [12]. Among commonly used SGLT2 inhibitors, Canagliflozin has the greatest potential for inhibiting SGLT1 receptors. In contrast, Empagliflozin and Ertugliflozin are the most selective for SGLT2 and have the lowest potential for interaction with SGLT1 [27]. Therefore, theoretically, to obtain the neuroprotective effect associated with SGLT1 inhibition in diabetic patients, Sotagliflozin and Canagliflozin should be preferred over Dapagliflozin, Empagliflozin, and Ertugliflozin.

Table 1. Comparison of pleiotropic effects of Sotagliflozin, Canagliflozin, Dapagliflozin, Empagliflozin, Ertugliflozin.

	Sotagliflozin	**Canagliflozin**	**Dapagliflozin**	**Empagliflozin**	**Ertugliflozin**
SGLT2 Selectivity over SGLT1	20 fold [28]	250 fold [28]	1200 fold [28]	2500 fold [28]	2500 fold [28]
Brain/Serum Ratio	n/a	0.3	0.3	0.5	n/a
AChE Inhibition	K_i 5.6μM [29]	The most potent, even called a dual inhibitor K_i 0.13 μM [29]	K_i 25.02μM [29]	K_i 0.177μM [30]	K_i 31.69μM [29]
BDNF Increase	n/a	n/a	n/a	Yes [31]	n/a
Anti-epileptic Potential	n/a	n/a	Yes [32]	n/a	n/a
CIMT Regression	n/a	n/a	Yes [33]	Yes [34]	n/a
Anti-inflammatory	n/a	Yes [35]	Yes [36]	Yes [37]	No I n/a [38]
Blood-brain Barrier Protection	n/a	n/a	n/a	Yes [37]	n/a

Table 1. *Cont.*

	Sotagliflozin	Canagliflozin	Dapagliflozin	Empagliflozin	Ertugliflozin
NLRP3 Inflammasome Inhibition	n/a	n/a	Yes [39]	Yes [40]	n/a
Promoting M2 Macrophages Polarization	n/a	Yes [41]	Yes [42]	Yes [43]	n/a
Oxidative Stress Reduction	Yes [44]	Yes [45]	Yes [46]	Yes [47]	Yes [48]
Neurovascular Unit Remodeling	n/a	n/a	n/a	Yes [49]	n/a
Cerebral Ischemia/Reperfusion Damage Reduction	n/a	n/a	n/a	Yes [50]	n/a
Reduced mTOR Signaling	n/a	Yes [51]	Yes [51]	Yes [52]	Yes [53]

In the central nervous system, there is also a place for selective SGLT2 inhibitors since, based on the results obtained by Erdogan MA. et al., Dapagliflozin significantly reduces seizure activity, both at the electrophysiological and clinical level, in a rat model of epilepsy [32]. It may be associated with a similar effect of glucose fasting-like metabolic switch as the one observed in ketogenic diets, which in some circumstances also improve brain seizure activity [54]. There is no clinical data comparing the efficacy of ketogenic diets and dapagliflozin therapy on brain epileptic activity; however, adhering to a ketogenic diet is difficult and has to be closely monitored. On the contrary, dapagliflozin is a safe drug widely used in diabetic patients. Interestingly, cognitive impairment shares the same risk factors as epilepsy and atherosclerosis, and commonly used anti-epileptic drugs such as phenytoin, carbamazepine, valproic acid are associated with increased cardiovascular risk [55]. Dapagliflozin may be a preferable flozin in diabetic patients with epilepsy as it has an anti-epileptic potential. Moreover, it significantly reduces cardiovascular risk and thus may prevent cognitive decline.

There is in vivo evidence for the expression of SGLT2 protein in choroid plexus epithelial cells and ependymal cells of the human brain [56]. This is crucial information indicating that SGLT2 may have an influence on the composition of the cerebrospinal fluid (CSF), whose role in the pathology of neurodegenerative disorders provides a new direction for research and requires further investigation [57].

There is growing evidence that apart from direct mechanisms of SGLT2 inhibitors in the central nervous system, they also exert a beneficial pleiotropic effect. In silico studies indicate that flozins have the molecular ability to inhibit acetylcholinesterase. Canagliflozin was even called a 'dual inhibitor of SGLT2 and AChE' as its estimated inhibition constant K_i (i.e., the concentration required to produce half-maximum inhibition) against AChE was 0.12859 μM [58]. It is clinically relevant as patients taking canagliflozin reach a serum drug concentration of 10μM, and the brain/serum ratio of canagliflozin is 0.3. Therefore, the amount of canagliflozin penetrating the brain (3 μM) is enough to inhibit AChE [17,59]. As for other SGLT2i, the K_i for inhibiting AChE is 0.177 μM for empagliflozin and 25.02 μM for dapagliflozin, and brain concentrations are 0.5 μM and 0.3 μM, respectively, so out of those two, only in the case of empagliflozin, brain concentration is enough to inhibit AChE (Table 1) [17,30,60]. Patients with Alzheimer's disease have a reduced amount of acetylcholine neurotransmitters in the brain, and acetylcholinesterase inhibitors including donepezil, rivastigmine, galantamine are commonly used to increase the acetylcholine level and improve cognition [61]. In a rat model of cognitive impairment induced by scopolamine, canagliflozin, similarly to galantamine, decreased AChE activity, increased acetylcholine M1 receptor (M1 mAChR) and monoamines levels. It also improved cognitive functions in the Y maze task and water maze task [62]. Canagliflozin has the greatest potential of inhibiting AChE and may be a preferable solution in patients with T2DM who would also benefit from the inhibition of acetylcholinesterase.

Another promising effect SGLT2i exert on the central nervous system was described by Lin B. et al., for empagliflozin, which significantly increased cerebral BDNF (Brain-derived neurotrophic factor) levels in db/db mice (Table 1). Moreover, this effect was accompanied by improvement in cognitive functions [31]. BDNF takes part in the growth, survival, and plasticity of neurons as well as in the modulation of neurotransmission. It is an important factor for the processes of learning and memorizing [63]. Interestingly, a significant decline of BDNF was observed in patients with T2DM, and it was associated with cognitive impairment, which was not observed in non-diabetic controls [64]. Surprisingly, BDNF is crucial not only for the central nervous system but also for atherosclerosis. Patients with DMAS (Diabetes Mellitus Accelerated Atherosclerosis) had a lower expression of BDNF, and it was negatively correlated with inflammation. In the same study, supplementation of BDNF in mice significantly reduced atherosclerotic lesions [65]. The anti-inflammatory properties of BDNF are probably associated with promoting M2 macrophages polarization via STAT3 [65]. SGLT2i may thus bring benefits to diabetic patients with atherosclerosis by preventing cognitive impairment associated with low levels of BDNF.

3. Atherosclerosis, Cognitive Impairment, and SGLT2i

The presence of cholesterol-rich plaques in the walls of large cerebral arteries is defined as Cerebral Atherosclerosis (CA). In previous studies, atherosclerotic lesions in intra- and extra-cranial arteries were associated with cognitive impairment and even dementia [2,66,67]. According to results obtained by Dearborn JL. et al., atherosclerotic plaques in the anterior cerebral artery occurred independently of vascular risk factors associated with increased prevalence of dementia (RPR 3.81 95%CI [1.57–9.23] $p = 0.003$) in elderly patients [2]. On the other hand, atherosclerosis in the posterior cerebral artery increased the risk of Mild Cognitive Impairment (MCI) (RPR 1.44 95% CI [1.04–1.98] $p = 0.027$) [2]. As demonstrated by another study, dementia occurred more frequently in patients with atherosclerotic calcifications in intra and extra-cranial arteries as opposed to coronary vessels [66]. Cerebral atherosclerosis and dementia are related to each other; however, the exact mechanism remains unknown. In reference to the proteomic sequencing of the dorsolateral prefrontal cortex of 438 humans performed by Wingo A.P. et al., CA was associated with reduced synaptic function, excess myelination, and axonal injury independently of ischemia [67]. Preventing atherosclerosis would contribute to the improvement in cognitive functions in elderly people. Results obtained by Sabia S. et al. show that cardiovascular health at the age of 50 years is crucial for further development of cognitive impairment [68]. As mentioned before, SGLT2i significantly reduce cardiovascular risk. They exert a pleiotropic anti-atherosclerotic effect by reducing vascular inflammation, oxidative stress and improving endothelial dysfunction [69]. In a previous study including diabetic patients, a three-month treatment with empagliflozin resulted in a significant regression of complex intima media thickness (cIMT) by 7.9%; $p < 0.0001$. Interestingly, this effect was significant just after one month of empagliflozin therapy [34]. CIMT is a relevant marker of early atherosclerosis, and it is often measured in the carotid arteries [70]. According to Feinkohl I. et al., cIMT is also a significant predictor of cognitive decline in patients with T2DM [71]. Future studies should evaluate the clinical relevance of the ability of SGLT2 to reduce atherosclerotic lesions and thus the impact on cognitive functions.

4. Inflammation

The inflammatory process in the central nervous system also referred to as neuroinflammation, is associated with a lot of pathologies, including cognitive dysfunction. In a study conducted by Suridjan I. et al., and including patients with Alzheimer's disease, the presence of neuroinflammation detected by [18F]-FEPPA was positively correlated with the level of cognitive decline [72]. There is growing evidence that the presence of inflammation outside the central nervous system (systemic inflammation) can also contribute to a decline in cognitive functions [73]. According to Walker K. et al., elevated inflammatory markers in middle adulthood resulted in significant cognitive decline after 20 years [74]. The neurovascular unit (NVU), which is composed of endothelial cells lining brain microvessels as well as neurons, microglia, astrocytes, and pericytes, mediates homeostasis by regulating traffic between blood and the neural environment. Systemic inflammation is associated with circulating proinflammatory cytokines, which impair the endothelium of brain microvessels, increase the permeability of the blood-brain barrier and change the phenotype of astrocytes and microglia into pro-inflammatory ones [75]. M1 activated microglia impair NVU by secreting proinflammatory cytokines, including TNF-α, IL-1β, IL-6, IL-18, which contribute to neurodegeneration by breaking neurotransmitters into bioactive metabolites, tau hyperphosphorylation, β-amyloid oligomerization, and complement activation [76,77]. In a mouse model of T2DM, empagliflozin had a protective effect, involving remodeling prevention on the neurovascular unit, the blood-brain barrier, pericytes, astrocytes, microglia, and oligodendrocytes [49]. The inflammatory process is also a key driver of atherosclerosis. In the CANTOS study, inhibition of interleukin-1β with canakinumab significantly reduced cardiovascular risk independently of lipid levels [78]. Proinflammatory cytokines including TNF-α, IL-1β, IL-6 are also a mediator of atherosclerosis since they activate endothelial cells, attract monocytes, and facilitate their adhesion by up-regulating MCP-1, ICAM, VCAM [79]. There is abundant evidence from animal studies showing that SGLT2 inhibitors slow down the progression of atherosclerosis and exert an anti-inflammatory effect by reducing the expression of proinflammatory cytokines, including TNF-α, IL-1β, IL-6, MCP-1, ICAM, VCAM [69]. In humans, the serum level of IL-6 dropped by 26.6% (p = 0.010) after 2 years of canagliflozin treatment [35].

NLRP3 (NOD-, LRR- and pyrin domain- containing protein 3) inflammasome activation is one of the key molecular pathways mediating inflammation as it leads to the release of IL-1β and IL-18 cytokines. It is a crucial element of the innate immune system activated not only by microbial infection or cellular damage but also by chronic inflammatory diseases, including atherosclerosis and Alzheimer's disease [80]. NLRP3 is an important mechanism that drives inflammation in atherosclerosis since activation of this pathway in arterial walls by lipoproteins triggers inflammatory response [81]. In a mouse model of atherosclerosis, the inhibition of the NLRP3 inflammasome by MCC950 resulted in a significant reduction in atherosclerotic lesions [82]. In Alzheimer's disease, NLRP3 inflammasome links systemic inflammation with neuroinflammation and impairs the removal of amyloid-beta by the microglia [83]. This effect may be clinically significant, as, in another study, the inhibition of NLRP3 by OLT1177 significantly improved cognitive impairment in a mouse model of Alzheimer's disease [84]. SGLT2 inhibitors may improve atherosclerosis and cognitive dysfunction via NLRP3 inflammasome inhibition (Table 1). As proven by Kim S. et al., in the ex vivo study in diabetic patients, empagliflozin significantly attenuated the inflammasome activity after 30 days of treatment [40].

Macrophages play a central role in atherosclerosis due to their foam cell formation in the vascular lesions. They are also an important factor in the pathology of cognitive impairment associated with Alzheimer's disease as their infiltration is increased in patients with AD being most abundant in the brain regions rich in Aβ plaques [85]. Macrophages are immune cells responsible for mediating chronic low-grade inflammation and residual cardiovascular risk, which remains after lipid reduction. They are characterized by an ability to change in response to the environment. There are two immunological types of macrophages, i.e., M1 and M2 macrophages. M1 proinflammatory macrophages secrete 1β, IL-6, and TNF-α, maintain a chronic inflammatory state, and promote atherogenesis. On the contrary, M2 macrophages have an anti-inflammatory and atheroprotective profile by secreting IL-1 receptor agonist, IL-10, and collagen [86]. SGLT2 inhibitors have been proven to strongly promote macrophage polarization towards M2 and thus alleviate inflammation and atherosclerosis (Table 1) [42]. In the central nervous system, M1 polarization of glial cells was associated with neurodegeneration [73]. M1 polarized macrophages activate

STAT-1, which is a proinflammatory transcription factor [87]. It can also be involved in cognitive impairment in Alzheimer's disease since it is activated by intracellular Tau accumulation. In a murine model, depletion of STAT-1 activation significantly reduced synaptic dysfunction and cognitive impairment associated with Tau accumulation [88]. Empagliflozin was proven to mitigate inflammation by downregulation of the JAK2/STAT1 pathway in macrophages [89]. Macrophages take part in cognitive impairment as perivascular macrophages (PVM) are the source of vascular oxidative stress by producing a large amount of free radicals near the neurovascular unit [90]. They also affect the permeability of the blood-brain barrier [91]. In previous studies, depletion of perivascular macrophages prevented short-term memory impairment in a murine model [92]. SGLT2 inhibitors may possibly attenuate atherosclerosis and cognitive impairment via macrophages by promoting M2 polarization and downregulating STAT-1 (Figure 2).

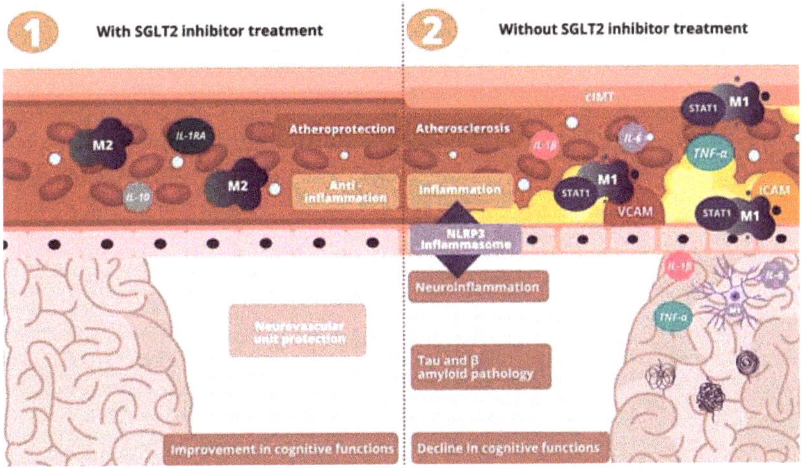

Figure 2. Influence of SGLT2 inhibitors on inflammation, atherosclerosis, and neuroinflammation. IL-1RA—Interleukin 1 Receptor Agonist, cIMT—carotid intima-media thickness, STAT1—Signal transducer and activator of transcription 1, VCAM—Vascular Cell Adhesion Molecule; ICAM-Intracellular Adhesion Molecule.

5. Oxidative Stress and Mitochondrial Dysfunction

A chronic inflammatory state also contributes to oxidative damage as it causes the release of reactive oxygen species (ROS) [93]. The overproduction of ROS or decrease in the anti-oxidant defense results in oxidative stress, which is a significant contributor to vascular diseases, including atherosclerosis, as it causes endothelial dysfunction, promotes remodeling and further enhances inflammation [94]. Oxidative stress is also associated with Aβ- or tau -induced neurotoxicity since it facilitates their aggregation, phosphorylation, and polymerization. These processes contribute to neurodegeneration which results in impaired synaptic plasticity, neuroinflammation, neurotransmitter imbalance, neuronal and synaptic loss leading to cognitive impairment [95]. In the previous study, the increased level of oxidative stress was associated with cognitive decline in a healthy population [96]. Interestingly, SGLT2 inhibitors were proven to ameliorate oxidative stress not only by maintaining a normal glucose level but also by reducing the generation of free radicals (Table 1) [97]. In patients with T2DM, empagliflozin significantly enhanced leukocyte expression of antioxidative enzymes including glutathione s-reductase and catalase and simultaneously reduced pro-oxidative myeloperoxidase after four months of treatment [47].

Mitochondrial function is crucial for maintaining neuronal homeostasis, as neurons are vulnerable to bioenergetic changes. Mitochondrial dysfunction plays an important role in the pathogenesis of neurodegenerative diseases; there is even a "Mitochondrial

Cascade hypothesis" in Alzheimer's Disease pathology [98]. In a murine model, depletion of AIF (apoptosis-inducing factor), which is a mitochondrial protein taking part in apoptosis and electron transport chain, was associated with serious disturbances in hippocampal-dependant spatial learning and memory [99]. In a rat model, taking dapagliflozin was associated with significant improvement in brain mitochondrial function, including decreased ROS production, mitochondrial swelling, and mitochondrial membrane depolarization [100]. The existing evidence supports the concept that SGLT2 may improve atherosclerosis and cognitive impairment by reduction in oxidative stress and improvement in mitochondrial dysfunction.

6. mTOR Signaling

mTOR (mechanistic/mammalian target of rapamycin) is a novel, promising molecular pathway linking metabolic diseases and cognitive impairment. It is a crucial cellular coordinator of systemic energy status and local nutrients. Chronic up-regulation of mTOR is present in an anabolic state (increased levels of glucose, amino acids, growth factors) associated with over-nutrition and lack of physical activity [101]. Continuous activation of mTOR causes endothelial cell dysfunction, which is not only a key point of atherosclerosis but also contributes to interruption in the blood-brain barrier [102]. Unrestrained mTOR up-regulation has also been linked to tau and amyloid β hyperphosphorylation and aggregation in Alzheimer's disease [103]. Moreover, chronic mTOR activation impairs lysosomal protein degradation, which supports the "Endo-Lysosomal Dysfunction" hypothesis of Alzheimer's Disease [104]. It is believed that restoring the circadian rhythm of mTOR activation would be beneficial in metabolic diseases and cognitive impairment. This effect can be achieved by increasing physical activity, reducing calories intake, or intermittent fasting. All the abovementioned interventions require the patient's determination and are difficult to obtain in real-life clinical practice. SGLT2 inhibitors are able to mimic those states by promoting catabolism and restoring mTOR cycling, thus decreasing cognitive impairment associated with metabolic diseases [105]. An interesting SGLT2i effect was noticed by Esterline R. et al.; SGLT2 inhibitors cause loss of glucose with urine, but simultaneously they activate glycogenolysis and gluconeogenesis and thus increase fasting endogenous glucose production, which occurs particularly at night. This effect contributes to switching metabolism from anabolic to catabolic depending not on glucose and insulin but on fatty acid oxidation and leads to a decrease in mTOR fuel: blood insulin and amino-acids. Nocturnal mTOR suppression is followed by daily activation, and this state allows maintaining mitochondrial and lysosomal homeostasis (Figure 3) [104]. Additionally, according to Packer M, SGLT2 inhibitors cause transcriptional changes in cells that occur during starvation, which is called "state of fasting mimicry" and include SIRT/AMPK activation and Akt/mTOR suppression (Figure 3). Moreover, taking flozins causes changes similar to an ischemic state, including HIF-2α activation which stimulates erythropoiesis, and patients with higher erythrocyte count benefited most from SGLT2i therapy. Interestingly those effects occurred also in cells, which do not express SGLT [106]. There is a lot of evidence that SGLT2 inhibitors are able to suppress mTOR (Table 1). Flozins, by restoring the circadian rhythm of mTOR activity, seem to bring benefits in patients with Alzheimer's Disease according to "Type 3 Diabetes Hypothesis", "Mitochondrial Cascade Hypothesis" and "Endo-Lysosomal Dysfunction Hypothesis" [105].

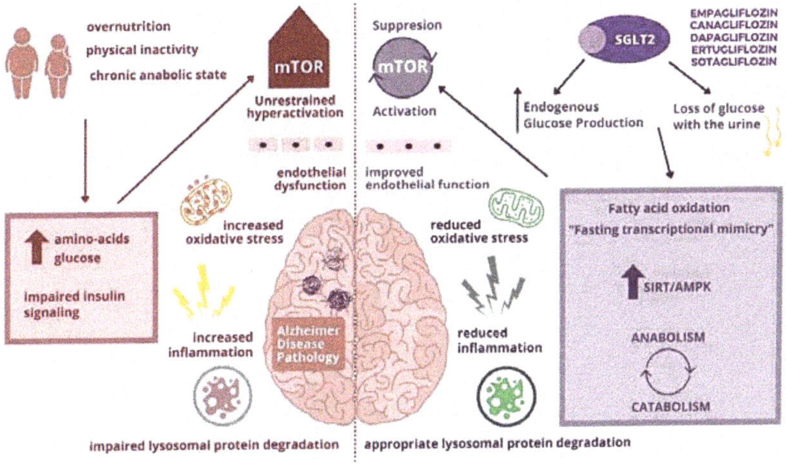

Figure 3. Influence of SGLT2 inhibitors on unrestrained activation of mTOR (mechanistic/mammalian target of rapamycin). AMPK-AMP-activated protein kinase, SIRT-Sirtuin.

7. Cerebrovascular Dysfunction

Cerebrovascular dysfunction is a pathological condition of the brain related to vascular pathology. A hyperglycemic state impairs the microvascular structure of the brain causing neurovascular remodeling, including loss of endothelial integrity, basement membrane thickening, loss of myelin and neurons, astrocytes and pericytes disturbance [107]. Such ultrastructural changes are associated with cognitive decline [108]. In a mouse model of T2DM, empagliflozin exerted a neuroprotective effect on neurovascular remodeling [49].

Cerebrovascular dysfunction is mainly associated with disturbed blood flow being either ischemia or bleeding. The presence of atherosclerotic lesions within arterial walls impairs cerebral blood flow and causes cerebrovascular dysfunction [109]. Most ischemic strokes are caused by atherosclerosis. According to a meta-analysis, the presence of carotid atherosclerosis was associated with an increased risk of recurrent stroke (OR: 2.87; 95% CI (2.42–3.37); $p < 0.00001$) [110]. Acute ischemic stroke leads to a critical limitation of blood supply, which results in neuronal cell death and cognitive decline. Cognitive impairment affects 20–80% of patients after acute brain ischemia [111]. Although SGLT2 inhibitors do not reduce the risk of ischemic stroke incidence, they affect the most important cerebrovascular risk factors, including hyperglycemia, hypertension, obesity, dyslipidemia, and atherosclerosis [112]. Hypertension is the most common risk factor of stroke [113]. SGLT2 inhibitors significantly lower systolic and diastolic blood pressure without reflex activation of the sympathetic nervous system and are even able to change the non-dipping to dipping circadian blood pressure profile. While the exact mechanism of the antihypertensive effect of SGLT2 inhibitors has not been clearly established, it is considered that the most important factors are osmotic diuresis (induced by glucosuria) and natriuresis. Other features of SGLT2 inhibitors that contribute to lowering blood pressure are suppression of the renin-angiotensin system, decreased activity of the sympathetic system, antioxidative activity, and improvement in endothelial cell function [114]. Moreover, SGLT2 inhibitors may improve brain damage and cognitive impairment in patients after a stroke. SGLT receptors are important in ischemia-reperfusion cerebral damage. As presented in a mouse model of subcortical white matter infarct with cognitive impairment, the knockout of the SGLT1 receptor was associated with a lower expression of proinflammatory cytokines and better cognitive performance [115]. SGLT1 receptors mediate sodium influx, which causes depolarization and contributes to neuronal cell death during ischemia. According to Yamazaki Y. et al., increased sodium influx via the SGLT1 receptor was associated with more exacerbated neuronal damage, which was not observed in SGLT-1 knockdown mice

(Figure 4) [116]. In a study assessing cerebral ischemia/reperfusion damage in a rat model, empagliflozin, in a dose-dependant manner, reduced neuronal death, infarct size and ameliorated cognitive impairment via HIF-1α/VEGF signaling [50]. SGLT2 inhibitors may preserve cognitive functions in diabetic patients by preventing neurovascular remodeling and reducing the well-known risk factors of stroke. They can also bring benefits to post-stroke patients by reducing inflammation, sodium influx, and HIF-1α/VEGF pathway.

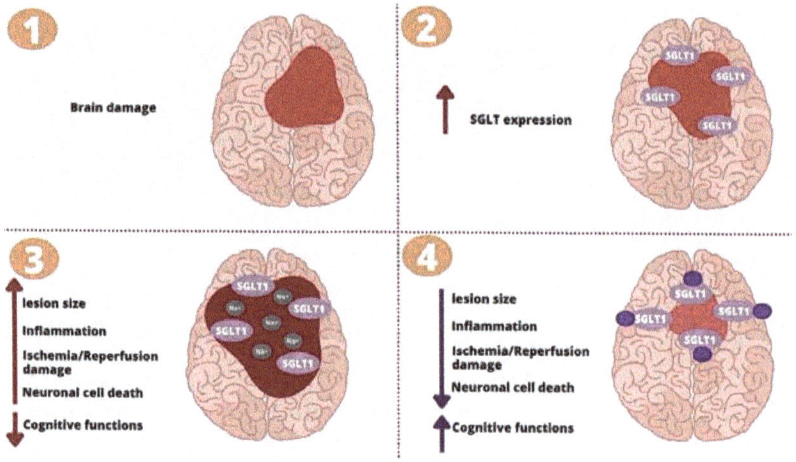

Figure 4. SGLT1 inhibition and ischemic brain damage. 1. Brain damage; 2. In the area of brain damage, there is an increase in the expression of SGLT1; 3. Sodium influx through SGLT1 receptors is associated with increased ischemia/reperfusion damage, lesion size, edema, inflammation, neuronal cell death, and decline in cognitive functions; 4. SGLT receptor blockage/knockdown was associated with improvement in damages caused by ischemia and ischemia/reperfusion damage.

8. The Effect of SGLT2i on Alzheimer's Disease Pathology

SGLT2 inhibitors can possibly bring benefits in patients with Alzheimer's Disease using the abovementioned mechanisms, including not only anti-inflammatory, anti-oxidative or atheroprotective effects, but also direct neuroprotective effects including BDNF increase and AChE inhibition. Additionally, SGLT2i can also be favorable for AD patients by improving brain insulin sensitivity [100]. Insulin resistance is present in 8 out of 10 patients suffering from Alzheimer's Disease [117]. Peripheral resistance to insulin also occurs in the CNS, as the glucose metabolic rate is reduced in the brains of AD patients in fluorodeoxyglucose positron emission tomography (FDG PET) [118,119]. Increased insulin level in the brain contributes to Alzheimer's Disease pathology, as the insulin-degrading enzyme (IDE) also takes part in degrading senile plaques, and in insulin resistance, it is involved in degrading insulin [117]. Moreover, insulin resistance is associated with activating GSK3-β (glycogen synthase kinase 3β) signaling, which takes part in tau phosphorylation and Aβ production and Aβ mediated neuronal damage [117,120]. SGLT2 inhibition reduced GSK3-β activity in hepatocytes [121]. In previous studies involving murine models, SGLT2i treatment caused a significant reduction in AD pathology, including tau phosphorylation and senile plaques density. This effect was associated with the improvement in cognitive functions, including memory and learning processes in the new object discrimination test and Morris water maze test [15].

9. Summary

Type 2 Diabetes Mellitus, atherosclerosis, and cognitive impairment still remain global health problems as they are chronic, incurable diseases leading to a reduction in life quality and expectancy. All these diseases share many pathological pathways. In the era of tailored-made therapies and novel drugs with numerous pleiotropic effects, it is very important to seek for shared molecular pathways of commonly occurring diseases and redefine indications for commonly used medications since such solutions may be beneficial for patients. In this review, we have discussed the role of SGLT2 inhibitors used in diabetic patients for the prevention of atherosclerosis and cognitive impairment. Flozins may bring positive effects in T2DM, atherosclerosis, and cognitive impairment through several mechanisms, including anti-inflammatory and anti-atherosclerotic properties, SGLT1 inhibition, AChE inhibition, reduction in oxidative stress, amelioration cerebrovascular remodeling and restoring a balance between catabolism and anabolism. However, long-term clinical trials are necessary to establish whether the above-mentioned mechanisms are clinically relevant since atheroprotective and neuroprotective effects will not be immediate and require a long-term SGLT2i intake. Currently, the University of Kansas Medical Center (NCT03801642) is conducting a clinical trial on dapagliflozin in patients with Alzheimer's disease.

Funding: This research received no external funding.

Conflicts of Interest: The authors declare no conflict of interest.

References

1. Einarson, T.R.; Acs, A.; Ludwig, C.; Panton, U.H. Prevalence of cardiovascular disease in type 2 diabetes: A systematic literature review of scientific evidence from across the world in 2007–2017. *Cardiovasc. Diabetol.* **2018**, *17*, 1–19. [CrossRef] [PubMed]
2. Dearborn, J.L.; Qiao, Y.; Suri, M.F.K.; Liu, L.; Mosley, T.H.; Alonso, A.; Knopman, D.S. Intracranial atherosclerosis and dementia The Atherosclerosis Risk in Communities (ARIC) Study. *Am. Acad. Neurol.* **2017**, *88*, 1556–1563.
3. Iadecola, C. Revisiting atherosclerosis and dementia. *Nat. Neurosci.* **2020**, *23*, 691–692. [CrossRef] [PubMed]
4. Bertoluci, M.C.; Rocha, V.Z. Cardiovascular risk assessment in patients with diabetes. *Diabetol. Metab. Syndr.* **2017**, *9*, 1–13. [CrossRef]
5. Nguyen, T.T.; Ta, Q.T.H.; Nguyen, T.K.O.; Nguyen, T.T.D.; Van Giau, V. Type 3 diabetes and its role implications in alzheimer's disease. *Int. J. Mol. Sci.* **2020**, *21*, 3165. [CrossRef] [PubMed]
6. Zhang, J.; Chen, C.; Hua, S.; Liao, H.; Wang, M.; Xiong, Y.; Cao, F. An updated meta-analysis of cohort studies: Diabetes and risk of Alzheimer's disease. *Diabetes Res. Clin. Pract.* **2017**, *124*, 41–47. [CrossRef] [PubMed]
7. Exalto, L.G.; Biessels, G.J.; Karter, A.J.; Huang, E.S.; Katon, W.J.; Minkoff, J.R.; Whitmer, R.A. Risk score for prediction of 10 year dementia risk in individuals with type 2 diabetes: A cohort study. *Lancet Diabetes Endocrinol.* **2013**, *1*, 183–190. [CrossRef]
8. Hsia, D.S.; Grove, O.; Cefalu, W.T. An Update on SGLT2 Inhibitors for the Treatment of Diabetes Mellitus. *Curr Opin Endocrinol Diabetes Obes* **2017**, *24*, 73–79. [CrossRef] [PubMed]
9. Steiner, S. Empagliflozin, cardiovascular outcomes, and mortality in type 2 diabetes. *Z. Gefassmedizin* **2016**, *13*, 17–18. [CrossRef]
10. Mahaffey, K.W.; Neal, B.; Perkovic, V.; De Zeeuw, D.; Fulcher, G.; Erondu, N.; Shaw, W.; Fabbrini, E.; Sun, T.; Li, Q.; et al. Canagliflozin for Primary and Secondary Prevention of Cardiovascular Events: Results from the CANVAS Program (Canagliflozin Cardiovascular Assessment Study). *Circulation* **2018**, *137*, 323–334. [CrossRef]
11. Wiviott, S.D.; Raz, I.; Bonaca, M.P.; Mosenzon, O.; Kato, E.T.; Cahn, A.; Silverman, M.G.; Zelniker, T.A.; Kuder, J.F.; Murphy, S.A.; et al. Dapagliflozin and Cardiovascular Outcomes in Type 2 Diabetes. *N. Engl. J. Med.* **2019**, *380*, 347–357. [CrossRef] [PubMed]
12. Bhatt, D.L.; Szarek, M.; Steg, P.G.; Cannon, C.P.; Leiter, L.A.; McGuire, D.K.; Lewis, J.B.; Riddle, M.C.; Voors, A.A.; Metra, M.; et al. Sotagliflozin in Patients with Diabetes and Recent Worsening Heart Failure. *N. Engl. J. Med.* **2021**, *384*, 117–128. [CrossRef]
13. Cannon, C.P.; Pratley, R.; Dagogo-Jack, S.; Mancuso, J.; Huyck, S.; Masiukiewicz, U.; Charbonnel, B.; Frederich, R.; Gallo, S.; Cosentino, F.; et al. Cardiovascular Outcomes with Ertugliflozin in Type 2 Diabetes. *N. Engl. J. Med.* **2020**, *383*, 1425–1435. [CrossRef] [PubMed]
14. Heerspink, H.J.L.; Stefánsson, B.V.; Correa-Rotter, R.; Chertow, G.M.; Greene, T.; Hou, F.-F.; Mann, J.F.E.; McMurray, J.J.V.; Lindberg, M.; Rossing, P.; et al. Dapagliflozin in Patients with Chronic Kidney Disease. *N. Engl. J. Med.* **2020**, *383*, 1436–1446. [CrossRef]
15. Hierro-bujalance, C.; Infante-garcia, C.; Marco, A.; Herrera, M.; Carranza-naval, M.J.; Suarez, J.; Alves-martinez, P.; Lubian-lopez, S.; Garcia-alloza, M. Empagliflozin reduces vascular damage and cognitive impairment in a mixed murine model of Alzheimer' s disease and type 2 diabetes. *Alzheimer's Res. Ther.* **2020**, *4*, 1–13.
16. McGill, J.B.; Subramanian, S. Safety of Sodium-Glucose Co-Transporter 2 Inhibitors. *Am. J. Cardiol.* **2019**, *124*, S45–S52. [CrossRef] [PubMed]
17. Tahara, A.; Takasu, T.; Yokono, M.; Imamura, M.; Kurosaki, E. Characterization and comparison of sodium-glucose cotransporter 2 inhibitors in pharmacokinetics, pharmacodynamics, and pharmacologic effects. *J. Pharmacol. Sci.* **2016**, *130*, 159–169. [CrossRef] [PubMed]
18. Shah, K.; DeSilva, S.; Abbruscato, T. The role of glucose transporters in brain disease: Diabetes and Alzheimer's disease. *Int. J. Mol. Sci.* **2012**, *13*, 12629–12655. [CrossRef] [PubMed]

19. Wright, E.M.; LOO, D.D.F.L.; Hirayama, B.A. Biology of human sodium glucose transporters. *Physiol. Rev.* **2011**, *91*, 733–794. [CrossRef] [PubMed]
20. Poppe, R.; Karbach, U.; Gambaryan, S.; Wiesinger, H.; Lutzenburg, M.; Kraemer, M.; Witte, O.W.; Koepsell, H. Expression of the Na+-D-glucose cotransporter SGLT1 in neurons. *J. Neurochem.* **1997**, *69*, 84–94. [CrossRef] [PubMed]
21. Koepsell, H. Glucose transporters in brain in health and disease. *Pflugers Arch. Eur. J. Physiol.* **2020**, *472*, 1299–1343. [CrossRef] [PubMed]
22. Enerson, B.E.; Drewes, L.R. The rat blood-brain barrier transcriptome. *J. Cereb. Blood Flow Metab.* **2006**, *26*, 959–973. [CrossRef]
23. Nguyen, T.; Wen, S.; Gong, M.; Yuan, X.; Xu, D.; Wang, C.; Jin, J.; Zhou, L. Dapagliflozin activates neurons in the central nervous system and regulates cardiovascular activity by inhibiting sglt-2 in mice. *Diabetes, Metab. Syndr. Obes. Targets Ther.* **2020**, *13*, 2781–2799. [CrossRef] [PubMed]
24. Gaur, A.; Pal, G.K.; Ananthanarayanan, P.H.; Pal, P. Role of Ventromedial hypothalamus in high fat diet induced obesity in male rats: Association with lipid profile, thyroid profile and insulin resistance. *Ann. Neurosci.* **2014**, *21*, 104–107. [CrossRef]
25. Oerter, S.; Förster, C.; Bohnert, M. Validation of sodium/glucose cotransporter proteins in human brain as a potential marker for temporal narrowing of the trauma formation. *Int. J. Legal Med.* **2019**, *133*, 1107–1114. [CrossRef] [PubMed]
26. Sebastiani, A.; Greve, F.; Gölz, C.; Förster, C.Y.; Koepsell, H.; Thal, S.C. RS1 (Rsc1A1) deficiency limits cerebral SGLT1 expression and delays brain damage after experimental traumatic brain injury. *J. Neurochem.* **2018**, *147*, 190–203. [CrossRef]
27. Malhotra, A.; Kudyar, S.; Gupta, A.; Kudyar, R.; Malhotra, P. Sodium glucose co-transporter inhibitors—A new class of old drugs. *Int. J. Appl. Basic Med. Res.* **2015**, *5*, 161. [CrossRef] [PubMed]
28. Cinti, F.; Moffa, S.; Impronta, F.; Cefalo, C.M.; Sun, V.A.; Sorice, G.P.; Mezza, T.; Giaccari, A. Spotlight on ertugliflozin and its potential in the treatment of type 2 diabetes: Evidence to date. *Drug Des. Devel. Ther.* **2017**, *11*, 2905–2919. [CrossRef] [PubMed]
29. Shakil, S. Molecular Interaction of Anti-Diabetic Drugs with Acetylcholinesterase and Sodium Glucose Co-Transporter 2. *J. Cell. Biochem.* **2017**, *118*, 3855–3865. [CrossRef]
30. Shaikh, S.; Rizvi, S.M.; Suhail, T.; Shakil, S.; Abuzenadah, A.; Anis, R.; Naaz, D.; Dallol, A.; Haneef, M.; Ahmad, A.; et al. Prediction of Anti-Diabetic Drugs as Dual Inhibitors Against Acetylcholinesterase and Beta-Secretase: A Neuroinformatics Study. *CNS Neurol. Disord.—Drug Targets* **2016**, *15*, 1216–1221. [CrossRef] [PubMed]
31. Lin, B.; Koibuchi, N.; Hasegawa, Y.; Sueta, D.; Toyama, K.; Uekawa, K.; Ma, M.J.; Nakagawa, T.; Kusaka, H.; Kim-Mitsuyama, S. Glycemic control with empagliflozin, a novel selective SGLT2 inhibitor, ameliorates cardiovascular injury and cognitive dysfunction in obese and type 2 diabetic mice. *Cardiovasc. Diabetol.* **2014**, *13*, 1–15. [CrossRef] [PubMed]
32. Erdogan, M.A.; Yusuf, D.; Christy, J.; Solmaz, V.; Erdogan, A.; Taskiran, E.; Erbas, O. Highly selective SGLT2 inhibitor dapagliflozin reduces seizure activity in pentylenetetrazol-induced murine model of epilepsy. *BMC Neurol.* **2018**, *18*, 1–8. [CrossRef]
33. Akhanli, P.; Hepsen, S.; Emre, A.I.; Duger, H.; Bostan, H.; Kizilgul, M.; Ucan, B.; Cakal, E. AEP816: 24-week impact of dapagliflozin treatment on body weight, body composition, and cardiac risk indicators of patients with type-2 diabetes mellitus. In *Endocrine Abstracts*; Bioscientifica: Bristol, UK, 2020.
34. Irace, C.; Casciaro, F.; Scavelli, F.B.; Oliverio, R.; Cutruzzolà, A.; Cortese, C.; Gnasso, A. Empagliflozin influences blood viscosity and wall shear stress in subjects with type 2 diabetes mellitus compared with incretin-based therapy. *Cardiovasc. Diabetol.* **2018**, *17*, 1–9. [CrossRef] [PubMed]
35. Heerspink, H.J.L.; Perco, P.; Mulder, S.; Leierer, J.; Hansen, M.K.; Heinzel, A.; Mayer, G. Canagliflozin reduces inflammation and fibrosis biomarkers: A potential mechanism of action for beneficial effects of SGLT2 inhibitors in diabetic kidney disease. *Diabetologia* **2019**, *62*, 1154–1166. [CrossRef] [PubMed]
36. Xue, L.; Yuan, X.; Zhang, S.; Zhao, X. Investigating the Effects of Dapagliflozin on Cardiac Function, Inflammatory Response, and Cardiovascular Outcome in Patients with STEMI Complicated with T2DM after PCI. *Evidence-Based Complement. Altern. Med.* **2021**, *2021*, 9388562. [CrossRef] [PubMed]
37. Ganbaatar, B.; Fukuda, D.; Shinohara, M.; Yagi, S.; Kusunose, K.; Yamada, H.; Soeki, T.; Hirata, K.-i.; Sata, M. Empagliflozin ameliorates endothelial dysfunction and suppresses atherogenesis in diabetic apolipoprotein E-deficient mice. *Eur. J. Pharmacol.* **2020**, *875*, 173040. [CrossRef] [PubMed]
38. Liu, H.; Sridhar, V.S.; Lovblom, L.E.; Lytvyn, Y.; Burger, D.; Burns, K.; Brinc, D.; Lawler, P.R.; Cherney, D.Z.I. Markers of Kidney Injury, Inflammation, and Fibrosis Associated with Ertugliflozin in Patients With CKD and Diabetes. *Kidney Int. Reports* **2021**, *6*, 2095–2104. [CrossRef] [PubMed]
39. Ye, Y.; Bajaj, M.; Yang, H.C.; Perez-Polo, J.R.; Birnbaum, Y. SGLT-2 Inhibition with Dapagliflozin Reduces the Activation of the Nlrp3/ASC Inflammasome and Attenuates the Development of Diabetic Cardiomyopathy in Mice with Type 2 Diabetes. Further Augmentation of the Effects with Saxagliptin, a DPP4 Inhibitor. *Cardiovasc. Drugs Ther.* **2017**, *31*, 119–132. [CrossRef] [PubMed]
40. Kim, S.R.; Lee, S.G.; Kim, S.H.; Kim, J.H.; Choi, E.; Cho, W.; Rim, J.H.; Hwang, I.; Lee, C.J.; Lee, M.; et al. SGLT2 inhibition modulates NLRP3 inflammasome activity via ketones and insulin in diabetes with cardiovascular disease. *Nat. Commun.* **2020**, *11*, 1–11. [CrossRef] [PubMed]
41. Lin, F.; Song, C.; Zeng, Y.; Li, Y.; Li, H.; Liu, B.; Dai, M.; Pan, P. Canagliflozin alleviates LPS-induced acute lung injury by modulating alveolar macrophage polarization. *Int. Immunopharmacol.* **2020**, *88*. [CrossRef]
42. Lee, S.G.; Lee, S.J.; Lee, J.J.; Kim, J.S.; Lee, O.H.; Kim, C.K.; Kim, D.; Lee, Y.H.; Oh, J.; Park, S.; et al. Anti-inflammatory effect for atherosclerosis progression by sodium-glucose cotransporter 2 (SGLT-2) inhibitor in a normoglycemic rabbit model. *Korean Circ. J.* **2020**, *50*, 443–457. [CrossRef] [PubMed]

43. Xu, L.; Nagata, N.; Chen, G.; Nagashimada, M.; Zhuge, F.; Ni, Y.; Sakai, Y.; Kaneko, S.; Ota, T. Empagliflozin reverses obesity and insulin resistance through fat browning and alternative macrophage activation in mice fed a high-fat diet. *BMJ Open Diabetes Res. Care* **2019**, *7*, 1–11. [CrossRef]
44. Bode, D.; Semmler, L.; Wakula, P.; Hegemann, N.; Primessnig, U.; Beindorff, N.; Powell, D.; Dahmen, R.; Ruetten, H.; Oeing, C.; et al. Dual SGLT-1 and SGLT-2 inhibition improves left atrial dysfunction in HFpEF. *Cardiovasc. Diabetol.* **2021**, *20*, 1–14. [CrossRef]
45. Hasan, R.; Lasker, S.; Hasan, A.; Zerin, F.; Zamila, M. Canagliflozin ameliorates renal oxidative stress and inflammation by stimulating AMPK—Akt—eNOS pathway in the isoprenaline - induced oxidative stress model. *Sci. Rep.* **2020**, 1–15. [CrossRef] [PubMed]
46. Zaibi, N.; Li, P.; Xu, S.Z. Protective effects of dapagliflozin against oxidative stress-induced cell injury in human proximal tubular cells. *PLoS ONE* **2021**, *16*, 1–17. [CrossRef]
47. Iannantuoni, F.; De Marañon, A.M.; Diaz-morales, N.; Falcon, R.; Hernandez-mijares, A.; Rovira-llopis, S. The SGLT2 Inhibitor Empagliflozin Ameliorates the Inflammatory Profile in Type 2 Diabetic Patients and Promotes an Antioxidant Response in Leukocytes. *J. Clin. Med.* **2019**, *8*, 1814. [CrossRef]
48. Croteau, D.; Luptak, I.; Chambers, J.M.; Hobai, I.; Panagia, M.; Pimentel, D.R.; Siwik, D.A.; Qin, F.; Colucci, W.S. Effects of sodium-glucose linked transporter 2 inhibition with ertugliflozin on mitochondrial function, energetics, and metabolic gene expression in the presence and absence of diabetes mellitus in mice. *J. Am. Heart Assoc.* **2021**, *10*. [CrossRef] [PubMed]
49. Hayden, M.R.; Grant, D.G.; Aroor, A.R.; Demarco, V.G. Empagliflozin Ameliorates Type 2 Diabetes-Induced Ultrastructural Remodeling of the Neurovascular Unit and Neuroglia in the Female db/db Mouse. *Brain Sci.* **2019**, *9*, 57. [CrossRef] [PubMed]
50. Bdel-Latif, R.G.; Rifaai, R.A.; Amin, E.F. Empagliflozin alleviates neuronal apoptosis induced by cerebral ischemia/reperfusion injury through HIF-1α/VEGF signaling pathway. *Arch. Pharm. Res.* **2020**, *43*, 514–525. [CrossRef] [PubMed]
51. Zhou, J.; Zhu, J.; Yu, S.; Ma, H.; Chen, J.; Ding, X.; Chen, G.; Liang, Y.; Zhang, Q. Sodium-glucose co-transporter-2 (SGLT-2) inhibition reduces glucose uptake to induce breast cancer cell growth arrest through AMPK/mTOR pathway. *Biomed. Pharmacother.* **2020**, *132*, 110821. [CrossRef] [PubMed]
52. Sun, X.; Han, F.; Lu, Q.; Li, X.; Ren, D.; Zhang, J.; Han, Y.; Xiang, Y.K.; Li, J. Empagliflozin Ameliorates Obesity-Related Cardiac Dysfunction by Regulating Sestrin2-Mediated AMPK-mTOR Signaling and Redox Homeostasis in High-Fat Diet—Induced Obese Mice. *Diabetes* **2020**, *69*, 1292–1305. [CrossRef] [PubMed]
53. Moellmann, J.; Mann, P.; Krueger, K.; Klinkhammer, B.; Boor, P.; Marx, N.; Lehrke, M. The SGLT2 inhibitor ertugliflozin causes a switch of cardiac substrate utilization leading to reduced cardiac mTOR-signaling, unfolded protein response and apoptosis. *Eur. Heart J.* **2021**, *42*, 3289. [CrossRef]
54. Szekeres, Z.; Toth, K.; Szabados, E. The effects of sglt2 inhibitors on lipid metabolism. *Metabolites* **2021**, *11*, 87. [CrossRef] [PubMed]
55. Hamed, S.A. Atherosclerosis in epilepsy: Its causes and implications. *Epilepsy Behav.* **2014**, *41*, 290–296. [CrossRef]
56. Chiba, Y.; Sugiyama, Y.; Nishi, N.; Nonaka, W.; Murakami, R.; Ueno, M. Sodium/glucose cotransporter 2 is expressed in choroid plexus epithelial cells and ependymal cells in human and mouse brains. *Neuropathology* **2020**, *40*, 482–491. [CrossRef]
57. Pearson, A.; Ajoy, R.; Crynen, G.; Reed, J.M.; Algamal, M.; Mullan, M.; Purohit, D.; Crawford, F.; Ojo, J.O. Molecular abnormalities in autopsied brain tissue from the inferior horn of the lateral ventricles of nonagenarians and Alzheimer disease patients. *BMC Neurol.* **2020**, *20*, 1–20. [CrossRef] [PubMed]
58. Rizvi, S.; Shakil, S.; Biswas, D.; Shakil, S.; Shaikh, S.; Bagga, P.; Kamal, M. Invokana (Canagliflozin) as a Dual Inhibitor of Acetylcholinesterase and Sodium Glucose Co-Transporter 2: Advancement in Alzheimer's Disease- Diabetes Type 2 Linkage via an Enzoinformatics Study. *CNS Neurol. Disord.—Drug Targets* **2014**, *13*, 447–451. [CrossRef]
59. Behnammanesh, G.; Durante, Z.E.; Peyton, K.J.; Martinez-Lemus, L.A.; Brown, S.M.; Bender, S.B.; Durante, W. Canagliflozin inhibits human endothelial cell proliferation and tube formation. *Front. Pharmacol.* **2019**, *10*. [CrossRef] [PubMed]
60. Shaikh, S.; Rizvi, S.M.D.; Shakil, S.; Riyaz, S.; Biswas, D.; Jahan, R. Forxiga (dapagliflozin): Plausible role in the treatment of diabetes-associated neurological disorders. *Biotechnol. Appl. Biochem.* **2016**, *63*, 145–150. [CrossRef]
61. Ferreira-Vieira, H.T.; Guimaraes, M.I.; Silva, R.F.; Ribeiro, F.M. Alzheimer's disease: Targeting the Cholinergic System. *Curr. Neuropharmacol.* **2016**, *14*, 101–115. [CrossRef]
62. Arafa, N.M.S.; Ali, E.H.A.; Hassan, M.K. Canagliflozin prevents scopolamine-induced memory impairment in rats: Comparison with galantamine hydrobromide action. *Chem. Biol. Interact.* **2017**, *277*, 195–203. [CrossRef] [PubMed]
63. Bathina, S.; Das, U.N. Brain-derived neurotrophic factor and its clinical Implications. *Arch. Med. Sci.* **2015**, *11*, 1164–1178. [CrossRef] [PubMed]
64. Zhen, Y.F.; Zhang, J.; Liu, X.Y.; Fang, H.; Tian, L.B.; Zhou, D.H.; Kosten, T.R.; Zhang, X.Y. Low BDNF is associated with cognitive deficits in patients with type 2 diabetes. *Psychopharmacology* **2013**, *227*, 93–100. [CrossRef] [PubMed]
65. Bi, C.; Fu, Y.; Li, B. Brain-derived neurotrophic factor alleviates diabetes mellitus-accelerated atherosclerosis by promoting M2 polarization of macrophages through repressing the STAT3 pathway. *Cell. Signal.* **2020**, *70*, 109569. [CrossRef] [PubMed]
66. Bos, D.; Vernooij, M.W.; De Bruijn, R.F.A.G.; Koudstaal, P.J.; Hofman, A.; Franco, O.H.; Van Der Lugt, A.; Ikram, M.A. Atherosclerotic calcification is related to a higher risk of dementia and cognitive decline. *Alzheimer's Dement.* **2015**, *11*, 639–647.e1. [CrossRef] [PubMed]

67. Wingo, A.P.; Fan, W.; Duong, D.M.; Gerasimov, E.S.; Dammer, E.B.; Liu, Y.; Harerimana, N.V.; White, B.; Thambisetty, M.; Troncoso, J.C.; et al. Shared proteomic effects of cerebral atherosclerosis and Alzheimer's disease on the human brain. *Nat. Neurosci.* **2020**, *23*, 696–700. [CrossRef]
68. Sabia, S.; Fayosse, A.; Dumurgier, J.; Schnitzler, A.; Empana, J.P.; Ebmeier, K.P.; Dugravot, A.; Kivimäki, M.; Singh-Manoux, A. Association of ideal cardiovascular health at age 50 with incidence of dementia: 25 Year follow-up of Whitehall II cohort study. *BMJ* **2019**, *366*, 1–10. [CrossRef] [PubMed]
69. Liu, Z.; Ma, X.; Ilyas, I.; Zheng, X.; Luo, S.; Little, P.J.; Kamato, D.; Sahebkar, A.; Wu, W.; Weng, J.; et al. Impact of sodium glucose cotransporter 2 (SGLT2) inhibitors on atherosclerosis: From pharmacology to pre-clinical and clinical therapeutics. *Theranostics* **2021**, *11*, 4502–4515. [CrossRef] [PubMed]
70. O'Leary, D.H.; Polak, J.F.; Kronmal, R.A.; Manolio, T.A.; Burke, G.L.; Wolfson, S.K. Carotid-Artery Intima and Media Thickness as a Risk Factor for Myocardial Infarction and Stroke in Older Adults. *N. Engl. J. Med.* **1999**, *340*, 14–22. [CrossRef]
71. Feinkohl, I.; Keller, M.; Robertson, C.M.; Morling, J.R.; Williamson, R.M.; Nee, L.D.; McLachlan, S.; Sattar, N.; Welsh, P.; Reynolds, R.M.; et al. Clinical and subclinical macrovascular disease as predictors of cognitive decline in older patients with type 2 diabetes: The Edinburgh type 2 diabetes study. *Diabetes Care* **2013**, *36*, 2779–2786. [CrossRef]
72. Suridjan, I.; Pollock, B.G.; Verhoeff, N.P.L.G.; Voineskos, A.N.; Chow, T.; Rusjan, P.M.; Lobaugh, N.J.; Houle, S.; Mulsant, B.H.; Mizrahi, R. In-vivo imaging of grey and white matter neuroinflammation in Alzheimer's disease: A positron emission tomography study with a novel radioligand, "18 F"-FEPPA. *Mol. Psychiatry* **2015**, *20*, 1579–1587. [CrossRef] [PubMed]
73. Walker, K.A.; Ficek, B.N.; Westbrook, R. Understanding the Role of Systemic Inflammation in Alzheimer's Disease. *ACS Chem. Neurosci.* **2019**, *10*, 3340–3342. [CrossRef] [PubMed]
74. Walker, K.A.; Gottesman, R.F.; Wu, A.; Knopman, D.S.; Gross, A.L.; Mosley, T.H.; Selvin, E.; Windham, B.G. Systemic inflammation during midlife and cognitive change over 20 years: The ARIC Study. *Neurology* **2019**, *92*, E1256–E1267. [CrossRef] [PubMed]
75. Rochfort, K.D.; Cummins, P.M. The blood-brain barrier endothelium: A target for pro-inflammatory cytokines. *Biochem. Soc. Trans.* **2015**, *43*, 702–706. [CrossRef] [PubMed]
76. Vogels, T.; Murgoci, A.N.; Hromádka, T. Intersection of pathological tau and microglia at the synapse. *Acta Neuropathol. Commun.* **2019**, *7*, 109. [CrossRef]
77. Wang, W.Y.; Tan, M.S.; Yu, J.T.; Tan, L. Role of pro-inflammatory cytokines released from microglia in Alzheimer's disease. *Ann. Transl. Med.* **2015**, *3*, 1–15. [CrossRef]
78. Ridker, P.M.; Everett, B.M.; Thuren, T.; MacFadyen, J.G.; Chang, W.H.; Ballantyne, C.; Fonseca, F.; Nicolau, J.; Koenig, W.; Anker, S.D.; et al. Antiinflammatory Therapy with Canakinumab for Atherosclerotic Disease. *N. Engl. J. Med.* **2017**, *377*, 1119–1131. [CrossRef] [PubMed]
79. Rooks, M. G and Garrett, W.S, 2016 The Role of Cytokines in the Development of Atherosclerosis. *Biochemistry* **2016**, *176*, 1358–1370. [CrossRef]
80. Kelley, N.; Jeltema, D.; Duan, Y.; He, Y. The NLRP3 Inflammasome: An Overview of Mechanisms of Activation and Regulation. *Int. J. Mol. Sci.* **2019**, *20*, 3328. [CrossRef] [PubMed]
81. Jin, Y.; Fu, J. Novel Insights into the NLRP3 Inflammasome in Atherosclerosis. *J. Am. Heart Assoc.* **2019**, *8*, 1–12. [CrossRef]
82. Van Der Heijden, T.; Kritikou, E.; Venema, W.; Van Duijn, J.; Van Santbrink, P.J.; Slütter, B.; Foks, A.C.; Bot, I.; Kuiper, J. NLRP3 Inflammasome Inhibition by MCC950 Reduces Atherosclerotic Lesion Development in Apolipoprotein E–Deficient Mice—Brief Report. *Arterioscler. Thromb. Vasc. Biol.* **2017**, *37*, 1457–1461. [CrossRef] [PubMed]
83. Tejera, D.; Mercan, D.; Sanchez-caro, J.M.; Hanan, M.; Greenberg, D.; Soreq, H.; Latz, E.; Golenbock, D.; Heneka, M.T. Systemic inflammation impairs microglial A b clearance through NLRP 3 inflammasome. *EMBO J.* **2019**, *38*, e101064. [CrossRef] [PubMed]
84. Lonnemann, N.; Hosseini, S.; Marchetti, C.; Skouras, D.B.; Stefanoni, D.; D'Alessandro, A.; Dinarello, C.A.; Korte, M. The NLRP3 inflammasome inhibitor OLT1177 rescues cognitive impairment in a mouse model of Alzheimer's disease. *Proc. Natl. Acad. Sci. USA* **2020**, *117*, 32145–32154. [CrossRef] [PubMed]
85. Lathe, R.; Sapronova, A.; Kotelevtsev, Y. Atherosclerosis and Alzheimer—Diseases with a common cause? Inflammation, oxysterols, vasculature. *BMC Geriatr.* **2014**, *14*, 1–30. [CrossRef]
86. Barrett, T.J. Macrophages in Atherosclerosis Regression. *Arterioscler. Thromb. Vasc. Biol.* **2020**, *40*, 20–33. [CrossRef] [PubMed]
87. Zhang, Z.; Li, X.G.; Wang, Z.H.; Song, M.; Yu, S.P.; Kang, S.S.; Liu, X.; Zhang, Z.; Xie, M.; Liu, G.P.; et al. δ-Secretase-cleaved Tau stimulates Aβ production via upregulating STAT1-BACE1 signaling in Alzheimer's disease. *Mol. Psychiatry* **2021**, *26*, 586–603. [CrossRef]
88. Li, X.; Hong, X.; Wang, Y.; Zhang, S.; Zhang, J.; Li, X.; Liu, Y.; Sun, D.; Feng, Q.; Ye, J.; et al. Tau accumulation triggers STAT 1-dependent memory deficits by suppressing NMDA receptor expression. *EMBO Rep.* **2019**, *20*, 1–18. [CrossRef]
89. Lee, N.; Heo, Y.J.; Choi, S.E.; Jeon, J.Y.; Han, S.J.; Kim, D.J.; Kang, Y.; Lee, K.W.; Kim, H.J. Anti-inflammatory Effects of Empagliflozin and Gemigliptin on LPS-Stimulated Macrophage via the IKK/NF- κ B, MKK7/JNK, and JAK2/STAT1 Signalling Pathways. *J. Immunol. Res.* **2021**, *2021*. [CrossRef] [PubMed]
90. Faraco, G.; Sugiyama, Y.; Lane, D.; Garcia-Bonilla, L.; Chang, H.; Santisteban, M.M.; Racchumi, G.; Murphy, M.; Van Rooijen, N.; Anrather, J.; et al. Perivascular macrophages mediate the neurovascular and cognitive dysfunction associated with hypertension. *J. Clin. Invest.* **2016**, *126*, 4674–4689. [CrossRef] [PubMed]
91. He, H.; Mack, J.J.; Güç, E.; Warren, C.M.; Squadrito, M.L.; Kilarski, W.W.; Baer, C.; Freshman, R.D.; McDonald, A.I.; Ziyad, S.; et al. Perivascular Macrophages Limit Permeability. *Arterioscler. Thromb. Vasc. Biol.* **2016**, *36*, 2203–2212. [CrossRef] [PubMed]

92. Kerkhofs, D.; Van Hagen, B.T.; Milanova, I.V.; Schell, K.J.; Van Essen, H.; Wijnands, E.; Goossens, P.; Blankesteijn, W.M.; Unger, T.; Prickaerts, J.; et al. Pharmacological depletion of microglia and perivascular macrophages prevents Vascular Cognitive Impairment in Ang II-induced hypertension. *Theranostics* **2020**, *10*, 9512–9527. [CrossRef]
93. Mittal, M.; Siddiqui, M.R.; Tran, K.; Reddy, S.P.; Malik, A.B. Reactive Oxygen Species in Inflammation and Tissue Injury. *Antioxid. Redox Signal.* **2014**, *20*, 1126–1167. [CrossRef] [PubMed]
94. Zalba, G. Oxidative Stress in Vascular Pathophysiology: Still Much to Learn. *Antioxidants* **2021**, *10*, 673. [CrossRef] [PubMed]
95. Huang, W.E.N.J.; Zhang, X.I.A.; Chen, W.E.I.W.E.I. Role of oxidative stress in Alzheimer' s disease (Review). *Biomed. Rep.* **2016**, *4*, 519–522. [CrossRef]
96. Hajjar, I.; Hayek, S.S.; Goldstein, F.C.; Martin, G.; Jones, D.P.; Quyyumi, A. Oxidative stress predicts cognitive decline with aging in healthy adults: An observational study. *J. neuroinflammation* **2018**, *15*, 1–7. [CrossRef] [PubMed]
97. Yaribeygi, H.; Atkin, S.L.; Butler, A.E. Sodium—Glucose cotransporter inhibitors and oxidative stress: An update. *J. Cell. Physiol.* **2019**, *234*, 3231–3237. [CrossRef] [PubMed]
98. Cenini, G.; Voos, W. Mitochondria as potential targets in Alzheimer disease therapy: An update. *Front. Pharmacol.* **2019**, *10*, 1–20. [CrossRef]
99. Khacho, M.; Clark, A.; Svoboda, D.S.; MacLaurin, J.G.; Lagace, D.C.; Park, D.S.; Slack, R.S. Mitochondrial dysfunction underlies cognitive defects as a result of neural stem cell depletion and impaired neurogenesis. *Hum. Mol. Genet.* **2017**, *26*, 3327–3341. [CrossRef] [PubMed]
100. Sa-nguanmoo, P.; Tanajak, P.; Kerdphoo, S.; Jaiwongkam, T.; Pratchayasakul, W.; Chattipakorn, N.; Chattipakorn, S.C. SGLT2-inhibitor and DPP-4 inhibitor improve brain function via attenuating mitochondrial dysfunction, insulin resistance, inflammation, and apoptosis in HFD-induced obese rats. *Toxicol. Appl. Pharmacol.* **2017**, *333*, 43–50. [CrossRef] [PubMed]
101. Mao, Z.; Zhang, W. Role of mTOR in Glucose and Lipid Metabolism. *Int. J. Mol. Sci.* **2018**, *19*, 2043. [CrossRef] [PubMed]
102. Uddin, S.; Bin-jumah, M.N. Multifarious roles of mTOR signaling in cognitive aging and cerebrovascular dysfunction of Alzheimer' s disease. *Iubmb Life* **2020**, *72*, 1843–1855. [CrossRef] [PubMed]
103. Van Skike, C.E.; Galvan, V. A Perfect sTORm: The Role of the Mammalian Target of Rapamycin (mTOR) in Cerebrovascular Dysfunction of Alzheimer ' s Disease: A Mini-Review. *Gerontology* **2018**, *64*, 205–211. [CrossRef]
104. Esterline, R.; Oscarsson, J.; Burns, J. *International Review of Neurobiology*, 1st ed.; Elsevier Inc.: Amsterdam, The Netherlands, 2020; pp. 113–140.
105. Stanciu, G.D.; Rusu, R.N.; Bild, V.; Filipiuc, L.E.; Tamba, B.I.; Ababei, D.C. Systemic actions of sglt2 inhibition on chronic mtor activation as a shared pathogenic mechanism between alzheimer's disease and diabetes. *Biomedicines* **2021**, *9*, 576. [CrossRef] [PubMed]
106. Packer, M. SGLT2 inhibitors produce cardiorenal benefits by promoting adaptive cellular reprogramming to induce a state of fasting mimicry: A paradigm shift in understanding their mechanism of action. *Diabetes Care* **2020**, *43*, 508–511. [CrossRef] [PubMed]
107. Al Hamed, F.A.; Elewa, H. Potential Therapeutic Effects of Sodium Glucose-linked Cotransporter 2 Inhibitors in Stroke. *Clin. Ther.* **2020**, *42*, e242–e249. [CrossRef]
108. Yan, C.; Zhou, Y.; Chen, Q.; Luo, Y.; Zhang, J.H.; Huang, H.; Shao, A. Dysfunction of the neurovascular unit in diabetes-related neurodegeneration. *Biomed. Pharmacother.* **2020**, *131*, 110656. [CrossRef]
109. Shabir, O.; Berwick, J.; Francis, S.E. Neurovascular dysfunction in vascular dementia, Alzheimer' s and atherosclerosis. *BMC Neurosci.* **2018**, *19*, 1–16. [CrossRef]
110. Liu, J.; Zhu, Y.; Wu, Y.; Liu, Y.; Teng, Z.; Hao, Y. Association of carotid atherosclerosis and recurrent cerebral infarction in the Chinese population: A meta-analysis. *Neuropsychiatr Dis Treat.* **2017**, *13*, 527–533. [CrossRef]
111. Sun, J.; Tan, L.; Yu, J. Post-stroke cognitive impairment: Epidemiology, mechanisms and management. *Ann. Transl. Med.* **2014**, *2*. [CrossRef]
112. Usman, M.S.; Siddiqi, T.J.; Memon, M.M.; Khan, M.S.; Rawasia, W.F.; Talha Ayub, M.; Sreenivasan, J.; Golzar, Y. Sodium-glucose co-transporter 2 inhibitors and cardiovascular outcomes: A systematic review and meta-analysis. *Eur. J. Prev. Cardiol.* **2018**, *25*, 495–502. [CrossRef] [PubMed]
113. Wajngarten, M.; Sampaio Silva, G. Hypertension and stroke: Update on treatment. *Eur. Cardiol. Rev.* **2019**, *14*, 111–115. [CrossRef] [PubMed]
114. Briasoulis, A.; Al Dhaybi, O.; Bakris, G.L. SGLT2 Inhibitors and Mechanisms of Hypertension. *Curr. Cardiol. Rep.* **2018**, *20*, 8–10. [CrossRef] [PubMed]
115. Ishida, N.; Saito, M.; Sato, S.; Koepsell, H.; Taira, E.; Hirose, M. SGLT1 participates in the development of vascular cognitive impairment in a mouse model of small vessel disease. *Neurosci. Lett.* **2020**, *727*, 134929. [CrossRef] [PubMed]
116. Yamazaki, Y.; Harada, S.; Wada, T.; Hagiwara, T.; Yoshida, S.; Tokuyama, S. Sodium influx through cerebral sodium-glucose transporter type 1 exacerbates the development of cerebral ischemic neuronal damage. *Eur. J. Pharmacol.* **2017**. [CrossRef] [PubMed]
117. Sim, A.Y.; Barua, S.; Kim, J.Y.; Lee, Y.H.; Lee, J.E. Role of DPP-4 and SGLT2 Inhibitors Connected to Alzheimer Disease in Type 2 Diabetes Mellitus. *Front. Neurosci.* **2021**, *15*, 1–11. [CrossRef]

118. Langbaum, J.B.S.; Chen, K.; Lee, W.; Reschke, C.; Bandy, D.; Fleisher, A.S.; Alexander, G.E.; Foster, N.L.; Weiner, M.W.; Koeppe, R.A.; et al. Categorical and correlational analyses of baseline fluorodeoxyglucose positron emission tomography images from the Alzheimer's Disease Neuroimaging Initiative (ADNI). *Neuroimage* **2009**, *45*, 1107–1116. [CrossRef] [PubMed]
119. Anthony, K.; Reed, L.J.; Dunn, J.T.; Bingham, E.; Hopkins, D.; Marsden, P.K.; Amiel, S.A. The Cerebral Basis for Impaired Control of Food Intake in. *Diabetes* **2006**, *55*, 2986–2992. [CrossRef]
120. Hernandez, F.; Lucas, J.J.; Avila, J. GSK3 and tau: Two convergence points in Alzheimer's disease. *J. Alzheimer's Dis.* **2013**, *33*, 141–144. [CrossRef]
121. Inaba, Y.; Hashiuchi, E.; Watanabe, H.; Kimura, K.; Sato, M.; Kobayashi, M.; Matsumoto, M.; Kitamura, T.; Kasuga, M.; Inoue, H. Hepatic Gluconeogenic Response to Single and Long-Term SGLT2 Inhibition in Lean/Obese Male Hepatic G6pc-Reporter Mice. *Endocrinology* **2019**, *160*, 2811–2824. [CrossRef]

molecules

MDPI

Review

Current Modulation of Guanylate Cyclase Pathway Activity—Mechanism and Clinical Implications

Grzegorz Grześk [1] and Alicja Nowaczyk [2,*]

1 Department of Cardiology and Clinical Pharmacology, Faculty of Health Sciences, Ludwik Rydygier Collegium Medicum in Bydgoszcz, Nicolaus Copernicus University in Toruń, 75 Ujejskiego St., 85-168 Bydgoszcz, Poland; g.grzesk@cm.umk.pl

2 Department of Organic Chemistry, Faculty of Pharmacy, Ludwik Rydygier Collegium Medicum in Bydgoszcz, Nicolaus Copernicus University in Toruń, 2 dr. A. Jurasza St., 85-094 Bydgoszcz, Poland

* Correspondence: alicja@cm.umk.pl; Tel.: +48-52-585-3904

Abstract: For years, guanylate cyclase seemed to be homogenic and tissue nonspecific enzyme; however, in the last few years, in light of preclinical and clinical trials, it became an interesting target for pharmacological intervention. There are several possible options leading to an increase in cyclic guanosine monophosphate concentrations. The first one is related to the uses of analogues of natriuretic peptides. The second is related to increasing levels of natriuretic peptides by the inhibition of degradation. The third leads to an increase in cyclic guanosine monophosphate concentration by the inhibition of its degradation by the inhibition of phosphodiesterase type 5. The last option involves increasing the concentration of cyclic guanosine monophosphate by the additional direct activation of soluble guanylate cyclase. Treatment based on the modulation of guanylate cyclase function is one of the most promising technologies in pharmacology. Pharmacological intervention is stable, effective and safe. Especially interesting is the role of stimulators and activators of soluble guanylate cyclase, which are able to increase the enzymatic activity to generate cyclic guanosine monophosphate independently of nitric oxide. Moreover, most of these agents are effective in chronic treatment in heart failure patients and pulmonary hypertension, and have potential to be a first line option.

Keywords: guanylate cyclase (GC); chronic heart failure (CHF); pulmonary arterial hypertension (PAH)

Citation: Grześk, G.; Nowaczyk, A. Current Modulation of Guanylate Cyclase Pathway Activity—Mechanism and Clinical Implications. *Molecules* **2021**, *26*, 3418. https://doi.org/10.3390/molecules26113418

Academic Editor: Jan Brezovsky

Received: 22 April 2021
Accepted: 2 June 2021
Published: 4 June 2021

1. Introduction

Since the beginning of the 21st century, the treatment of metabolic disturbances-related diseases of the cardiovascular system has become deeper. Previously, the target of treatment was rather clinical, whereas now, the clinical answer is important but the tools have changed; now, they are generally metabolic. For years, GCs had seemed to be an homogenic and tissue nonspecific enzyme, whereas within the last few years, in light of preclinical and clinical trials, it became an interesting an target for pharmacological intervention. This review will focus on the role of direct and indirect modulation of guanylate cyclases in cardiovascular pharmacology.

2. Guanylate Cyclases

In mammals, there are two key types of guanylate cyclases (GC), classified according to localization of enzymes in the cell. The first is called guanylate cyclase-coupled receptor or membrane-bound guanylate cyclase (mGC). The second is completely intracellular, soluble (sGC). Agonists for mGC are peptides, such as natriuretic peptides type A, B, C, whereas for sGC, they are gaseous mediators, such as nitric oxide and carbon monoxide [1].

In detail, there are four soluble guanylate cyclase subunits, marked $\alpha 1$, $\alpha 2$, $\beta 1$ and $\beta 2$, and transmembrane forms named with consecutive letters of the alphabet, from A to G (Table 1). Dimer is a typical and minimal form of catalytic unit [2,3]. Transmembrane forms exist as homodimers, whereas soluble forms are heterodimers. One of the mGCs, type C, seems to be different—homotrimer [2–5].

Table 1. Guanylyl cyclases: activators, tissue expression and physiological effects.

Guanylyl Cyclase	Tissue Expression	Physiological Activator	Key Effects
Soluble α1	Cardiovascular system, platelets, brain	NO, CO	Vasodilation, angiogenesis, inhibition of platelet aggregation
Soluble α2	Cardiovascular system, brain	NO, CO	Vasodilation, angiogenesis
Soluble β1	Cardiovascular system, platelets, brain	NO, CO	Vasodilation, angiogenesis inhibition of platelet aggregation, intestinal motility
Soluble β2	Gastrointestinal tract, liver, kidney	NO, CO	Apoptosis, inhibition of anti-apoptotic endothelin pathway
GC-A	Cardiovascular system (vascular smooth muscle, heart), lung, kidney, adrenal, adipose tissue	ANP, BNP	Vasodilation, angiogenesis, regulation of hypertrophy, remodeling processes
GC-B	Cardiovascular system (vascular smooth muscle, endothelium, heart), lung, bone, brain, liver, uterus, follicle	CNP	Vasodilation, angiogenesis. regulation of hypertrophy, remodeling processes, cartilage homeostasis and endochondral bone formation, regulation of female fertility
GC-C	Intestinal epithelium	Guanylin, uroguanylin and bacterial heat-stable enterotoxin	Regulation of colonic epithelial cell proliferation
GC-D	Olfactory bulb	Guanylin, uroguanylin, CO_2/HCO_3	guanylin- and uroguanylin-dependent olfactory signaling, food and odor preference response (mices)
GC-E	Retina, pineal gland	guanylyl cyclase activator proteins	Vision process
GC-F	Retina	guanylyl cyclase activator proteins	Vision process
GC-G	Olfactory bulb, lung, intestine, skeletal muscle, testes	Pheromones, CO_2/HCO_3	detection of the volatile alarm pheromones, kidney, ischemia/reperfusion preconditioning

Soluble GCs (Figure 1, EC 4.6.1.2) were found in many different tissues, especially brain, cardiovascular system, kidney and lungs [5]. All four units—α1, α2, β1 and β2—were identified in humans. At the amino acid level, the α1 subunit found in humans is about 34% identical to the β1 subunit, whereas the α2 subunit is 48% homologous to the α1 subunit [6–8]. Experiments performed on mice suggest that α1 is the major subunit in platelets and lungs. Meanwhile, α2 subunits are responsible for about 6% of activity of sGCs in vasculature, but in response to NO in mice, lacking α1 is sufficient to achieve maximal vascular smooth muscle relaxation [8]. Further, β1 contains several interesting binding domains, such as about 200 residues in the aminoterminal heme prosthetic group and about 250 residues of carboxyl-terminal GC domain. In this condition, compared to the β1 isoform, β2 subunit has an additional 86 carboxyl-terminal amino acids sequence for isoprenylation or carboxymethylation [9]. The relation between sCG and hemoglobin is interesting. The β1 subunit is the axial ligand of the pentacoordinated reduced iron center of heme. The binding place, His-105, is located at the amino terminus of the β1 subunit (Figure 1). This kind of binding is necessary for both NO- and CO-dependent activation. NO binds to the heme ring at sixth position. It breaks the bond between the iron and axial histidine to form a five-coordinated ring with NO in the fifth position. sGC can be activated by other gaseous mediator CO, but it binds heme to form a six-coordinated complex [10]. This interaction can partially explain the hyperreactivity of vascular smooth muscle after blood transfusions. Disruption of β1 subunit leads to significant reduction in NO-dependent vascular relaxation and platelet aggregation, whereas disruption of α1 subunit leads to loss of platelet aggregation only. The male mice lacking β1 subunit are infertile. Homozygous knockout animals presented gastrointestinal obstruction similar to the cGMP dependent protein kinase G (PKG). Molecular studies suggest that sGC is one of the most important enzymes in the cardiovascular system and targets for possible pharmacological intervention. Increased vascular resistance in cases with reduced NO bioavailability secondary to the endothelial damage can be effectively bypassed by direct intervention at the sGC level. Mergia et al. [8] confirmed that GC activation is sufficient to mediate vasorelaxation not only at higher NO concentrations, but by direct enzyme stimulation. The results of study presented by Wedel et al. suggested that mutation of six conserved histidine residues reduced—but did not abolish—nitric oxide stimulation, whereas a change of His-105 to phenylalanine in the beta 1 subunit yielded a heterodimer that retained basal cyclase activity but failed to respond to nitric oxide supporting thesis that direct activation can be more effective option than heme-related intervention [10]. The results presented by Friebe et al. confirmed the crucial role of sGC as a receptor for NO in different smooth muscle reactivity related settings [11]. The loss of cGMP-dependent protein kinase I abolishes nitric oxide dependent relaxation of smooth muscle, resulting in severe vascular and intestinal dysfunctions confirming role of sGC pathway in relaxation of smooth muscle [12], especially signalling pathway mediated by IP3 receptor associated cGMP-dependent protein kinase type I substrate which is highly expressed in smooth muscle of cardiovascular and gastrointestinal tissue is essential for smooth muscle relaxation by NO/cGMP and ANP/cGMP [13]. The GC pathway, especially sGC, is crucial enzyme mediating relaxation of different types of smooth muscles [14,15]; thus, it is a very interesting target for achieving therapeutic goals, especially in diseases secondary to atherosclerosis process with common endothelial dysfunction and decreased NO bioavailability.

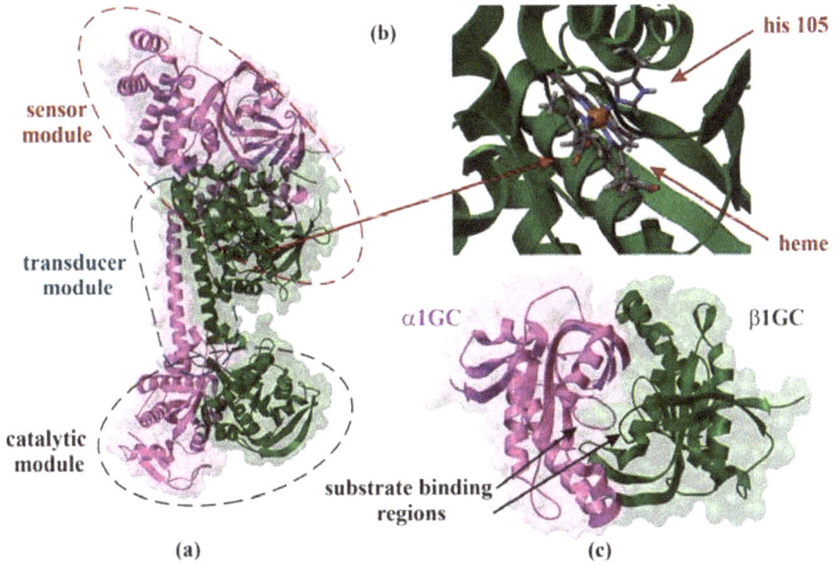

Figure 1. X-ray structure of soluble guanylate cyclase (sGC). Domain organization of the human α1β1GC heterodimer (PDB ID: 6JT1, 3.9 Å) (**a**) [16], interaction side view between heme and histidine 105 (his 105) (**b**) and α1β1GC catalytic domains that resembles the Chinese yin-yang symbol with both subunits arranged in a head-to-tail conformation (PDB ID: 4NI2, 1.9 Å) (**c**) [17].

Guanylate cyclase-coupled receptors (mGC) are activated by peptides such as atrial natriuretic peptides (NP). The first type of mGC is called GC-A and is activated by NP type A (ANP) and B (BNP). The lack of ANP stimulation leads to cardiovascular hypertrophy with hypertensive vessel response, whereas isolated BNP deficiency is a situation leading to hypertrophy without hyperreactivity of vascular smooth muscle cells [18–21]. GC type B (GC-B) is activated by NP type C (CNP). Structurally, it is similar to the GC-A, but predominantly localized in bone and ovary tissue make the key actions in stimulation of endochondral ossification required for long bone growth and oocyte maturation. Because of its localization in the cardiovascular system, smooth muscle cells and fibroblasts GC-B seem to be one of the most important mGCs in heart failure [18,22–28]. GC type C is activated by different peptide agonists: guanylin and uroguanylin. GC-C present on apical membrane of epithelial cells is a target for heat stable enterotoxins leading by elevation of intracellular cGMP concentration and PKG-dependent phosphorylation of the cystic fibrosis transmembrane regulator to increased Cl^- secretion in gut [29]. An animal model of mice lacking functional GC-C resistance to heat stable endotoxin (Salmonella enterica serovar Typhimurium) was found [30]. Inhibition of guanylin stimulation increased colonic epithelial cell proliferation with no influence on vessel smooth muscle cells contractility and sodium excretion. In this condition, uroguanylin signaling inhibition decreased the ability to excrete an enteral sodium and chlorides ions load and induced salt-independent hypertension [31,32]. The influence on the process of epithelial cells proliferation seems to be a possible therapeutic target, i.e., in the treatment of colon cancer [29,33,34]. Type D of GC was found in the olfactory system. GC-D can be activated by peptides guanylin and uroguanylin, but not heat stable enterotoxins and additionally by carbon dioxide and bicarbonate. In mice, GC-D participates in food preference response [35–37]. GCs type E and F are involved in the process of producing vision. Both types are expressed in retina and GC-E additionally in pineal gland. Inactivation of enzymes leads to rod and cone dystrophy and blindness [38,39]. GC-G was found in rat small intestine. The structure is similar to NP receptors, but elevation of activity of GC was not dependent on ANP, BNP, CNP and heat stable enterotoxins. Some authors suggest bicarbonate as an activator [40]. In mice, GC-G serves as an unusual receptor in Grueneberg ganglion of the anterior nasal region neurons mediating the detection of the volatile alarm pheromones especially substance 2-sec-butyl-4,5-dihydrothiazole [41,42].

Animal studies suggested the significant role of modulation of GC function in pathogenesis of diseases especially of the cardiovascular system, intestinal, skeletal, visual system and fertility. There are some possibilities of pharmacological intervention. An increase in the activity of GC may be achieved directly or indirectly. Direct pharmacological intervention is the simplest way to modify receptor or enzyme answers. sGCs can be activated by NO or NO donors such as sodium nitroprusside; thus, modulation of vascular smooth muscle reactivity was used in different clinical settings such as arterial hypertension and pulmonary arterial hypertension (PAH) to achieve rapid blood pressure stabilization in heart failure patients. This pathway of the modulation of vessel function was effective for different contraction models [43–45] and different clinical settings [46–50]. In this condition, the source of NO can be nitric oxide produced by nitric oxide synthase or drug and, thus, exogenous NO or NO-donor.

The key molecule in this system is cGMP. The produced cGMP is responsible for numerous effects in cells. Most of them are guided by PKG pathway. Activation of PKG is responsible for the activation of myosin phosphatase, which, in turn, leads to the release of calcium from intracellular stores in smooth muscle cells, finally leading to vascular smooth muscle relaxation. Phosphorylation by the PKG of vasodilator-stimulated phosphoprotein (VASP) is responsible for the decrease in platelet activation level and the activation of a number of transcription factors which can lead to changes in gene expression, which, in turn, can alter the response of the cell to a variety of stimuli [12–15].

3. NO Production

Nitric oxide synthase is an enzyme that catalyzes the synthesis of nitric oxide in two different steps. The first one is the oxidation of L-arginine to Nω-hydroxy-L-arginine; then, the substrate under the influence of NOS and oxygen is decomposed into L-citrulline, accompanied by the release of nitric oxide from vascular endothelial cells. Three basic types of nitric oxide synthase have been distinguished, now called NOS-1, NOS-2 and NOS-3. In the recently used nomenclature, they were designated NOS-1: nNOS (neuronal NOS), NOS-2: iNOS (inducible NOS) and NOS-3: eNOS (endothelial NOS), respectively. Type 1 synthase is localized primarily in the central and peripheral nervous system, skeletal muscles, pancreatic islets, endometrium and nephron dense macula. The basic physiological tasks of NOS-1 include modulating nerve transmission and regulating the function of the nephron or regulating intestinal peristalsis. Nitric oxide produced by NOS-1 can also act as a neurotransmitter, especially in the vegetative system known as non-adrenergic non-cholinergic (NANC). Type 2 synthase is located mainly in macrophages, cardiac striated muscle cells, liver, smooth muscle and vascular endothelium, and is synthesized as part of the response to infection, inflammation or sepsis, under the influence of inflammatory cytokines (mainly interleukin-1, interferon-γ or TNF-α). The activated enzyme remains active for several hours, synthesizing significant amounts of nitric oxide [51]. Nitric oxide produced by NOS-3 plays primarily a role as a regulator of muscle tone in the local vascular endothelial-vascular muscular system. It is also a factor that inhibits the adhesion and aggregation of platelets and angiogenesis. The role of NOS-3, as an element initiating the activation of NOS-2 under the influence of lipopolysaccharides, is emphasized. In experimental studies on the hyporeactivity of vessels treated with lipopolysaccharides, it was suggested that synthase located in the vascular endothelium was involved as the first link in the development of vascular hyporeactivity in sepsis [46]. In studies on isolated animal tissues exposed to short exposure to lipopolysaccharides, a statistically significant inhibition of NOS-2 expression was demonstrated in the case of a previous blockage of NOS-3 activity. Such results suggest that nitric oxide synthesized by NOS-3 may be a mediator of inflammation in sepsis [52] and confirmed results presented by Grześk in 2001 [46] and 2003 [48]. The results confirm the results of subsequent experiments, which showed that the lack of NOS-3 prevents from full expression of NOS-2 in the presence of lipopolysaccharides, which suggests that in the pathogenesis of sepsis there is primary activation of NOS-3, followed by the released nitric oxide being a pro-inflammatory stimulus for expression NOS 2 [53].

4. Pharmacological Intervention

There are several possible options leading to increase in cGMP concentrations. The first one is related to the use of analogues of ANP and BNP. The second is the increasing ANP and BNP by inhibition of degradation of peptides. The third one leads to increase in cGMP concentration by inhibition of its degradation by inhibition of phosphodiesterase type 5. The last option is the increasing concentration of cGMP by additional direct activation of sGC (Figure 2).

At the clinical level, pharmacological intervention seems to be dedicated for all clinical settings with low bioavailability of nitric oxide. In clinical medicine, there is a huge family of diseases with a vascular endothelium as one of the core symptoms. The depressed GC-pathway signaling is common in a family of atherosclerosis related diseases such as coronary artery disease, heart failure and hypertension, but also diabetes and hypercholesterolemia. It explains why side effects are very rare during the stimulation of this pathway, but, if are they present, are related to the overstimulation in non-target tissues. The overproduction of NO is seen especially in acute diseases such as septic shock. The common side effects are low blood pressure, blurred vision, confusion, dizziness, faintness or lightheadedness when getting up suddenly from a lying or sitting position, pale skin, sweating, trouble breathing, unusual bleeding or bruising, unusual tiredness or weakness.

On the other hand, the predominant therapeutic effect for all studies and all therapeutic pathways is the same: to decrease mortality, hospitalization rate and increase quality of life.

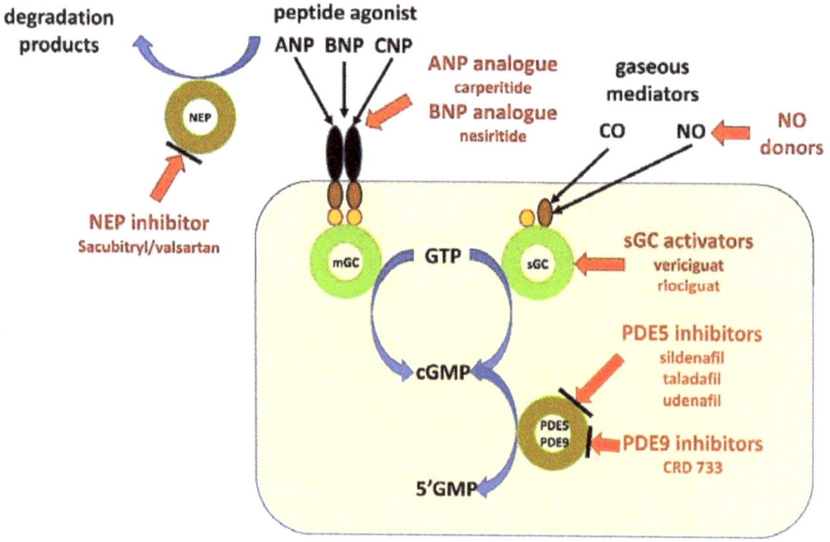

Figure 2. Schematic illustration of pharmacological intervention in guanylate cyclase/cyclic GMP pathway. Guanylate cyclase-coupled receptor, membrane-bound guanylyl cyclase (mGC); soluble guanylate cyclase (sGC); natriuretic peptides type A, B and C (ANP, BNP and CNP); neprilysin (NEP); gaseous mediators–nitric oxide (NO) and carbon monoxide (CO); cyclic guanosine monophosphate (cGMP); guanosine triphosphate (GTP); guanosine monophosphate (GMP); phosphodiesterase type x (PDEx).

4.1. Natriuretic Peptides Analogues

According to the current guidelines, pharmacological intervention with NO or NO-donors as stimulators of sGC are considered only for short-time actions, whereas in chronic treatment, these are not recommended [54–56]. What is interesting is the possibility of activation of mGC, located in cells of the cardiovascular system; thus, types activated by NPs type A, B and C GC-A and GC-B can be stimulated by physiological agonists, ANP, BNP and CNP, but with the analogs too. The first attempt at this kind of intervention was made after the discovery of analogues of NPs: carperitide, analogue of ANP and nesiritide, an analogue of BNP. Carperitide is a recombinant α-human atrial natriuretic peptide, leading to vasodilation. It is indicated for the treatment of patients with acute heart failure (including acute exacerbation of chronic heart failure). Moreover, carperitide was approved by the Pharmaceuticals and Medical Devices Agency of Japan (PMDA). Nesiritide is the recombinant form of BNP. Nesiritide works to facilitate cardiovascular fluid homeostasis through the counterregulation of the renin–angiotensin–aldosterone system, stimulating cGMP, leading to smooth muscle cell relaxation. Both mechanisms were important in the prevention of progression in the exacerbation of heart failure and chronic kidney disease. Nesiritide was investigated as a pharmacological agent indicated in acute decompensated congestive heart failure. It was registered in the United States Food and Drug Administration (FDA) for this purpose in 2001 after initial non-approval. Mitaka et al. [57] analyzed the risk of cardiovascular and renal effects of carperitide and nesiritide for preventing and treating acute kidney injury in cardiovascular surgery patients. A meta-analysis showed that carperitide infusion significantly decreased peak serum creatinine levels, incidence of arrhythmia and renal replacement therapy. The meta-analysis also showed that carperitide or nesiritide infusion significantly decreased the length of intensive care unit stay and hospital stay vs. controls. The authors concluded that NP treatment is an interesting option to preserve postoperative renal function in cardiovascular surgery patients [57]. Sezai et al. [58] investigated the efficacy of carperitide treatment for high-risk patients undergoing coronary artery bypass grafting (CABG). In a randomized controlled trial of 367 high-risk patients undergoing CABG, the primary endpoint was major adverse cardiovascular and cerebrovascular events. There was no significant difference in survival between the carpetide and placebo groups ($p = 0.1651$), but no patient from the carperitide group started hemodialysis after operation, but 7 patients did in the placebo group and the dialysis rate was significantly lower in the carperitide group ($p = 0.0147$). Serum creatinine and BNP were also significantly lower in the carperitide group at 1 year postoperatively. The authors concluded that in the early postoperative period, carperitide has a cardiorenal protective effect that prevents postoperative cardiovascular and cerebrovascular events and hemodialysis. Perioperative low-dose carperitide infusion was found useful in high-risk patients undergoing on-pump CABG [58]. Zhao et al. [59] prepared a meta-analysis of the efficacy and safety of nesiritide in patients with acute myocardial infarction and heart failure. The results of trials involving 870 participants were included in the meta-analysis. Nesiritide treatment significantly increased left ventricular ejection fraction, cardiac index and 24 and 72 h urine volumes. Additionally, pulmonary capillary wedge pressure, right atrial pressure and BNP and N-terminal brain natriuretic peptide (NT-proBNP) levels were significantly decreased in patients treated with nesiritide, compared with those treated with control drugs ("control drugs" were optimal pharmacotherapy according to guidelines). The authors concluded that nesiritide appeared to improve cardiac function and, moreover, was safe for patients [59]. The results of large clinical trials presented by O'Conor et al. in 2011 failed to show a difference between nesiritide and placebo on mortality or rehospitalization rate in this group of patients [60]. Other studies suggest that protective effect is non-significant or borderline [61]; thus, large placebo-controlled studies must be performed to clarify the role of these agents in clinical medicine.

Therapeutic stimulation with analogues of NP is interesting, but, unfortunately, in all performed studies, populations were rather small and not homogenous. The multifactor etiology of heart failure can explain why the presented results were different. All the studies confirmed the safety of that therapeutic option and its efficacy in laboratory and echocardiographic parameters describing disease progress, highly suggesting that this therapeutic option must be considered. To clearly describe the parameters such as mortality and hospitalizations rate, large placebo-controlled studies must be performed to describe the role of NPs analogues in the treatment of heart failure.

4.2. Inhibition of Neprilysin

The second therapeutic option is the inhibition of degradation of NPs into inactive metabolites; thus, real tissue concentration becomes higher. Neprilysin (NEP, EC 3.4.24.11) is key enzyme responsible for degradation of vasoactive peptides, such as ANP, BNP and CNP, but also adrenomedullin, angiotensin I and II, bradykinin and vasoactive intestinal peptide. Some of these peptides, i.e., NPs or bradykinin, are responsible for vascular tone regulation and modulation of remodeling in cardiovascular system, especially in heart failure. The spectrum of NEP actions is wider and includes peptides involved in neurodegenerative diseases (i.e., amyloid β, neurotensin), inflammation processes (i.e., neurokinin A, calcitonin gene-related peptide), mitomitogenesis, angiogenesis and hypothalamic-pituary axis. McMurray et al. [62] published results of the PARADIGM-HF trial. The study drug, sacubitril/valsartan, was compared to the standard according to the current guidelines of therapy, including enalapril and angiotensin converting enzyme inhibitor. The study was a prospective, randomized, double-blind trial of 9,419 patients with NYHA class II-IV, heart failure and reduced left ventricular ejection fraction, with confirmation by elevated NP levels. The key exclusion criteria included symptomatic hypotension, SBP < 100 mm Hg, serum potassium >5.2 mmol/L, eGFR < 30 mL/min or a history of angioedema. The trial concluded early after meeting a pre-specified stopping point for compelling clinical benefit.

After a median follow-up of 27 months, the sacubitril/valsartan group of patients had a 20% reduction in the combined endpoint of cardiovascular death or HF hospitalization. All-cause mortality was also significantly lower in the valsartan/sacubitril group (17% vs. 19.8%) [62]. Clinical beneficial effect is predominantly dependent on ANP increase and partially BNP, whereas there are no changes in CNP levels [63,64]. Meta-analysis from clinical trials suggest the presence of a beneficial effect only in patients with reduced EF, whereas in patients with EF > 45%, the effect is not significant [65,66]. Additional beneficial effects were present during dual path treatment including NEP inhibition and angiotensin converting enzyme [67]. The benefits of the treatment are partially dose-dependent. Patients with dose reduction effects were similar to the target dose group [68]. According to the current guidelines of the European Society of Cardiology, the top target is the treatment of heart failure with reduced ejection fraction patients. The spectrum of sacubitril action is much wider and includes the possibility of arterial hypertension treatment [69] and treatment of chronic kidney disease, especially in heart failure subjects [70]. Moreover, recently, a drug was approved by the FDA for the treatment of heart failure with preserved ejection fraction. In animal models, NEP plays a role in pathogenesis of several amyloid deposition diseases such as age-related macular degeneration, cerebral amyloid angiopathy or sensorimotor axonal polyneuropathy. As heart failure is a disease affecting elderly groups, neurological benefits are valuable [71,72]. Studies performed with NEP inhibitors clearly presented the relation between benefits and side effects. Pharmacological intervention was very effective and safe; thus, NEP inhibitors became one of key groups in the treatment of heart failure with a high possibility of an increase in their role in next guidelines.

Currently, NEP inhibition represents a powerful therapeutic tool in treating chronic heart failure, but data suggest a potential role for the use of that pathway in a broader spectrum of cardiovascular and non-cardiovascular disease.

4.3. *Inhibition of Phosphodiesterases*

In humans, three PDEs are selective and involved in cGMP actions. There are PDE5 located especially in cardiovascular system, PDE6 found in the retina and PDE9 present in heart muscle and brain. In this condition, modulation of PDE5 and PDE9 function is interesting as a cardiovascular therapeutic option [73–75].

The family of PDE5 inhibitors was discovered as a drug for heart failure treatment. The key metabolic path was related to an increase in cGMP concentration, as PDE5 is responsible for specific cGMP degradation. Currently, PDE5 inhibitors are an important therapeutic option in the treatment of pulmonary hypertension and their concentration is the highest in pulmonary circulation. PDE5 inhibitors are effective in the treatment of pulmonary arterial hypertension, both primary and associated with systemic connective tissue disease, in adults and children [76–79]. Pulmonary arterial hypertension is characterized by a reduction in the production of NO in the endothelium with a simultaneous increase in the expression and activity of PDE type 5 in smooth muscle cells of the pulmonary arteries [76]. In the SUPER study (Sildenafil Use in Pulmonary Arterial Hypertension), 12 week treatment with sildenafil in 278 patients with pulmonary arterial hypertension in WHO functional class II or III compared to placebo was associated with an extension of 6 min walk distance and a decrease in pulmonary vascular resistance [80]. Similar properties were also demonstrated by tadalafil, which was confirmed in the PHIRST (Pulmonary Arterial Hypertension and Response to Tadalafil) study [81]. According to the current guidelines of pharmacotherapy with PDE5 inhibitors is cornerstone of pulmonary hypertension therapy [77,78]. In heart failure with reduced ejection fraction, there are only some small clinical trials. A hemodynamic effect was confirmed. Sildenafil decreased both resting and stress pulmonary pressure, pulmonary resistance, increased cardiac index, right ventricle ejection fraction and improved peak oxygen consumption [82]. Unfortunately, PDE5 were not effective in the treatment of heart failure with preserved ejection fraction [83]. Some studies and case reports describe the effectiveness of PDE5 before and after heart transplant in patients with pulmonary hypertension secondary to left ventricle heart failure [84]. PDE5 inhibitors, by stimulating the GCs pathways, show a relatively selective vasodilator activity to the pulmonary arteries, and thus are one of the basic groups used in pharmacotherapy of pulmonary hypertension. Moreover, they can reverse their pathological remodeling and directly increase the contractility of the overloaded right ventricle. Although data from clinical trials are limited, it appears that these drugs may become an attractive and clinically beneficial therapeutic option for patients with heart failure and secondary pulmonary hypertension.

PDE9 inhibition increases cGMP signaling and attenuates stress-induced hypertrophic heart disease in preclinical studies. In the mouse transverse aortic constriction pressure overload heart failure model, a PDE9 inhibitor, CRD-733 treatment reversed existing LV hypertrophy, significantly improved left ventricle ejection fraction and attenuated left atrial dilation. CRD-733 prevented elevations in left ventricle end diastolic pressures [85]. These findings support future investigation into the therapeutic potential of CRD-733 in human heart failure [85–87]. Inhibition of brain PDE9 may improve synaptic plasticity, behavior; thus, PDE9 inhibitors have been advanced into initial clinical studies to assess the potential to improve cognitive function in patients with Alzheimer's disease and schizophrenia [75,88].

The inhibition of PDE5 is commonly used as an element in multi-compound therapy of pulmonary hypertension and impotence, whereas historically, the primary target, treatment of heart failure due to side effects, failed because of low tissue selectivity in the cardiovascular system. In this condition, due to localization inside heart muscle cells and the brain, pharmacotherapy with novel PDE9 inhibitors seems to be very promising not only in cardiology, but in geriatrics too. According to the results of first studies, there is a huge chance for an effective and safe therapeutic option for both heart failure and dementia patients.

4.4. Direct Activation of Soluble Guanylate Cyclase

Modulators of sGC have been developed to target this important signaling cascade in the cardiovascular system. sGC stimulators display a dual directional action, synergistic effect with endogenous NO and direct stimulation of the native form of the enzyme independently of NO, resulting in increased cGMP production. sGC activators are able to activate the dysfunctional heme-free sGC, resulting in increased cGMP production even in reduced NO bioavailability [89,90]. In patients treated because of atherosclerosis dependent diseases such as heart failure, coronary artery disease, arterial hypertension and many others, the cornerstone of disease is endothelial dysfunction leading to depressed NO production; thus, heme-dependent activation of sGC and production of cGMP will be reduced. In that condition, there is only one possibility to stabilize cGMP levels; it is direct stimulation of sGC by its activators.

Riociguat is the first sGC stimulator to have made a successful transition from animal experiments to controlled clinical studies in patients [91]. After clinical evaluation, riociguat was accepted for the treatment of pulmonary arterial hypertension and chronic thromboembolic pulmonary hypertension. In pulmonary arterial hypertension patients, riociguat significantly improved exercise capacity and secondary efficacy endpoints in patients with pulmonary arterial hypertension. The 6 min walk distance had significantly increased by a mean of 30 m in the riociguat group and had decreased by a mean of 6 m in the placebo group. Riociguat improved the 6 min walk distance both in patients who were receiving no other treatment for the disease and in those who were receiving endothelin-receptor antagonists or prostanoids. There were significant hemodynamic improvements in pulmonary vascular resistance, NT-proBNP levels, WHO functional class, time to clinical worsening and Borg dyspnea score [92]. Patients with chronic thromboembolic pulmonary hypertension similar relations were observed in a riociguat group of patients: improvement in 6 min walk test, decrease in pulmonary vascular resistance, NT-proBNP levels, WHO functional class, quality of life [93]. Because of pharmacokinetic profile (short half lifetime) application of riociguat in other cardiovascular indications, such as heart failure, is limited [94].

Heart failure as clinical indication for vericiguat treatment was evaluated in clinical trials. One of the first of them was the SOCRATES-REDUCED study [95]. The key target was to determine the dosage and safety of vericiguat, a soluble guanylate cyclase stimulator, in patients with worsening chronic heart failure and reduced left ventricular ejection fraction. A total of 456 patients, clinically stable with ejection fraction less than 45% and a worsening chronic HF event. Vericiguat did not have a statistically significant effect on change in NT-proBNP level at 12 weeks but was well-tolerated. In the VICTORIA study, phase 3, randomized, double-blind, placebo-controlled trial, 5050 patients with chronic heart failure and an ejection fraction of less than 45% were enrolled. Patients were randomized to vericiguat or placebo, in addition to current guideline-based medical therapy. Among patients with high-risk heart failure, the incidence of death from cardiovascular causes or hospitalization for heart failure was lower among those who received vericiguat than among those who received placebo [96]. Moreover, results of studies in patients with chronic heart failure and preserved ejection fraction suggest that vericiguat treatment in current regimen is not effective, but continuation of large clinical trials is necessary [97,98]. Among patients with CHF with recent decompensation, a novel strategy of sGC activation was effective. Vericiguat compared with placebo was effective in reducing cardiovascular death or hospitalization for heart failure, but with no reduction in all-cause mortality. In this condition, vericiguat may represent a novel treatment option in heart failure patients with recent decompensation.

Clinical trial confirmed efficacy of small molecule sGC activator vericiguat in patients with heart failure with reduced ejection fraction. Due to the unequivocal results, it can be expected that this therapeutic option will be included in the nearest guidelines for the treatment of heart failure with reduced left ventricular systolic function. Unfortunately, treatment of heart failure with preserved systolic function has been difficult to date, as there is practically no therapeutic option with proven effectiveness. It is necessary to continue clinical trials conducted in relatively large and homogeneous populations in order to obtain conclusive results.

5. Conclusions and Perspective

Treatment based on modulation of GCs pathway function is one of the most promising technologies in pharmacology. Pharmacological intervention is not only effective and safe, but also provides a stable increase in the basal concentration of cGMP. The target for all therapeutic options is similar: to increase in cGMP level. The effect can be achieved by stimulation of guanylate cyclase-coupled receptors on cell surface with analogues of NPs, inhibition of degradation of cGMP with blockade of dependent enzymes PDE5 and PDE9 and inhibition of degradation of NPs into inactive metabolites by inhibition of neprilysin or direct stimulation of sGC. For all therapeutic options, benefits in laboratory and echocardiographic findings in cardiovascular diseases were confirmed.

Especially interesting is the role of sGC stimulators and sGC activators, able to increase the enzymatic activity of sGC to generate cGMP independently of NO. Moreover, most of these agents are effective in chronic treatment in heart failure patients and pulmonary hypertension and have a potential to be a first line option especially in patients with recurrent exacerbations. Additionally, the possibility to block PDE9 in heart failure and dementia patients is very interesting. The confirmation of mortality and hospitalization rate reduction was clearly presented for sGC activator, neprilysin inhibitor in heart failure patients and PDE5 inhibitors in pulmonary hypertension patients. For all groups of patients, it is necessary to continue clinical trials conducted in large and homogeneous populations in order to obtain conclusive results to modify and extend indications for current and novel agents.

The modulation of the GC pathway presents the potential to be a key therapeutic option in patients with atherosclerosis-related diseases, pulmonary hypertension and diseases with reduced cognitive function in elderlies.

Author Contributions: G.G. and A.N. have equally contributed to the present paper. All authors have read and agreed to the published version of the manuscript.

Funding: This research received no external funding.

Institutional Review Board Statement: Not applicable.

Informed Consent Statement: Not applicable.

Data Availability Statement: Not applicable.

Conflicts of Interest: The authors declare no conflict of interest.

Abbreviation

cAMP	Cyclic Adenosine Monophosphate
CO	carbon monoxide
FDA	US Food and Drug Administration
GC	guanylate cyclase
GC-A	guanylate cyclase type A
GC-B	guanylate cyclase type B
GC-C	guanylate cyclase type C
GC-D	guanylate cyclase type D
GC-E	guanylate cyclase type E
GC-F	guanylate cyclase type F
GC-G	guanylate cyclase type G
sGC	soluble guanylate cyclase
mGC	guanylate cyclase-coupled receptor or membrane-bound guanylyl cyclase
GMP	guanosine monophosphate
cGMP	cyclic guanosine monophosphate
GTP	guanosine triphosphate
LPS	lipopolysaccharide/endotoxin
NP	natriuretic peptide
ANP	natriuretic peptide type A
BNP	natriuretic peptide type B
CNP	natriuretic peptide type C
NANC	non-adrenergic, non-cholinergic
NEP	neprilysin
NO	nitric oxide
NOS	nitric oxide synthase
NOS-1	neuronal nitric oxide synthase
NOS-2	cytokine-inducible nitric oxide synthase
NOS-3	endothelial nitric oxide synthase
PAH	pulmonary arterial hypertension
PDE5	Phosphodiesterase type 5
PDE9	Phosphodiesterase type 9
PKG	cGMP dependent protein kinase G
SNP	sodium nitroprusside
TNFα	tumor necrosis factor α
NT-proBNP	N-terminal pro-brain natriuretic peptide
VASP	vasodilator-stimulated phosphoprotein

References

1. Dove, S. Mammalian Nucleotidyl Cyclases and Their Nucleotide Binding Sites. *Handb. Exp. Pharmacol.* **2017**, *238*, 49–66.
2. Liu, Y.; Ruoho, A.E.; Rao, V.D.; Hurley, J.H. Catalytic mechanism of the adenylyl and guanylyl cyclases: Modeling and mutation-al analysis. *Proc. Natl. Acad. Sci. USA* **1997**, *94*, 13414–13419. [CrossRef]
3. Thompson, D.K.; Garbers, D.L. Dominant negative mutations of the guanylyl cyclase-A receptor. Extracellular domain dele-tion and catalytic domain point mutations. *J. Biol. Chem.* **1995**, *270*, 425–430. [CrossRef]
4. Manning, G.; Whyte, D.B.; Martinez, R.; Hunter, T.; Sudarsanam, S. The Protein Kinase Complement of the Human Genome. *Science* **2002**, *298*, 1912–1934. [CrossRef]
5. Potter, L.R. Guanylyl cyclase structure, function and regulation. *Cell. Signal.* **2011**, *23*, 1921–1926. [CrossRef]
6. Giuili, G.; Scholl, U.; Bulle, F.; Guellaën, G. Molecular cloning of the cDNAs coding for the two subunits of soluble guanylyl cyclase from human brain. *FEBS Lett.* **1992**, *304*, 83–88. [CrossRef]
7. Harteneck, C.; Wedel, B.; Koesling, D.; Malkewitz, J.; Böhme, E.; Schultz, G. Molecular cloning and expression of a new al-pha-subunit of soluble guanylyl cyclase. Interchangeability of the alpha-subunits of the enzyme. *FEBS Lett.* **1991**, *292*, 217–222.
8. Mergia, E.; Friebe, A.; Dangel, O.; Russwurm, M.; Koesling, D. Spare guanylyl cyclase NO receptors ensure high NO sensitivity in the vascular system. *J. Clin. Investig.* **2006**, *116*, 1731–1737. [CrossRef]
9. Yuen, P.S.T.; Potter, L.R.; Garbers, D.L. A new form of guanylyl cyclase is preferentially expressed in rat kidney. *Biochemistry* **1990**, *29*, 10872–10878. [CrossRef] [PubMed]
10. Wedel, B.; Humbert, P.; Harteneck, C.; Foerster, J.; Malkewitz, J.; Bohme, E.; Schultz, G.; Koesling, D. Mutation of His-105 in the beta 1 subunit yields a nitric oxide-insensitive form of soluble guanylyl cyclase. *Proc. Natl. Acad. Sci. USA* **1994**, *91*, 2592–2596. [CrossRef] [PubMed]
11. Friebe, A.; Mergia, E.; Dangel, O.; Lange, A.; Koesling, D. Fatal gastrointestinal obstruction and hypertension in mice lacking nitric oxide-sensitive guanylyl cyclase. *Proc. Natl. Acad. Sci. USA* **2007**, *104*, 7699–7704. [CrossRef]
12. Pfeifer, A.; Klatt, P.; Massberg, S.; Ny, L.; Sausbier, M.; Hirneiß, C.; Wang, G.; Korth, M.; Aszódi, A.; Andersson, K.; et al. Defective smooth muscle regulation in cGMP kinase I-deficient mice. *EMBO J.* **1998**, *17*, 3045–3051. [CrossRef] [PubMed]
13. Desch, M.; Sigl, K.; Hieke, B.; Salb, K.; Kees, F.; Bernhard, D.; Jochim, A.; Spiessberger, B.; Höcherl, K.; Feil, R.; et al. IRAG determines nitric oxide- and atrial natriuretic peptide-mediated smooth muscle relaxation. *Cardiovasc. Res.* **2010**, *86*, 496–505. [CrossRef] [PubMed]
14. Carvajal, J.A.; Germain, A.M.; Huidobro-Toro, J.P.; Weiner, C.P. Molecular mechanism of cGMP-mediated smooth muscle relaxation. *J. Cell. Physiol.* **2000**, *184*, 409–420. [CrossRef]
15. Rajfer, J.; Aronson, W.J.; Bush, P.A.; Dorey, F.J.; Ignarro, L.J. Nitric Oxide as a Mediator of Relaxation of the Corpus Cavernosum in Response to Nonadrenergic, Noncholinergic Neurotransmission. *N. Engl. J. Med.* **1992**, *326*, 90–94. [CrossRef]
16. Kang, Y.; Liu, R.; Wu, J.-X.; Chen, L. Structural insights into the mechanism of human soluble guanylate cyclase. *Nature* **2019**, *574*, 206–210. [CrossRef]
17. Seeger, F.; Quintyn, R.; Tanimoto, A.; Williams, G.J.; Tainer, J.A.; Wysocki, V.H.; Garcin, E.D. Interfacial Residues Promote an Optimal Alignment of the Catalytic Center in Human Soluble Guanylate Cyclase: Heterodimerization Is Required but Not Sufficient for Activity. *Biochemistry* **2014**, *53*, 2153–2165. [CrossRef]
18. Suga, S.; Nakao, K.; Hosoda, K.; Mukoyama, M.; Ogawa, Y.; Shirakami, G.; Arai, H.; Saito, Y.; Kambayashi, Y.; Inouye, K.; et al. Receptor selectivity of natriuretic peptide family, atrial natriuretic peptide, brain natriuretic peptide, and C-type natriuretic peptide. *Endocrinology* **1992**, *130*, 229–239. [CrossRef] [PubMed]
19. Vesely, D.L. Atrial Natriuretic Peptide Prohormone Gene Expression: Hormones and Diseases That Upregulate its Expression. *IUBMB Life* **2002**, *53*, 153–159. [CrossRef]
20. Gupta, D.K.; Wang, T.J. Natriuretic Peptides and Cardiometabolic Health. *Circ. J.* **2015**, *79*, 1647–1655. [CrossRef]
21. Tamura, N.; Ogawa, Y.; Chusho, H.; Nakamura, K.; Nakao, K.; Suda, M.; Kasahara, M.; Hashimoto, R.; Katsuura, G.; Mukoyama, M.; et al. Cardiac fibrosis in mice lacking brain natriuretic peptide. *Proc. Natl. Acad. Sci. USA* **2000**, *97*, 4239–4244. [CrossRef]
22. Moyes, A.J.; Hobbs, A.J. C-Type Natriuretic Peptide: A Multifaceted Paracrine Regulator in the Heart and Vasculature. *Int. J. Mol. Sci.* **2019**, *20*, 2281. [CrossRef] [PubMed]
23. Yasoda, A.; Ogawa, Y.; Suda, M.; Tamura, N.; Mori, K.; Sakuma, Y.; Chusho, H.; Shiota, K.; Tanaka, K.; Nakao, K. Natriuretic peptide regulation of endochondral ossification. Evidence for possible roles of the C-type natriuretic peptide/guanylyl cyclase-B pathway. *J. Biol. Chem.* **1998**, *273*, 11695–11700. [CrossRef]
24. Zhang, M.; Su, Y.-Q.; Sugiura, K.; Xia, G.; Eppig, J.J. Granulosa Cell Ligand NPPC and Its Receptor NPR2 Maintain Meiotic Arrest in Mouse Oocytes. *Science* **2010**, *330*, 366–369. [CrossRef]
25. He, M.; Zhang, T.; Yang, Y.; Wang, C. Mechanisms of Oocyte Maturation and Related Epigenetic Regulation. *Front. Cell Dev. Biol.* **2021**, *9*. [CrossRef] [PubMed]
26. Santhekadur, P.K.; Kumar, D.P.; Seneshaw, M.; Mirshahi, F.; Sanyal, A.J. The multifaceted role of natriuretic peptides in metabolic syndrome. *Biomed. Pharmacother.* **2017**, *92*, 826–835. [CrossRef] [PubMed]
27. Nagase, M.; Katafuchi, T.; Hirose, S.; Fujita, T. Tissue distribution and localization of natriuretic peptide receptor subtypes in stroke-prone spontaneously hypertensive rats. *J. Hypertens.* **1997**, *15*, 1235–1243. [CrossRef] [PubMed]
28. Meng, J.; Chen, W.; Wang, J. Interventions in theB-type natriuretic peptide signalling pathway as a means of controlling chronic itch. *Br. J. Pharmacol.* **2020**, *177*, 1025–1040. [CrossRef]

29. Hamra, F.K.; Forte, L.R.; Eber, S.L.; Pidhorodeckyj, N.V.; Krause, W.J.; Freeman, R.H.; Chin, D.T.; Tompkins, J.A.; Fok, K.F.; Smith, C.E. Uroguanylin: Structure and activity of a second endogenous peptide that stimulates intestinal guanylate cyclase. *Proc. Natl. Acad. Sci. USA* **1993**, *90*, 10464–10468. [CrossRef]
30. Amarachintha, S.; Harmel-Laws, E.; Steinbrecher, K.A. Guanylate cyclase C reduces invasion of intestinal epithelial cells by bacterial pathogens. *Sci. Rep.* **2018**, *8*, 1521. [CrossRef]
31. Steinbrecher, K.A.; Wowk, S.A.; Rudolph, J.A.; Witte, D.P.; Cohen, M.B. Targeted Inactivation of the Mouse Guanylin Gene Results in Altered Dynamics of Colonic Epithelial Proliferation. *Am. J. Pathol.* **2002**, *161*, 2169–2178. [CrossRef]
32. Lorenz, J.N.; Nieman, M.; Sabo, J.; Sanford, L.P.; Hawkins, J.A.; Elitsur, N.; Gawenis, L.R.; Clarke, L.L.; Cohen, M.B. Uroguanylin knock-out mice have increased blood pressure and impaired natriuretic response to enteral NaCl load. *J. Clin. Investig.* **2003**, *112*, 1244–1254. [CrossRef] [PubMed]
33. Rappaport, J.A.; Waldman, S.A. An update on guanylyl cyclase C in the diagnosis, chemoprevention, and treatment of colorectal cancer. *Expert Rev. Clin. Pharmacol.* **2020**, *13*, 1125–1137. [CrossRef]
34. Dye, F.S.; Larraufie, P.; Kay, R.; Darwish, T.; Rievaj, J.; Goldspink, D.A.; Meek, C.L.; Middleton, S.J.; Hardwick, R.H.; Roberts, G.; et al. Characterisation of proguanylin expressing cells in the intestine—Evidence for constitutive luminal secretion. *Sci. Rep.* **2019**, *9*, 15574. [CrossRef]
35. Arakawa, H.; Kelliher, K.R.; Zufall, F.; Munger, S.D. The Receptor Guanylyl Cyclase Type D (GC-D) Ligand Uroguanylin Promotes the Acquisition of Food Preferences in Mice. *Chem. Senses* **2013**, *38*, 391–397. [CrossRef]
36. Kenemuth, J.K.; Hennessy, S.P.; Hanson, R.J.; Hensler, A.J.; Coates, E.L. Investigation of nasal CO_2 receptor transduction mechanisms in wild-type and GC-D knockout mice. *Chem. Senses.* **2013**, *38*, 769–781. [CrossRef] [PubMed]
37. Zufall, F.; Munger, S.D. Receptor guanylyl cyclases in mammalian olfactory function. *Mol. Cell. Biochem.* **2010**, *334*, 191–197. [CrossRef] [PubMed]
38. Gill, J.S.; Georgiou, M.; Kalitzeos, A.; Moore, A.T.; Michaelides, M. Progressive cone and cone-rod dystrophies: Clinical features, molecular genetics and prospects for therapy. *Br. J. Ophthalmol.* **2019**, *103*, 711–720. [CrossRef] [PubMed]
39. Fain, G.L.; Sampath, A.P. Light responses of mammalian cones. *Pflügers Arch. Eur. J. Physiol.* **2021**, *473*, 1–14. [CrossRef]
40. Chao, Y.-C.; Cheng, C.-J.; Hsieh, H.-T.; Lin, C.-C.; Chen, C.-C.; Yang, R.-B. Guanylate cyclase-G, expressed in the Grueneberg ganglion olfactory subsystem, is activated by bicarbonate. *Biochem. J.* **2010**, *432*, 267–273. [CrossRef]
41. Chao, Y.-C.; Fleischer, J.; Yang, R. Guanylyl cyclase-G is an alarm pheromone receptor in mice. *EMBO J.* **2018**, *37*, 39–49. [CrossRef]
42. Calvo-Ochoa, E.; Byrd-Jacobs, C.A.; Fuss, S.H. Diving into the streams and waves of constitutive and regenerative olfactory neurogenesis: Insights from zebrafish. *Cell Tissue Res.* **2021**, *383*, 227–253. [CrossRef]
43. Grześk, E.; Tejza, B.; Wiciński, M.; Malinowski, B.; Szadujkis-Szadurska, K.; Baran, L.; Kowal, E.; Grześk, G. Effect of pertussis toxin on calcium influx in three contraction models. *Biomed. Rep.* **2014**, *2*, 584–588. [CrossRef] [PubMed]
44. Szadujkis-Szadurska, K.; Grzesk, G.; Szadujkis-Szadurski, L.; Gajdus, M.; Matusiak, G. Role of acetylcholine and calcium ions in three vascular contraction models: Angiotensin II, phenylephrine and caffeine. *Exp. Ther. Med.* **2012**, *4*, 329–333. [CrossRef]
45. Grześk, E.; Darwish, N.; Stolarek, W.; Wiciński, M.; Malinowski, B.; Burdziński, I.; Grześk, G. Effect of reperfusion on vascular smooth muscle reactivity in three contraction models. *Microvasc. Res.* **2019**, *121*, 24–29. [CrossRef] [PubMed]
46. Grześk, G.; Szadujkis-Szadurski, L. Pharmacometric analysis of alpha1-adrenoceptor function in rat tail artery pretreated with lipopolysaccharides. *Pol. J. Pharmacol.* **2001**, *53*, 605–613.
47. Bloch-Bogusławska, E.; Grześk, E.; Grześk, G. Comparison of the post-mortem interval on the effect of vascular responses to the activation of ionotropic and metabotropic receptors. *Biomed. Rep.* **2015**, *3*, 230–234. [CrossRef]
48. Grześk, G.; Szadujkis-Szadurski, L. Physiological antagonism of angiotensin II and lipopolysaccharides in early endotoxemia: Pharmacometric analysis. *Pol. J. Pharmacol.* **2003**, *55*, 753–762. [PubMed]
49. Szadujkis-Szadurska, K.; Grzesk, G.; Szadujkis-Szadurski, L.; Gajdus, M.; Matusiak, G. Role of nitric oxide and cGMP in the mod-ulation of vascular contraction induced by angiotensin II and Bay K8644 during ischemia/reperfusion. *Exp. Ther. Med.* **2013**, *5*, 616–620. [CrossRef] [PubMed]
50. Slupski, M.; Szadujkis-Szadurski, L.; Grześk, G.; Wlodarczyk, Z.; Masztalerz, M.; Piotrowiak, I.; Jasinski, M.; Szadujkis-Szadurski, R.; Szadujkis-Szadurska, K. Guanylate Cyclase Activators Influence Reactivity of Human Mesenteric Superior Arteries Retrieved and Preserved in the Same Conditions as Transplanted Kidneys. *Transplant. Proc.* **2007**, *39*, 1350–1353. [CrossRef]
51. Alderton, W.K.; Cooper, C.E.; Knowles, R.G. Nitric oxide synthases: Structure, function and inhibition. *Biochem. J.* **2001**, *357*, 593–615. [CrossRef]
52. Vo, P.A.; Lad, B.; Tomlinson, J.A.; Francis, S.; Ahluwalia, A. Autoregulatory Role of Endothelium-derived Nitric Oxide (NO) on Lipopolysaccharide-induced Vascular Inducible NO Synthase Expression and Function. *J. Biol. Chem.* **2005**, *280*, 7236–7243. [CrossRef]
53. Connelly, L.; Madhani, M.; Hobbs, A.J. Resistance to endotoxic shock in endothelial nitric-oxide synthase (eNOS) knock-out mice: A pro-inflammatory role for eNOS-derived no in vivo. *J. Biol. Chem.* **2005**, *280*, 10040–10046. [CrossRef]
54. Piepoli, M.F.; Hoes, A.W.; Agewall, S.; Albus, C.; Brotons, C.; Catapano, A.L.; Cooney, M.T.; Corrà, U.; Cosyns, B.; Deaton, C.; et al. 2016 European Guidelines on cardiovascular disease prevention in clinical practice: The Sixth Joint Task Force of the European Society of Cardiology and Other Societies on Cardiovascular Disease Prevention in Clinical Practice (constituted by representatives of 10 societies and by invited experts) Developed with the special contribution of the European Association for Cardiovascular Prevention & Rehabilitation (EACPR). *Eur. Heart J.* **2016**, *37*, 2315–2381. [PubMed]

55. Ponikowski, P.; Voors, A.A.; Anker, S.D.; Bueno, H.; Cleland, J.G.F.; Coats, A.J.S.; Falk, V.; González-Juanatey, J.R.; Harjola, V.P.; Jankowska, E.A.; et al. 2016 ESC Guidelines for the diagnosis and treatment of acute and chronic heart failure: The Task Force for the diagnosis and treatment of acute and chronic heart failure of the European Society of Cardiology (ESC) Developed with the special contribution of the Heart Failure Association (HFA) of the ESC. *Eur. Heart J.* **2016**, *37*, 2129–2200.
56. Cuspidi, C.; Tadic, M.; Grassi, G.; Mancia, G. Treatment of hypertension: The ESH/ESC guidelines recommendations. *Pharmacol. Res.* **2018**, *128*, 315–321. [CrossRef]
57. Mitaka, C.; Kudo, T.; Haraguchi, G.; Tomita, M. Cardiovascular and renal effects of carperitide and nesiritide in cardiovascular surgery patients: A systematic review and meta-analysis. *Crit. Care* **2011**, *15*, R258. [CrossRef] [PubMed]
58. Sezai, A.; Nakata, K.-I.; Iida, M.; Yoshitake, I.; Wakui, S.; Hata, H.; Shiono, M. Results of Low-Dose Carperitide Infusion in High-Risk Patients Undergoing Coronary Artery Bypass Grafting. *Ann. Thorac. Surg.* **2013**, *96*, 119–126. [CrossRef] [PubMed]
59. Zhao, X.; Zhang, D.Q.; Song, R.; Zhang, G. Nesiritide in patients with acute myocardial infarction and heart failure: A meta-analysis. *J. Int. Med. Res.* **2020**, *48*, 300060519897194. [CrossRef]
60. O'Connor, C.; Starling, R.; Hernandez, A.; Armstrong, P.; Dickstein, K.; Hasselblad, V.; Heizer, G.; Komajda, M.; Massie, B.; McMurray, J.; et al. Effect of Nesiritide in Patients with Acute Decompensated Heart Failure. *N. Engl. J. Med.* **2011**, *365*, 32–43. [CrossRef] [PubMed]
61. Van Deursen, V.M.; Hernandez, A.F.; Stebbins, A.; Hasselblad, V.; Ezekowitz, J.A.; Califf, R.M.; Gottlieb, S.S.; O'Connor, C.M.; Starling, R.C.; Tang, W.H.; et al. Nesiritide, renal function, and associated outcomes during hospitaliza-tion for acute decompensated heart failure: Results from the Acute Study of Clinical Effectiveness of Nesiritide and Decompensated Heart Failure (ASCEND-HF). *Circulation* **2014**, *130*, 958–965. [CrossRef] [PubMed]
62. McMurray, J.J.; Packer, M.; Desai, A.S.; Gong, J.; Lefkowitz, M.P.; Rizkala, A.R.; Rouleau, J.L.; Shi, V.C.; Solomon, S.D.; Swedberg, K.; et al. Angiotensin–Neprilysin Inhibition versus Enalapril in Heart Failure. *N. Engl. J. Med.* **2014**, *371*, 993–1004. [CrossRef]
63. Grodin, J.L.; Liebo, M.J.; Butler, J.; Metra, M.; Felker, G.M.; Hernandez, A.F.; Voors, A.A.; McMurray, J.J.; Armstrong, P.W.; O'Connor, C.; et al. Prognostic Implications of Changes in Amino-Terminal Pro–B-Type Natriuretic Peptide in Acute Decompensated Heart Failure: Insights From ASCEND-HF. *J. Card. Fail.* **2019**, *25*, 703–711. [CrossRef]
64. Ibrahim, N.E.; McCarthy, C.P.; Shrestha, S.; Gaggin, H.K.; Mukai, R.; Szymonifka, J.; Apple, F.S.; Burnett, J.C.; Iyer, S.; Januzzi, J.L. Effect of Neprilysin Inhibition on Various Natriuretic Peptide Assays. *J. Am. Coll. Cardiol.* **2019**, *73*, 1273–1284. [CrossRef] [PubMed]
65. Solomon, S.D.; McMurray, J.J.; Anand, I.S.; Ge, J.; Lam, C.S.; Maggioni, A.P.; Martinez, F.; Packer, M.; Pfeffer, M.A.; Pieske, B.; et al. Angiotensin–Neprilysin Inhibition in Heart Failure with Preserved Ejection Fraction. *N. Engl. J. Med.* **2019**, *381*, 1609–1620. [CrossRef]
66. Solomon, S.D.; McMurray, J.J.V.; PARAGON-HF Steering Committee and Investigators. Angiotensin-Neprilysin Inhibition in Heart Failure with Preserved Ejection Fraction: Reply. *N. Engl. J. Med.* **2020**, *382*, 1182–1183.
67. Solomon, S.D.; Claggett, B.; McMurray, J.J.; Hernandez, A.F.; Fonarow, G. Combined neprilysin and renin-angiotensin system inhibition in heart failure with reduced ejection fraction: A meta-analysis. *Eur. J. Heart Fail.* **2016**, *18*, 1238–1243. [CrossRef] [PubMed]
68. Vardeny, O.; Claggett, B.; Packer, M.; Zile, M.R.; Rouleau, J.; Swedberg, K.; Teerlink, J.R.; Desai, A.S.; Lefkowitz, M.; Shi, V.; et al. Prospective Comparison of ARNI with ACEI to Determine Impact on Global Mortality and Morbidity in Heart Failure (PARADIGM-HF) Investigators. Efficacy of sacubitril/valsartan vs. enalapril at lower than target doses in heart failure with reduced ejection fraction: The PARADIGM-HF trial. *Eur. J. Heart Fail.* **2016**, *18*, 1228–1234. [PubMed]
69. Ruilope, L.M.; Dukat, A.; Böhm, M.; Lacourcière, Y.; Gong, J.; Lefkowitz, M.P. Blood-pressure reduction with LCZ696, a novel du-al-acting inhibitor of the angiotensin II receptor and neprilysin: A randomised, double-blind, placebo-controlled, active comparator study. *Lancet* **2010**, *375*, 1255–1266. [CrossRef]
70. Voors, A.A.; Gori, M.; Liu, L.C.Y.; Claggett, B.; Zile, M.; Pieske, B.; McMurray, J.J.V.; Packer, M.; Shi, V.; Lefkowitz, M.P.; et al. Renal effects of the angiotensin receptor neprilysin inhibitor LCZ696 in patients with heart failure and preserved ejection fraction. *Eur. J. Heart Fail.* **2015**, *17*, 510–517. [CrossRef]
71. Campbell, D.J. Long-term neprilysin inhibition—Implications for ARNIs. *Nat. Rev. Cardiol.* **2017**, *14*, 171–186. [CrossRef] [PubMed]
72. Riddell, E.; Vader, J.M. Potential Expanded Indications for Neprilysin Inhibitors. *Curr. Heart Fail. Rep.* **2017**, *14*, 134–145. [CrossRef]
73. Cote, R.H. Characteristics of Photoreceptor PDE (PDE6): Similarities and differences to PDE5. *Int. J. Impot. Res.* **2004**, *16*, S28–S33. [CrossRef]
74. Maryam, A.; Vedithi, S.C.; Khalid, R.R.; Alsulami, A.F.; Torres, P.H.M.; Siddiqi, A.R.; Blundell, T.L. The Molecular Organization of Human cGMP Specific Phosphodiesterase 6 (PDE6): Structural Implications of Somatic Mutations in Cancer and Retinitis Pigmentosa. *Comput. Struct. Biotechnol. J.* **2019**, *17*, 378–389. [CrossRef]
75. Ribaudo, G.; Memo, M.; Gianoncelli, A. A Perspective on Natural and Nature-Inspired Small Molecules Targeting Phosphodiesterase 9 (PDE9): Chances and Challenges against Neurodegeneration. *Pharmaceuticals* **2021**, *14*, 58. [CrossRef]
76. Montani, D.; Günther, S.; Dorfmüller, P.; Perros, F.; Girerd, B.; Garcia, G.; Jaïs, X.; Savale, L.; Artaud-Macari, E.; Price, L.C.; et al. Pulmonary arterial hypertension. *Orphanet. J. Rare Dis.* **2013**, *8*, 97. [CrossRef]

77. Barnes, H.; Brown, Z.; Burns, A.; Williams, T. Phosphodiesterase 5 inhibitors for pulmonary hypertension. *Cochrane Database Syst. Rev.* **2019**, *1*, CD012621. [CrossRef]
78. Mayeux, J.D.; Pan, I.Z.; Dechand, J.; Jacobs, J.A.; Jones, T.L.; McKellar, S.H.; Beck, E.; Hatton, N.D.; Ryan, J.J. Management of Pulmonary Arterial Hypertension. *Curr. Cardiovasc. Risk Rep.* **2021**, *15*, 1–24. [CrossRef] [PubMed]
79. Frank, B.S.; Ivy, D.D. Diagnosis, Evaluation and Treatment of Pulmonary Arterial Hypertension in Children. *Children* **2018**, *5*, 44. [CrossRef]
80. Galiè, N.; Ghofrani, A.; Torbicki, A.; Barst, R.J.; Rubin, L.J.; Badesch, D.; Fleming, T.; Parpia, T.; Burgess, G.; Branzi, A.; et al. Sildenafil Citrate Therapy for Pulmonary Arterial Hypertension. *N. Engl. J. Med.* **2005**, *353*, 2148–2157. [CrossRef] [PubMed]
81. Galiè, N.; Brundage, B.H.; Ghofrani, H.A.; Oudiz, R.J.; Simonneau, G.; Safdar, Z.; Shapiro, S.; White, R.J.; Chan, M.; Beardsworth, A.; et al. Tadalafil therapy for pulmonary arterial hypertension. *Circulation* **2009**, *119*, 2894–2903. [CrossRef]
82. Lewis, G.D.; Lachmann, J.; Camuso, J.; Lepore, J.J.; Shin, J.; Martinovic, M.E.; Systrom, D.M.; Bloch, K.D.; Semigran, M.J. Sildenafil im-proves exercise hemodynamics and oxygen uptake in patients with systolic heart failure. *Circulation* **2007**, *115*, 59–66. [CrossRef] [PubMed]
83. Redfield, M.M.; Chen, H.H.; Borlaug, B.A.; Semigran, M.J.; Lee, K.L.; Lewis, G.; LeWinter, M.M.; Rouleau, J.L.; Bull, D.A.; Mann, D.L.; et al. Effect of phosphodiesterase-5 inhibition on exercise capacity and clinical status in heart failure with preserved ejection fraction: A randomized clinical trial. *JAMA* **2013**, *309*, 1268–1277. [CrossRef]
84. Pons, J.; Leblanc, M.-H.; Bernier, M.; Cantin, B.; Bourgault, C.; Bergeron, S.; Proulx, G.; Morin, J.; Nalli, C.; O'Connor, K.; et al. Effects of chronic sildenafil use on pulmonary hemodynamics and clinical outcomes in heart transplantation. *J. Heart Lung Transplant.* **2012**, *31*, 1281–1287. [CrossRef] [PubMed]
85. Richards, D.A.; Aronovitz, M.J.; Liu, P.; Martin, G.L.; Tam, K.; Pande, S.; Karas, R.H.; Bloomfield, D.M.; Mendelsohn, M.E.; Blanton, R.M. CRD-733, a Novel PDE9 (Phosphodiesterase 9) Inhibitor, Reverses Pressure Overload-Induced Heart Failure. *Circ. Heart Fail.* **2021**, *14*, e007300. [CrossRef]
86. Pinilla-Vera, M.; Hahn, V.S.; Kass, D.A. Leveraging Signaling Pathways to Treat Heart Failure with Reduced Ejection Fraction. *Circ. Res.* **2019**, *124*, 1618–1632. [CrossRef]
87. Kokkonen-Simon, K.M.; Saberi, A.; Nakamura, T.; Ranek, M.J.; Zhu, G.; Bedja, D.; Kuhn, M.; Halushka, M.K.; Lee, D.I.; Kass, D.A. Marked disparity of microRNA modulation by cGMP-selective PDE5 versus PDE9 inhibitors in heart disease. *JCI Insight.* **2018**, *3*, e121739. [CrossRef] [PubMed]
88. Patel, N.S.; Klett, J.; Pilarzyk, K.; Lee, D.I.; Kass, D.; Menniti, F.S.; Kelly, M.P. Identification of new PDE9A isoforms and how their expression and subcellular compartmentalization in the brain change across the life span. *Neurobiol. Aging* **2018**, *65*, 217–234. [CrossRef]
89. Stasch, J.-P.; Hobbs, A. NO-Independent, Haem-Dependent Soluble Guanylate Cyclase Stimulators. *Handb. Exp. Pharmacol.* **2009**, *191*, 277–308.
90. Schmidt, H.H.H.W.; Schmidt, P.M.; Stasch, J.-P. NO- and Haem-Independent Soluble Guanylate Cyclase Activators. *Handb. Exp. Pharmacol.* **2009**, *191*, 309–339.
91. Stasch, J.P.; Evgenov, O.V. Soluble guanylate cyclase stimulators in pulmonary hypertension. *Handb. Exp. Pharmacol.* **2013**, *218*, 279–313. [PubMed]
92. Ghofrani, H.-A.; Galiè, N.; Grimminger, F.; Grünig, E.; Humbert, M.; Jing, Z.-C.; Keogh, A.M.; Langleben, D.; Kilama, M.O.; Fritsch, A.; et al. Riociguat for the Treatment of Pulmonary Arterial Hypertension. *N. Engl. J. Med.* **2013**, *369*, 330–340. [CrossRef] [PubMed]
93. Ghofrani, H.-A.; D'Armini, A.M.; Grimminger, F.; Hoeper, M.; Jansa, P.; Kim, N.H., Mayer, E.; Simonneau, G.; Wilkins, M.R.; Fritsch, A.; et al. Riociguat for the Treatment of Chronic Thromboembolic Pulmonary Hypertension. *N. Engl. J. Med.* **2013**, *369*, 319–329. [CrossRef] [PubMed]
94. Frey, R.; Mück, W.; Unger, S.; Artmeier-Brandt, U.; Weimann, G.; Wensing, G. Single-Dose Pharmacokinetics, Pharmacodynamics, Tolerability, and Safety of the Soluble Guanylate Cyclase Stimulator BAY 63-2521: An Ascending-Dose Study in Healthy Male Volunteers. *J. Clin. Pharmacol.* **2008**, *48*, 926–934. [CrossRef] [PubMed]
95. Gheorghiade, M.; Greene, S.J.; Butler, J.; Filippatos, G.; Lam, C.S.; Maggioni, A.P.; Ponikowski, P.; Shah, S.J.; Solomon, S.D.; Kraigher-Krainer, E.; et al. Effect of Vericiguat, a Soluble Guanylate Cyclase Stimulator, on Natriuretic Pep-tide Levels in Patients with Worsening Chronic Heart Failure and Reduced Ejection Fraction: The Socrates-Reduced Randomized Trial. *JAMA* **2015**, *314*, 2251–2262. [CrossRef] [PubMed]
96. Armstrong, P.W.; Pieske, B.; Anstrom, K.J.; Ezekowitz, J.; Hernandez, A.F.; Butler, J.; Lam, C.S.; Ponikowski, P.; Voors, A.A.; Jia, G.; et al. Vericiguat in Patients with Heart Failure and Reduced Ejection Fraction. *N. Engl J. Med.* **2020**, *382*, 1883–1893. [CrossRef] [PubMed]
97. Filippatos, G.; Maggioni, A.P.; Lam, C.S.; Pieske-Kraigher, E.; Butler, J.; Spertus, J.; Ponikowski, P.; Shah, S.J.; Solomon, S.D.; Scalise, A.V.; et al. Vericiguat in patients with worsening chronic heart failure and preserved ejection fraction: Results of the Soluble Guanylate Cyclase Stimulator in Heart Failure Patients with Preserved EF (Socrates-Preserved) Study. *Eur. Heart J.* **2017**, *38*, 1119–1127.
98. Armstrong, P.W.; Lam, C.S.P.; Anstrom, K.J.; Ezekowitz, J.; Hernandez, A.F.; O'Connor, C.M.; Pieske, B.; Ponikowski, P.; Shah, S.J.; Solomon, S.D.; et al. Effect of Vericiguat vs Placebo on Quality of Life in Patients with Heart Failure and Preserved Ejection Fraction: The Vitality-HFpEF Randomized Clinical Trial. *JAMA* **2020**, *324*, 1512–1521. [CrossRef] [PubMed]

molecules MDPI

Review

The Effects of Statins on Neurotransmission and Their Neuroprotective Role in Neurological and Psychiatric Disorders

Michał Kosowski [1,*], Joanna Smolarczyk-Kosowska [2], Marcin Hachuła [1], Mateusz Maligłówka [1], Marcin Basiak [1], Grzegorz Machnik [1], Robert Pudlo [2] and Bogusław Okopień [1]

[1] Department of Internal Medicine and Clinical Pharmacology, Medical University of Silesia, Medyków 18, 40-752 Katowice, Poland; d200998@365.sum.edu.pl (M.H.); mmaliglowka@sum.edu.pl (M.M.); mbasiak@sum.edu.pl (M.B.); gmachnik@sum.edu.pl (G.M.); bokopien@sum.edu.pl (B.O.)

[2] Department of Psychiatry, Faculty of Medical Sciences in Zabrze, Medical University of Silesia, 40-055 Katowice, Poland; joanna.smolarczyk@med.sum.edu.pl (J.S.-K.); rpudlo@sum.edu.pl (R.P.)

* Correspondence: mkosowski@sum.edu.pl; Tel.: +48-32-208-85-10

Abstract: Statins are among the most widely used drug classes in the world. Apart from their basic mechanism of action, which is lowering cholesterol levels, many pleiotropic effects have been described so far, such as anti-inflammatory and antiatherosclerotic effects. A growing number of scientific reports have proven that these drugs have a beneficial effect on the functioning of the nervous system. The first reports proving that lipid-lowering therapy can influence the development of neurological and psychiatric diseases appeared in the 1990s. Despite numerous studies about the mechanisms by which statins may affect the functioning of the central nervous system (CNS), there are still no clear data explaining this effect. Most studies have focused on the metabolic effects of this group of drugs, however authors have also described the pleiotropic effects of statins, pointing to their probable impact on the neurotransmitter system and neuroprotective effects. The aim of this paper was to review the literature describing the impacts of statins on dopamine, serotonin, acetylcholine, and glutamate neurotransmission, as well as their neuroprotective role. This paper focuses on the mechanisms by which statins affect neurotransmission, as well as on their impacts on neurological and psychiatric diseases such as Parkinson's disease (PD), Alzheimer's disease (AD), vascular dementia (VD), stroke, and depression. The pleiotropic effects of statin usage could potentially open floodgates for research in these treatment domains, catching the attention of researchers and clinicians across the globe.

Keywords: dopamine; acetylcholine; glutamate; BDNF; serotonin; neurotransmitters; statins; neurodegenerative diseases; stroke; depression

Citation: Kosowski, M.; Smolarczyk-Kosowska, J.; Hachuła, M.; Maligłówka, M.; Basiak, M.; Machnik, G.; Pudlo, R.; Okopień, B. The Effects of Statins on Neurotransmission and Their Neuroprotective Role in Neurological and Psychiatric Disorders. *Molecules* **2021**, *26*, 2838. https://doi.org/10.3390/molecules26102838

Academic Editors: Grzegorz Grześk and Alicja Nowaczyk

Received: 10 April 2021
Accepted: 10 May 2021
Published: 11 May 2021

1. Introduction

Statins are the most widespread group of lipid-lowering drugs in the world [1]. For this reason, they are recommended for the primary and secondary prevention of cardiovascular events [2]. For many years, other effects of this group of drugs have been well known, which are primarily focused on anti-inflammatory activity [3,4]. The first scientific reports on the impacts of antilipid therapy on psychiatric and neurological diseases appeared in the 1990s. In 1990, Muldoon et al. proved that cholesterol-lowering therapy increases the risk of death in men as a result of accidents and suicide [5]. Subsequent reports also showed a relationship between cholesterol levels and the occurrence of anxiety, depression, and related suicide [6,7]. Moreover, despite very ambiguous results concerning these effects, meta-analyses have shown that statins reduce depressive symptoms and the frequency of hospitalization caused by intensification of these symptoms [8,9]. At the same time, reports began to appear in which researchers described the relationship between cholesterol level and the symptom severity in neurodegenerative diseases such as Alzheimer's disease (AD) and Parkinson's disease (PD) [10,11]. These observations prompted researchers to look for a potential mechanism of action by which statins act on neurotransmitter systems to influence neurological and psychiatric disorders.

This study aims to systematize the current knowledge about the potential mechanisms by which statins affect cholinergic, dopaminergic, glutaminergic, and serotonergic transmission, as well as the impact of these interactions on the development and progression of neurodegenerative diseases and psychiatric disorders. Obviously, the effects of statins on neurological diseases through their lowering of the amount of total cholesterol and antiatherosclerotic effects seem not to be overlooked. However, in our manuscript, we only focus on their effects on neurotransmission and their neuroprotective role, because this topic is still a subject of discussion among scientists and requires further clinical research [12,13]. In this publication, we try to systematically review the current scientific data from international reports. For this purpose, the PubMed databases were reviewed in order to isolate reports according to the following key phrases: "statins and neurotransmission", "lipid signaling and neurotransmission", "statins and neurodegenerative diseases", and "statins and psychiatric disorders".

2. Statins–Structure and Permeability

Statins are drugs whose primary mechanism of action is to inhibit 3-hydroxy-3-methylglutaryl coenzyme A reductase (HMGCR). This is related to the ability of the pharmacophore, which for all statins is a dihydroheptanoic acid, to lower HMGCR activity. However, it is not a pharmacophore but rather the covalently related hydrophobic ring system that determines the chemical properties of individual statins, such as their solubility or pharmacokinetic properties.

Statins are divided into two categories: type 1, natural or semi-synthetic (these include lovastatin, simvastatin, and pravastatin); and type 2, otherwise known as fully synthetic [14]. One of the differences between the types of statins is their ability to bind to HMGCR. Type 2 statins, such as atorvastatin and rosuvastatin, are able to interact more strongly with HMGCR due to their greater hydrogen binding capacity [15]. The second difference is their different hydrophilicity. Lovastatin, simvastatin, fluvastatin, pitavastatin, and cerivastatin are more lipophilic, while rosuvastatin and pravastatin are more hydrophilic. This feature is very important in the context of the pleiotropic effects of this group of drugs. Lipophilic statins have a greater ability to passively pass from blood to tissues, including the ability to cross the blood–brain barrier (BBB). This results, among other things, in a greater severity of side effects. Hydrophilic statins, due to the necessity to penetrate inside the cells by active transport, show a more hepatoselective effect, which means that other effects, apart from lipid-lowering activity, are less intense. Recent studies confirm this difference in the ability to produce pleiotropic effects after taking type 1 and type 2 statins [16].

In summary, the basic differences between the two types of statins consist of their differences in chemical structure, which result in different pharmacokinetics for both types and the ability to penetrate into different types of tissues. Thereby, this results in the differentially expressed capacity to induce pleiotropic effects by different types of statins, including actions on the central nervous system (CNS).

3. Statins and Dopaminergic Neurotransmission

3.1. Structure and Synthesis of Dopamine

The chemical 4-(2-aminoethyl)-1,2-benzenediol, known as dopamine (DA), is one of the most important neurotransmitters in the human nervous system. It is synthesized from phenylalanine (Phe), which is converted by phenylalanine hydroxylase (PH) to tyrosine (Tyr), which is a precursor of several important bioactive molecules. Two enzymes are involved in the conversion of Tyr to DA: L-tyrosine hydroxylase (TH), used as a marker for dopamine-producing cells, and levo-dopa decarboxylase (DOPA DEC). DA synthesized in cells can be used and is then degraded, but in some cells with dopamine beta-hydroxylase

(DAβH), such as adrenal gland cells, it takes part in the synthesis of norepinephrine (NA). The detailed synthesis and degradation process is shown in Figure 1.

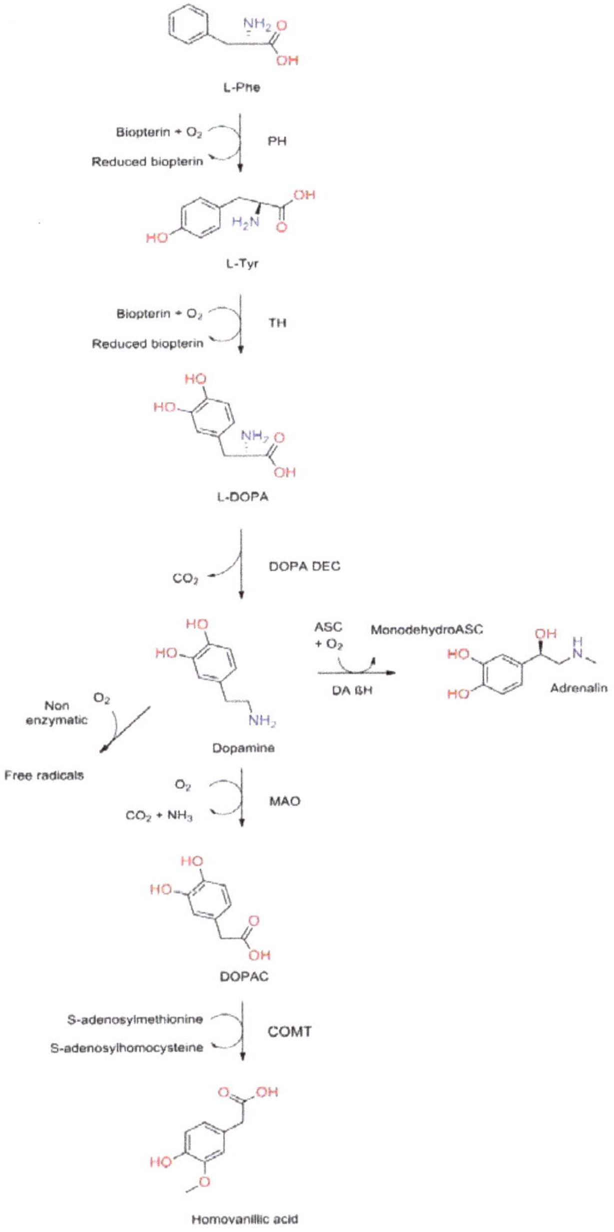

Figure 1. Dopamine synthesis and degradation pathways. L-Phe, L-phenylalanine; PH, phenylalanine hydroxylase; L-Tyr, L-tyrosine; TH, tyrosine hydroxylase; L-DOPA, levo-dopa; DOPA DEC, L-DOPA decarboxylase; ASC, ascorbic acid; DA βH, dopamine β-hydroxylase; MAO, monoamine oxidase; DOPAC, 3,4-dihydroxyphenylacetic acid; COMT, catechol-o-methyltransferase.

In the CNS, the process described above is carried out by groups of neurons called dopaminergic neurons, which can be found in many different parts of the CNS but are mostly concentrated in the substantia nigra pars compacta (SNpc). These neurons are responsible for receiving signals traveling from the striatum, then processing them and further transmitting them to other parts of the CNS, such as the globus pallidus (GP), thalamus, or substantia nigra pars reticulata (SNpr). DA, through the signaling pathways described above, participates in many processes regulated by the CNS, from the control of motor functions to cognition. Its action is based on two well-known mechanisms. The first one, called wiring transmission, involves the release of DA by neurons into the synaptic cleft, which then the released neurotransmitter acts on receptors in the postsynaptic membrane. The second mechanism, which is much more interesting, is called volume transmission, in which DA released from the presynaptic membrane reaches the extracellular space and binds to the dopaminergic receptors of neurons, which are not in direct contact with the cell from which it is released [17–19].

3.2. *Dopamine Receptors*

So far, five dopamine receptors (D1, D2, D3, D4, and D5) have been described. They belong to the G-protein-coupled receptor (GPCR) family. It is considered that the binding of DA to these receptors leads to changes in the concentration of cyclic adenosine monophosphate (cAMP), which changes the activity of kinase DA- and cAMP-regulated phosphoprotein of 32 kDa molecular weight (DARPP32), which is a key protein in dopaminergic neurotransmission. This is mediated by G proteins associated with the individual dopaminergic receptors. The Gs protein, associated with D1 and D5 receptors, causes the activation of adenylate cyclase (AC), which causes an increase in cAMP concentration, while the Gi protein, associated with D2, D3, and D4 receptors, causes inactivation of AC and a decrease in cAMP concentration [20]. This process is shown in Figure 2. Importantly, dopamine receptors can be found not only in the brain, but also in other types of tissues, which leads to the conclusion that DA is more than just a neurotransmitter [21–23].

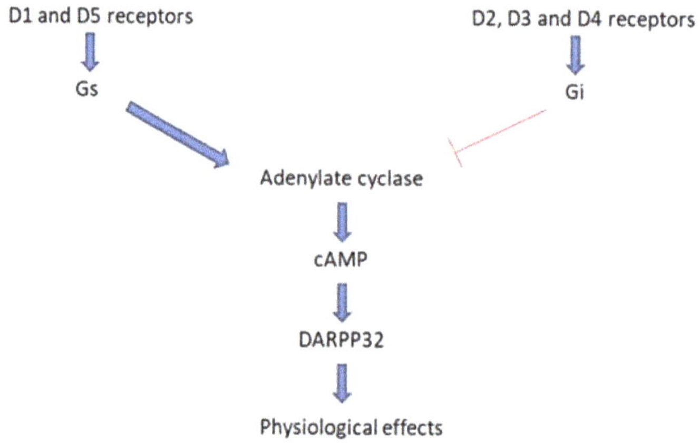

Figure 2. Mechanism of action of dopaminergic receptors. The binding of dopamine to the D1 and D5 receptors causes the activation of adenylate cyclase (AC) via the Gs protein. Activation of AC causes an increase in the concentration of cyclic adenosine monophosphate (cAMP), which results in an increase in the concentration of DA- and cAMP-regulated phosphoprotein of 32 kDa molecular weight (DARPP32), which penetrates into the cell nucleus, inducing a physiological response of the cell to dopamine. The reverse reaction is caused by the binding of dopamine to the D2, D3, and D4 receptors, which causes the inhibition of AC through the Gi protein.

Researchers have repeatedly described the presence of different variants of dopamine receptors and many polymorphisms of the genes encoding these receptors. Importantly, some of these polymorphisms may be associated with some types of addiction, such as alcohol or drug addiction [24–27]. The variety of DA's effects and the variety of drugs affecting dopaminergic transmission come from the ability of dopamine receptors to form complexes in which they combine with each other or with other types of membrane receptors. Importantly, each of the heteromers formed in this way transmits a different signal inside the cell after activation by DA, so each has a different physiological role and pharmacological properties [28,29]. Examples of such heteromers are homeotropic heteromers D1–D3 [30], D2–D3 [31], D2–D5 [32], and D2–D4 [33] and heterotropic heteromers A1–D1 [34], A2A–D2 [35], D1–H3 [36], D2–H3 [37] and D4-adrenergic [38]. The presence of these heteromers is important not only in physiological mechanisms, such as the regulation of melatonin production by the pineal gland [39], but also in the pathogenesis of diseases such as PD. One of the main causes of this disease is the antagonism between dopaminergic transmission and purinergic regulation of neurotransmitter release caused by the presence of A1–D1 and A2A–D2 heteromers [40,41].

3.3. *Cholesterol and Dopaminergic Transmission*

Because disorders of dopaminergic transmission were found to be among the main causes of PD development, researchers have also described other mechanisms that are responsible for such disorders. One of the described mechanisms is a disorder of DA release and reuptake regulated by the dopamine transporter (DAT) and vesicular monoamine transporter 2 (VMAT2) proteins. These proteins are key regulators of DA release into the synaptic cleft. Because the structure of DAT consists of two conserved cholesterol-like molecules, it is suggested that the protein may interact directly with cholesterol. In the absence of cholesterol, changes occur in the conformation of this protein that enhance DA reuptake, and in the presence of bound cholesterol these conformational changes are inhibited [42]. Moreover, cholesterol strengthens H-bonds, which bind DA and levo-dopa (L-DOPA) to the cell membrane, influencing their metabolism [43]. It is worth noting that the relationship between cholesterol and DA is not one-sided. Excess DA is responsible for the increase in cholesterol synthesis by activating the c-Jun N-terminal kinase (JNK3)/sterol regulatory element-binding protein 2 (SREBP2) signaling pathway in astrocyte colonies [44].

Another described mechanism by which cholesterol levels may influence the development of PD is an increased concentration of oxysterols produced from cholesterol. Evidence from studies shows that an elevated concentration of 24-hydroxycholesterol (24-OHC) in the cerebrospinal fluid of patients suffering from PD correlates with the worst prognosis [45]. Accordingly, it has been proposed that 24-OHC becomes a biomarker in PD. Other studies also indicate the effect of 27-hydroxycholesterol (27-OHC), another oxysterol. In dopaminergic neurons, this causes an increase in α-synuclein concentration by inhibiting proteasomes and activating the liver X receptors (LXRs) [46,47]. Moreover, 27-OHC induces inhibition of the estrogen receptor, which leads to inhibition of the expression of TH, and thus slows down the synthesis of DA [48].

The last mechanism by which cholesterol metabolism may affect neurodegenerative processes within dopaminergic neurons is related to the relationship between cholesterol and accumulated α-synuclein deposits [49]; α-synuclein is a protein whose overexpression may inhibit the transport and release of neurotransmitters from synaptic vesicles [50]. The α-synuclein molecule is made up of 140 amino acids and can be broken down into three domains: the *N*-terminal lipid-binding α-helix, the amyloid-binding central domain (known as NAC), and the *C*-terminal acidic tail. Importantly, its structure is characterized by a tandem repeat in the α-helix similar to those found in apolipoproteins. It follows that this protein has a structure similar to apolipoproteins [51,52]. The two cholesterol binding domains thus give the α-synuclein molecule a strong tendency to bind to lipid membranes, especially in cholesterol-rich regions. Moreover, studies conducted in vitro and in animal models show that α-synuclein could play a role in cholesterol transport [53–55]. Studies have reported that cholesterol may affect the interaction between α-synucelin oligomers and the cell membrane, which leads to membrane destruction, and thus cell death [56]. Moreover, with a low concentration of apolipoprotein E (APOE), α-synuclein is more prone to aggregation, which suggests that these two proteins may be competitively bound to cholesterol [57]. The mechanisms described above are illustrated in Figure 3.

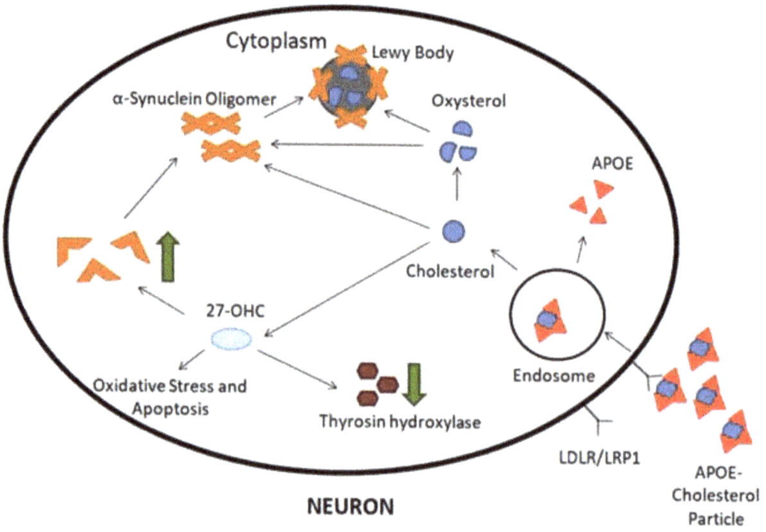

Figure 3. Cholesterol metabolism in Parkinson's disease. After endocytosis of apolipoprotein E (APOE)-cholesterol particles, cholesterol is metabolized to 27-hydroxylcholesterol (27-OHC) and other oxysterols. Furthermore, 27-OHC can increase α-synuclein synthesis, downregulate tyrosine hydroxylase (TH) activity, and cause oxidative stress and apoptosis. In addition, excessive cholesterol and oxysterol can promote α-synuclein aggregation, and aggregated α-synuclein will eventually form Lewy bodies (LBs).

It is important to emphasize that the last two described mechanisms concerning oxysterols and the deposition of α-synuclein are responsible for neurodegeneration not only within dopaminergic neurons, but also within other types of neurons, which may result in the occurrence of diseases such as AD [58,59] or Lewy body dementia (LBD) [60].

3.4. *Influence of Statins on Dopaminergic Transmission*

Due to the above-described mechanisms involving the influence of cholesterol on neurodegenerative processes and dopaminergic transmission, researchers' attention has been drawn to the influence of lipid-lowering therapy with statins on the course of neurodegenerative diseases such as PD and AD. Studies show that chronic statin treatment exerts an anti-inflammatory effect, inhibits oxidative stress, and has a preventive effect on apoptosis of neurons, including dopaminergic neurons [61,62]. This effect is mainly focused on inhibiting the release of pro-inflammatory cytokines and the activation of nuclear factor kappa-light-chain-enhancer of activated B (NF-κB) cells [61]. It has also been proven in cell models that simvastatin, by inhibiting *N*-methyl-*D*-aspartate receptor 1 (NMDAR1), inhibits the inflammatory process within nerve cells [63]. Another mechanism by which statins inhibit neurodegenerative processes is in vitro reduction of beta-amyloid (Aβ) concentration in nerve cells [64], as well as activation of a disintegrin and metalloproteinase domain-containing protein 10 (ADAM10) and increased activity of phospholipid transporter (PLTP), which reduces the concentration of plasma-phosphorylated tau181 (p-tau181) [65]. So far, however, there are no reports describing the influence of statins on the process of dopaminergic transmission by modifying cholesterol levels. All preclinical effects of statins on the process of neurotransmission and neuroprotection discussed in this article are summarized in the Table S1.

In connection with the above-described mechanisms, many clinical trials have been conducted to determine the effects of lipid-lowering therapy on the course of PD and AD. In the case of AD, previous studies have shown that statin therapy reduces the risk of AD by up to 70% [66,67]. However, later studies showed no correlation between this therapy and the risk of dementia [68]. These differences may be caused not only by differences in disease severity between patients, but also by the different chemical properties of the statins. For example, lipophilic statins, due to the ease of crossing BBB, show a stronger effect than hydrophilic ones in inhibiting the progression of AD [69]. In the case of PD research, the divergence is even greater. According to a meta-analysis prepared by Sheng et al., most observational studies show that statins can reduce the risk of PD by up to 26% [70], while several clinical studies have shown that statins are harmful to patients suffering from PD. Studies on the efficacy of statins for the prevention of PD and AD are summarized in Table 1.

Table 1. Studies on the efficacy of statins for prevention of Alzheimer's disease (AD) and Parkinson'sdisease (PD).

Statins	Model	Group Size	Effects	References
All types	Rotterdam study	6992	Reduced risk of late-onset AD	Haag et al. [71]
	Prospective study	15,291	Incerased risk of PD	Huang et al. [72]
	Retrospective case–control analysis	2322	Lipophilic statins increased risk of PD and hydrophilic statins did not affect incidence of PD	Liu et al. [73]
	Population-based cohort study	232,877	Statins did not affect incidence of PD	Rozani et al. [74]
	Meta-analysis	3,845,303	Statins, especially atorvastatin, reduced risk of PD	Yan et al. [75]
	Meta-analysis	3,513,209	Decreased risk of PD	Bai et al. [76]
	Meta-analysis	2,787,249	Statins reduced risk of PD	Sheng et al. [70]
Atorvastatin	Randomized controlled trial	640	No therapeutic effect in AD	Feldman et al. [77]
	Randomized controlled trial	63	AD progressed slowly	Sparks et al. [78]
Lovastatin	Randomized controlled trial	160	Decreased serum Aβ	Friedhoff et al. [79]

Because of these uncertainties regarding the research on groups of patients with PD and AD, well-designed controlled trials are needed to clearly demonstrate the effects of these groups of drugs on neurodegenerative diseases.

4. Statins and Cholinergic Neurotransmission

4.1. Cholinergic Transmission in Pathogenesis of Vascular Dementia

Vascular dementia (VD) is the second most frequent subtype of cognitive disorders after AD [80]. Chronic cerebral hypoperfusion (CCH), the crucial factor, which is caused by negative modification of cerebral blood vessels and associated with the initiation and progression of VD, results in numerous molecular changes inside the brain cells and neuronal junctions, including neurotransmitter and lipid metabolism disturbance, mitochondrial dysfunction, alteration of growth factors, neuroinflammation, and overproduction of reactive oxygen species (ROS) [81].

Acetylcholine (ACh) plays an important role in the physiological functioning of the CNS. The neuronal synthesis of Ach from choline and acetyl-CoA is catalyzed by acetylcholine transferase enzyme (ChAT). Subsequently, Ach, transported in vesicles with the involvement of vesicular acetylcholine transporter (VAChT), is released into the synaptic cleft, where it can bind to receptors. Within the synapse, ACh is degraded by acetylcholinesterase (AChE), resulting in the formation of acetic acid and choline, a precursor for the synthesis of new ACh [82,83].

There are two types of ACh receptors: metabotropic muscarinic receptors (mAChRs) and ionotropic nicotinic receptors (nAChRs). The family of mACHRs contains five subtypes of GPCR, M1–M5. The larger group, with pentameric nAChRs made up of α and β subunits, contains nonselective cation channels. The effects of binding ACh to cholinergic receptors can result in stimulation or inhibition of neuronal signaling, depending on the receptor subtype and its location on a pre- or postsynaptic membrane [84–86].

The basal forebrain cholinergic system, comprising the medial septal nucleus, the nucleus of the diagonal band of Broca, and the nucleus basalis of Meynert, is widely accepted as a crucial structure of cognitive functions. It is involved in the regulation of memory, attention, and emotions [87]. There is some evidence that cholinergic mechanisms are also responsible for the control of cerebral blood flow [88,89]. This may partially explain the pathogenesis of VD and deterioration in the course of disease. The ongoing neuroinflammation in patients with VD may also be attenuated by activation of the cholinergic system (α7 nAChRs) [90].

Ischemic lesions observed in various areas of the brain in patients with VD can cause decreased amounts of ACh, gamma-aminobutyric acid (GABA), or DA [81]. The most profound deficits of common cholinergic markers, such as ChAT, AChE, and VAChT, appear in the temporal cortex and hippocampus [91]. However, the latest research suggests that more evident loss of cholinergic function occurs in the brains of patients with mixed dementia [92]. A decreased Ach level is also observed in cerebrospinal fluid [93,94].Findings concerning changes in cholinergic receptor numbers are contradictory for mAChRs [95,96]. The amount of nAChRs seems to be preserved in VD [97]. The cholinergic reductions observed in the course of VD may be responsible for the cognitive impairment [98].

4.2. Influence of Statins on Cholinergic Transmission

Statins, due to their pluripotential pleiotropic effects on brain cells and vessels beyond lipid-lowering actions, have been widely tested as drugs for the treatment of VD [99]. In L-methionine-induced VD, the use of simvastatin ameliorated behavioral status and increased the amount of ACh in the brain tissue of rats [100]. These encouraging observations have not been seen in human patients with VD. Moreover, some studies indicated potential harmful effects of statin therapy on neuropsychological tests of attention and psychomotor speed [101]. Recent assessments of randomized, placebo-controlled trials did not confirm the clinical significance of these observations [102]. Although statin therapy is useful in primary and secondary prevention of vascular incidents, including strokes, to date there is no conclusive proof that statins have a major influence on the prevention, incidence, or progression of VD [80,103].

5. Statins and Glutamatergic Neurotransmission

5.1. Structure and Synthesis of Glutamate

Glutamate (Glu), the anion of glutamic acid, acts as a neurotransmitter. It is the major excitatory transmitter within the human nervous system, accounting for over 85% of the synaptic connections in the CNS. Glu can be produced de novo from α-ketoglutaric acid as part of the citric acid cycle. In CNS, Glu is synthesized in the glutamate–glutamine cycling mechanism. These reactions occur in presynaptic neurons or glial cells. Glu is transported within presynaptic neurons by vesicular glutamate transporters and then released into the synaptic cleft. Inside the synaptic cleft, anions of glutamic acid can bind several different postsynaptic receptor types, named according to their agonists: kainite receptor (KAR), α-amino-3-hydroxy-5-methyl4-isoxazole propionic acid receptor (AMPAR), and N-methyl-D-aspartate receptor (NMDAR). Glu binds to these receptors with different affinity and induces differential effects on target postsynaptic neurons [104,105]. For this part of the review, we would like to focus on NMDARs.

5.2. N-Methyl-D-Aspartate Receptor

Belonging to the neurotransmitter receptors, NMDARs constitute the largest subclass of glutamate-gated ion channels in human excitatory synapses, which have a main part in neuroplasticity, neuronal development, and learning and memory processes [106]. NMDARs are heteromeric molecules formed of one obligatory GluN1 (also referred to asNR1) incorporated with various constellations of GluN2 (also named NR2) and GluN3 subunits, which take several variants: the single GluN1 subunit with eight isoforms, four GluN2 subunits (GluN2A–GluN2D), and two GluN3 subunits. Both the GluN1 and GluN2 subunits participate in the development of the NMDAR ion channel. Each NMDAR has a similar membrane subunit topology, which is dominated by a large extracellular N-terminus, a membrane region containing three transmembrane segments, a re-entrant loop, and an extracellular loop between the transmembrane segments. Intracellularly, it is situated in a carboxyl (C) domain of various sizes, and miscellaneous proteins interact in this site [107–111].

NMDAR is extraordinary in that the opening of the channel requires the merging of two different agonists, Glu and glycine (Gly). Glu binds to the GluN2 subunit, while the binding site for Gly, the co-agonist, is located on the GluN1 subunits. The NMDAR ion channel is permeable to monovalent cations, such as Na^+ and K^+, and divalent cations, especially Ca^{2+}. It is regulated by voltage-dependent Mg^{2+} blockade. Accordingly, both depolarization of the postsynaptic neurons and presynaptic release of Glu is needed for maximal current flow through the NMDAR channel. The concentration of Gly in most synapses is usually enough to allow for efficient NMDAR activation [108,110–113]. NMDAR is mainly located at dendritic spines, where through specific interactions it connects to intracellular molecules of the postsynaptic multiprotein network known as the postsynaptic density (PSD); for the subunit GluN1thisis neurofilament light protein (NF-L), while for GluN2 these are PSD-95, PSD-93, and synapse-associated protein 102(SAP102). In addition to their function as PSD cytoskeleton proteins, PSD-95 and SAP102 are involved in transporting newly synthesized NMDA receptors to the PSD. Build or behavior irregularities for these molecules could disturb receptor signaling, interfere with NMDAR trafficking, and finally affect neurotransmission [107]. The number of NMDARs can be modified, which contributes to the mechanism regulating synaptic efficacy and their remodeling [114]. With disorder in the NMDA signal pathway, glutamatergic transmission could exacerbate brain diseases, including psychiatric, neurodegenerative, and excitotoxic disorders [112].

5.3. *Role of Glutamatergic Transmission in the Pathogenesis of Stroke*

Excitotoxicity is a pathological process that causes cell death as the result of the toxic actions of excitatory amino acids. Considering that Glu is the main excitatory neurotransmitter in the human CNS, excitotoxicity typically refers to the trauma and death of neurons that occur from prolonged exposition to Glu. It comes from overloading the cell with ions, mainly calcium, which is notably neurotoxic and leads to the activation of enzymes that degrade proteins, nucleic acids, and other components of the cell. It is considered that Ca^{2+} inflow through NMDA channels is a common pathway of neuronal cell death. Excess levels of Glu in the CNS are associated with increased intracellular calcium ions levels, which cause a rise in their concentration in sensitive organelles such as mitochondria and the endoplasmic reticulum (ER) [115]. The mitochondrial uptake of calcium results in the production of ROS [116].

Stroke is a major cause of death, causing approximately 9% of deaths worldwide. Up to 80% of the global burden of stroke is attributed to ischemic stroke. This is a type of stroke characterized by a temporary or permanent reduction in blood perfusion due to embolic or thrombotic occlusion in cerebral arteries. Most cases of focal ischemia result from occlusion of the middle cerebral artery [117]. There is evidence that stroke leads to the release of large amounts of Glu, which activates NMDARs, and that glutamate-induced excitotoxicity participates in the neuronal death observed after stroke [118]. The first step of excitotoxicity during acute ischemia is a sudden increase of Glu levels in the ischemic region of the brain. Activation of NMDARs does not always lead to excitotoxicity. There is evidence that this receptor has dual effects, depending on the subunit subpopulation. GluN2A tends to promote neuronal survival and protects the brain against excitotoxic injury, whereas the GluN2B subunit promotes neuronal death. Cerebral ischemia triggering excessive activation of NMDARs induces rapid and specific upregulation of GluN2B [119].

Previous studies found that the excitotoxic process connected with acute ischemia is responsible for redistributed microtubule-associated proteins (MAP2) and loss of microtubule stability as a consequence. Normally these proteins are engaged in the regulation of vesicle transport during the creation or recovery of neuronal pathways [120]. Complexes of cadherin or catenins and actin are involved in maintaining the structure of the scaffolding proteins. Cerebral ischemia leads to structural damage of the cytoskeleton mediated by RhoGTPasas imbalance, Ras homolog family member A (RhoA) activation, and inactivation of Ras-related C3 botulinum toxin substrate (Rac), related to the rupture of adhesion. A study by Cespedes-Rubio showed that RhoA activity is increased in cell death processes due to excitotoxicity [121]. The inflammatory response induced by ischemia triggers the activation of signaling pathways, finally leading to neuronal cell death. There is evidence confirming that the phosphatidylinositol 3-kinase (PI3K)-protein kinase B (Akt) signaling pathway is one of the serious signaling paths taking part in neuronal apoptosis. Glycogen synthase kinase-3β (GSK-3β) is an important protein downstream of Akt. Sustained activation of GSK-3β is pro-apoptotic in cerebral ischemia because it leads to hyperphosphorylation of tau, with consequent microtubule destabilization [122].

5.4. *Influence of Statins on Glutamatergic Transmission and Their Neuroprotective Effect*

Researchers continue to look for new effects of statin treatment in stroke, in primary and secondary prevention and in the acute phase of ischemia. Statins exert protective effects in vivo and in experimental models of stroke. Recent meta-analyses showed that statin therapy significantly reduces the overall risk and mortality rate of stroke, in both primary and secondary prevention, which confirms that accurate control of the lipid profile is needed [123,124]. Beyond their effects on the lipid profile, statins are also credited with pleiotropic effects. Among the pleiotropic effects reported in cerebral ischemia is improved endothelial function, stabilized atherosclerotic plaque, impaired inflammation with a concomitant decrease in ROS, and inhibition of the thrombogenic response [125]. Increasingly, studies are examining the effects of statin treatment on NMDARs and the process of excitotoxicity after acute ischemia. The precise mechanisms involved in these actions are not completely known. Studies indicate that NMDA channels are involved in the neuroprotective mechanism induced by statins to promote neuronal recovery after cerebral focal ischemia.

Gutierrez-Vargas et al. examined the influence of a high dose of atorvastatin on NMDA receptors after cerebral ischemia in laboratory rats. This work suggests that atorvastatin protects neurons after ischemia, restoring the balance of subunits by decreasing GluN2B upregulation [106]. Additionally, the same study described that treatment with atorvastatin improves the adhesion protein complex of NMDARs associated with PSD-95, influences Akt activation in promoting cell survival, and in turn promotes synaptic plasticity. Statins inhibit the synthesis of valid isoprenoids, such as farnesyl pyrophosphate (FPP) and geranylgeranyl pyrophosphate (GGPP), which are important intermediates for the post-translational modification of Rho GTPases, leading to the modulation of various cellular functions, e.g., decreased structural damage of the cytoskeleton [125]. Additionally, Gutierrez-Vargas et al. proved that atorvastatin used after ischemic stroke influences the recovery of the actin cytoskeleton and stabilizes microtubules by increased activity of Rac and RhoA reduction [126]. Another mechanism of neuroprotection by statins involves their influence on inflammation through a number of proinflammatory cytokines. Tuttolomondo et al., in the first human randomized trial, proved that early administration of high-dose atorvastatin caused a significantly lower serum level of inflammatory markers and may be related to a better prognosis after stroke [127]. Additionally, Campos-Martorell et al. showed that simvastatin used after acute ischemia had an influence on decreased oxidative stress [128]. Brain-derived neurotrophic factor (BDNF) induces neuronal proliferation and synaptogenesis and is also involved in the regulation of neurogenesis. After injury, it takes part in the recovery of neuronal tissue. Cerebral ischemia decreased levels of BDNF [129]. Atorvastatin used in the treatment of cerebral ischemia in animals led to recovered BDNF levels [106].

Considering that cerebral ischemia is one of the major global health problems with great costs for rehabilitation and recovery, more effective and accessible methods are needed to immediately reduce postischemic injury. Statins meet these criteria: they are cheap and easily available. Experimental models, experiments on rats, and preclinical studies have shown that they influence neuronal cells differently and could be used to reduce neurodegeneration after stroke. The above studies prove that large multi-center clinical studies are needed.

6. Statins and Serotoninergic Neurotransmission

6.1. Structure and Synthesis of Serotonin

Serotonin (5-HT) is one of the oldest neurotransmitters; it is estimated that its receptors appeared 700–800 million years ago in unicellular eukaryotes, such as Paramecium caudatum [130]. It is a monoamine produced within both the CNS and the peripheral nervous system (PNS). In the CNS, serotonergic neurons can be found in the dorsalraphe nucleus (DRN) and median raphe nucleus (MRN) [131]. In the PNS, it is synthesized in the gastrointestinal (GI) system by gut neurons and enterochromaffin cells. The substrate for its production is tryptophan and the synthesis process follows the scheme shown in Figure 4 [132].

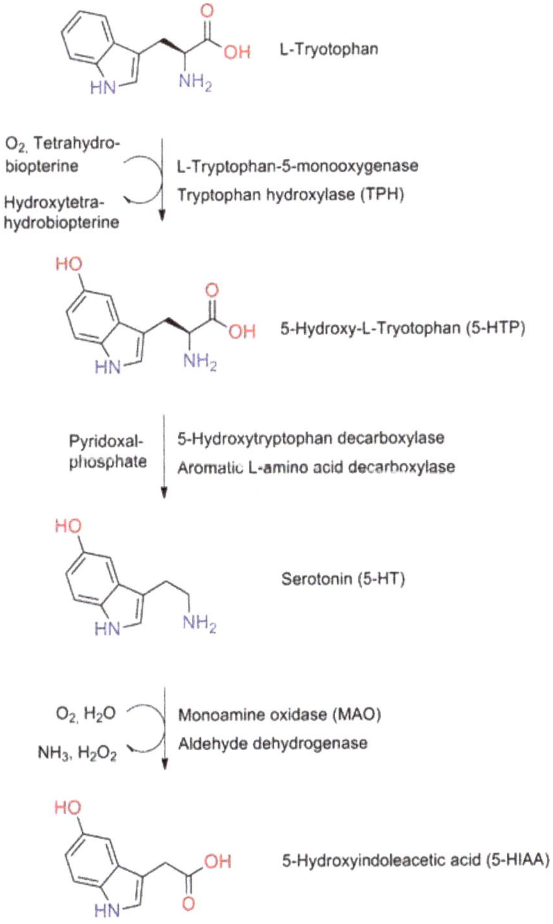

Figure 4. Serotonin synthesis and degradation pathways.

In the CNS, serotonergic neurons from DRN and MRN communicate with various areas within the cerebral cortex, limbic system, midbrain, and cerebellum [133]. Serotonin communication occurs mainly through volume transmission (VT) in the extracellular space and the cerebrospinal fluid (CSF). Serotonin travels from the source to target cells (neurons and astroglia) through energy gradients, leading to its diffusion and convection [134]. By interacting with its receptors, 5-HT is responsible for the regulation of many processes important for life, which include perception, mood, anxiety, aggression, cognitive functions, attention, sexual functions, and the circadian rhythm [131,135,136].

6.2. Serotonin Receptors and Transporters

Thirteen G-protein-coupled heptahelial serotonin receptors (5-HTRs) and one ligand-gated ion channel have been identified and are divided into seven distinct classes (5-$HT_{1–7}$) [132,134]. All 5-HTRs are heteroreceptors associated with the postsynaptic membrane on nonserotonergic neurons. Presynaptically located autoreceptors (5-$HT_{1A,1B,1D}$) respond to the regulation of 5-HT release through negative feedback and influence the neuronal firing rate. The 5-HTRs are located within the CNS, PNS, and other tissues, and the exact mechanisms of their action and the effects of stimulation are presented in Table 2 [132,137].

Table 2. Serotonin (5-HT) receptor subtypes. CNS, central nervous system; cAMP, cyclic adenosine monophosphate; AC, adenylate cyclase; GIT, gastrointestinal tract; IP3, inositol-1,4,5-triphosphate; PKC, protein kinase C.

Receptor	Location	Mechanism of Action	Functions
5-HT_{1A}	CNS	Decreased cAMP concentration by inhibition of AC	Learning and memory, depression, anxiety-like behaviors
5-HT_{1B}	CNS, vascular smooth muscle	Decreased cAMP concentration by inhibition of AC	Aggression, antimigraine effects and vasoconstriction, depression and anxiety-like behaviors
5-HT_{1C}	CNS, limfocytes	Not completely understood	Not completely understood
5-HT_{1D}	CNS, vascular smooth muscle	Decreased cAMP concentration by inhibition of AC	Pain perception, antimigraine effects, and vasoconstriction
5-HT_{1E}	CNS	Decreased cAMP concentration by inhibition of AC	Not completely understood
5-HT_{1F}	CNS, uterus, heart, GIT	Decreased cAMP concentration by inhibition of AC	Pain perception, antimigraine effects, andanxiety-like behaviors
5-HT_{2A}	CNS, PNS, thrombocytes, smooth muscles	Enhanced AC activity and IP3	Pain perception, sensorimotor, motivation, emotionalregulation, vasoconstriction, smooth muscles cell constriction, thrombocyte aggregation
5-HT_{2B}	CNS, stomach	Enhanced PKC activity and IP3	Anxiety-like behaviors, smooth muscle cell constriction
5-HT_{2C}	CNS, limfocytes	Enhanced PKC activity and IP3	Anxiogenesis, sexual behavior, pain perception, regulation of serotonergic neuron activity
5-HT_3	CNS, PNS	Opening of Na^+, Ca^{2+}, and K^+ channels, depolarization of plasma membrane	Vomiting reflex, anxiety-like behaviors
5-HT_4	CNS, PNS	Increased cAMP concentration by activation of AC	Anxiety-like behaviors, learning and memory
5-HT_{5A}	CNS	Decreased cAMP concentration by inhibition of AC	Learning and memory, emotional behaviors, acquisition of adaptive behavior, circadian rhythm
5-HT_6	CNS, leukocytes	Increased cAMP concentration by activation of AC	Anxiety-like behaviors, learning and memory, cognition
5-HT_7	CNS, GIT, vascular smooth muscles	Increased cAMP concentration by activation of AC	Regulation of sleep and circadian rhythm, thermoregulation, learning and memory, regulation of 5-HT release

One of the new concepts of depression is that disturbances in integrated allosteric receptor–receptor interactions in highly sensitive 5-HT_{1A} heteroreceptor complexes may contribute to the induction of major depression (MD). For example, disruption or dysfunction in 5-HT_{1A}-FGFR1 heteroreceptor complexes in the suture–hippocampal serotonin neuron systems may contribute to the development of MD [134].

Another important membrane protein involved in serotonergic transmission is the serotonin reuptake transporter (SERT). It is responsible for the removal of free 5-HT from the synaptic cleft, which directly affects the duration of 5-HTR activation. Some transporter-regulatory proteins, such as syntaxin 1A (Syn1A) and secretory carrier membrane protein 2 (SCAMP2), are involved in regulating the activity of SERT [138]. It is also known that some polymorphisms in the SERT gene are associated with the occurrence of depression, anxiety disorders, autism, and suicidality [139]; therefore, the process of 5-HT reuptake has become one of the most important points in therapy for depression disorders.

6.3. Influence of Statins on Serotoninergic Transmission

Due to the influence of statins on neurodegenerative diseases and cognitive disorders known from many studies, consideration was also given to their potential influence on psychiatric disorders. A possible mechanism of their action is to increase serotonin reuptake through the SERT receptor in a manner independent of the cholesterol synthesis pathway, as described in animal models [140]. The range of concentrations in which statins increase SERT uptake is wide and includes concentrations achieved in acute systemic treatment [140,141]. Such a mechanism would suggest a potential effect of intensifying or inducing depressive symptoms. However, a cohort study of the Swedish population published in 2020 suggested that the incidence of depressive disorders in the group of people taking statins was lower than in the general population [142].

Possible mechanisms underlying the antidepressant effects of statins may include anti-inflammatory, antioxidant, and lipid-lowering properties [143]. The potential anti-inflammatory effects of statins include lowering C-reactive protein (CRP) levels [144] andantioxidant activity [145], inhibiting the production of pro-inflammatory cytokines by monocytes [146], inhibiting lymphocytes by blocking the function of antigen-1 leukocytes (LFA-1) [147], and blocking T-cell activation [148]. The antidepressant mechanism of statins may also be related to their antiatherosclerotic effect and their influence on damage to small white matter vessels, which underlies the hypothesis of vascular depression [149]. Such injuries may predispose people to depression, accelerate its course, and reduce the effectiveness of antidepressants [143].

Despite the mechanisms described above and the retrospective studies conducted so far, the influence of statins on the incidence of depressive disorders is still unclear and requires further research.

7. Conclusions

To date, researchers have described a number of mechanisms by which cholesterol influences neuronal transmission. These mechanisms can also be influenced by statins, which has been confirmed in animal and cellular models. Additionally, many retrospective studies have described the beneficial effects of this group of drugs on neurological diseases and psychiatric disorders. So far, however, there have been no clinical trials that have unequivocally proven their beneficial effects on the diseases described in our paper. This opens up a wide field for researchers, especially as statins still remain one of the most widely used drug groups in the general population.

Supplementary Materials: The following are available online. Table S1: Preclinical effects of statins on neurotransmission and neuroprotection.

Author Contributions: Conceptualization, M.K. and J.S.-K.; methodology, M.K. and J.S.-K.; resources, M.K., J.S.-K., M.H., M.B., M.M., and G.M.; writing—original draft preparation, M.K., J.S.-K., M.H., and M.M.; writing—review and editing, M.K., M.B., R.P., and B.O.; supervision, R.P. and B.O.; project administration, M.K., J.S.-K., and M.B. All authors have read and agreed to the published version of the manuscript.

Funding: This research was funded by Medical University of Silesia, grant number PCN-1-185/N/9/O.

Institutional Review Board Statement: Not applicable.

Informed Consent Statement: Not applicable.

Data Availability Statement: Not applicable.

Conflicts of Interest: The authors declare no conflict of interest.

References

1. Koushki, K.; Shahbaz, S.K.; Mashayekhi, K.; Sadeghi, M.; Zayeri, Z.D.; Taba, M.Y.; Banach, M.; Al-Rasadi, K.; Johnston, T.P.; Sahebkar, A. Anti-inflammatory Action of Statins in Cardiovascular Disease: The Role of Inflammasome and Toll-Like Receptor Pathways. *Clin. Rev. Allergy Immunol.* **2021**, *60*, 175–199. [CrossRef]
2. Rabar, S.; Harker, M.; O'Flynn, N.; Wierzbicki, A.S.; On behalf of the Guideline Development Group. Lipid modification and cardiovascular risk assessment for the primary and secondary prevention of cardiovascular disease: Summary of updated NICE guidance. *BMJ* **2014**, *349*, g4356. [CrossRef]
3. Altaf, A.; Qu, P.; Zhao, Y.; Wang, H.; Lou, D.; Niu, N. NLRP3 inflammasome in peripheral blood monocytes of acute coronary syndrome patients and its relationship with statins. *Coron. Artery Dis.* **2015**, *26*, 409–421. [CrossRef]
4. de Bont, N.; Netea, M.G.; Rovers, C.; Smilde, T.; Demacker, P.N.; van der Meer, J.W.; Stalenhoef, A.F. LPS-induced cytokine pro-duction and expression of LPS-receptors by peripheral blood mononuclear cells of patients with familial hypercholesterolemia and the effect of HMG-CoA reductase inhibitors. *Atherosclerosis* **1998**, *139*, 147–152. [CrossRef]
5. Muldoon, M.F.; Manuck, S.B.; Matthews, K.A. Lowering cholesterol concentrations and mortality: A quantitative review of primary prevention trials. *BMJ* **1990**, *301*, 309–314. [CrossRef] [PubMed]
6. Huang, T.-L.; Wu, S.-C.; Chiang, Y.-S.; Chen, J.-F. Correlation between serum lipid, lipoprotein concentrations and anxious state, depressive state or major depressive disorder. *Psychiatry Res.* **2003**, *118*, 147–153. [CrossRef]
7. Vevera, J.; Zukov, I.; Morcinek, T.; Papezová, H. Cholesterol concentrations in violent and non-violent women suicide attempters. *Eur. Psychiatry* **2003**, *18*, 23–27. [CrossRef]
8. Parsaik, A.K.; Singh, B.; Hassan, M.M.; Singh, K.; Mascarenhas, S.S.; Williams, M.D.; Lapid, M.I.; Richardson, J.W.; West, C.P.; Rummans, T.A. Statins use and risk of depression: A systematic review and meta-analysis. *J. Affect. Disord.* **2014**, *160*, 62–67. [CrossRef]
9. Yatham, M.S.; Yatham, K.S.; Ravindran, A.V.; Sullivan, F. Do statins have an effect on depressive symptoms? A systematic review and meta-analysis. *J. Affect. Disord.* **2019**, *257*, 55–63. [CrossRef] [PubMed]
10. Corrigan, F.; Van Rhijn, A.; Ijomah, G.; McIntyre, F.; Skinner, E.; Horrobin, D.; Ward, N. Tin and fatty acids in dementia. *Prostaglandins, Leukot. Essent. Fat. Acids.* **1991**, *43*, 229–238. [CrossRef]
11. Dexter, D.T.; Holley, A.E.; Flitter, W.D.; Slater, T.F.; Wells, F.R.; Daniel, S.E.; Lees, A.J.; Jenner, P.; Marsden, C.D. Increased levels of lipid hydroperoxides in the parkinsonian substantia nigra: An HPLC and ESR study. *Mov. Disord.* **1994**, *9*, 92–97. [CrossRef]
12. Kivipelto, M.; Solomon, A. Cholesterol as a risk factor for Alzheimer's disease—Epidemiological evidence. *Acta Neurol. Scand. Suppl.* **2006**, *185*, 50–57. [CrossRef]
13. Wei, Q.; Wang, H.; Tian, Y.; Xu, F.; Chen, X.; Wang, K. Reduced Serum Levels of Triglyceride, Very Low Density Lipoprotein Cholesterol and Apolipoprotein B in Parkinson's Disease Patients. *PLoS ONE* **2013**, *8*, e75743. [CrossRef]
14. Schachter, M. Chemical, pharmacokinetic and pharmacodynamic properties of statins: An update. *Fundam. Clin. Pharmacol.* **2004**, *19*, 117–125. [CrossRef]
15. Davidson, M.H. Rosuvastatin: A highly efficacious statin for the treatment of dyslipidaemia. *Expert Opin. Investig. Drugs.* **2002**, *11*, 125–141. [CrossRef]
16. Irwin, J.C.; Fenning, A.S.; Vella, R.K. Statins with different lipophilic indices exert distinct effects on skeletal, cardiac and vascular smooth muscle. *Life Sci.* **2020**, *242*, 117225. [CrossRef]
17. Fuxe, K.; Borroto-Escuela, D.O. Volume transmission and receptor-receptor interactions in heteroreceptor complexes: Understanding the role of new concepts for brain communication. *Neural Regen. Res.* **2016**, *11*, 1220–1223. [CrossRef]
18. Fuxe, K.; Agnati, L.F.; Marcoli, M.; Borroto-Escuela, D.O. Volume Transmission in Central Dopamine and Noradrenaline Neurons and Its Astroglial Targets. *Neurochem. Res.* **2015**, *40*, 2600–2614. [CrossRef] [PubMed]
19. Zoli, M.; Torri, C.; Ferrari, R.; Jansson, A.; Zini, I.; Fuxe, K.; Agnati, L.F. The emergence of the volume transmission concept. *Brain Res. Rev.* **1998**, *26*, 136–147. [CrossRef]
20. Alexander, S.P.; Christopoulos, A.; Davenport, A.P.; Kelly, E.; Mathie, A.; Peters, J.A.; Veale, E.L.; Armstrong, J.F.; Faccenda, E.; Harding, S.D.; et al. The concise guide to pharmacology 2019/20: G protein-coupled receptors. *Br. J. Pharmacol.* **2019**, *176*, 21–141.
21. Ricci, A.; Mignini, F.; Tomassoni, D.; Amenta, F. Dopamine receptor subtypes in the human pulmonary arterial tree. *Auton. Autacoid Pharmacol.* **2006**, *26*, 361–369. [CrossRef]
22. Hussain, T.; Lokhandwala, M.F. Renal Dopamine Receptors and Hypertension. *Exp. Biol. Med.* **2003**, *228*, 134–142. [CrossRef] [PubMed]
23. Aslanoglou, D.; Bertera, S.; Sánchez-Soto, M.; Benjamin Free, R.; Lee, J.; Zong, W.; Xue, X.; Shrestha, S.; Brissova, M.; Logan, R.W.; et al. Dopamine regulates pancreatic glucagon and insulin secretion via adrenergic and dopaminergic receptors. *Transl. Psychiatry* **2021**, *11*, 59. [CrossRef]
24. Kranzler, H.R.; Edenberg, H.J. Pharmacogenetics of Alcohol and Alcohol Dependence Treatment. *Curr. Pharm. Des.* **2010**, *16*, 2141–2148. [CrossRef] [PubMed]

25. Le Foll, B.; Gallo, A.; Le Strat, Y.; Lu, L.; Gorwood, P. Genetics of dopamine receptors and drug addiction: A comprehensive review. *Behav. Pharmacol.* **2009**, *20*, 1–17. [CrossRef] [PubMed]
26. Smith, L.; Watson, M.; Gates, S.; Ball, D.; Foxcroft, D. Meta-Analysis of the Association of the Taq1A Polymorphism with the Risk of Alcohol Dependency: A HuGE Gene-Disease Association Review. *Am. J. Epidemiol.* **2007**, *167*, 125–138. [CrossRef]
27. Tyndale, R.F. Genetics of alcohol and tobacco use in humans. *Ann. Med.* **2003**, *35*, 94–121. [CrossRef]
28. Franco, N.; Franco, R. Understanding the Added Value of G-Protein-Coupled Receptor Heteromers. *Scientifica* **2014**, *2014*, 362937. [CrossRef]
29. Franco, R.; Casadó, V.; Cortés, A.; Ferrada, C.; Mallol, J.; Woods, A.; Lluís, C.; Canela, E.I.; Ferre, S. Basic Concepts in G-Protein-Coupled Receptor Homo- and Heterodimerization. *Sci. World J.* **2007**, *7*, 48–57. [CrossRef]
30. Marcellino, D.; Ferré, S.; Casadó, V.; Cortés, A.; Le Foll, B.; Mazzola, C.; Drago, F.; Saur, O.; Stark, H.; Soriano, A.; et al. Identification of dopamine D1-D3 receptor heteromers: Indications for a role of synergistic D1-D3 receptor interactions in the striatum. *J. Biol. Chem.* **2008**, *283*, 26016–26025. [CrossRef]
31. Scarselli, M.; Novi, F.; Schallmach, E.; Lin, R.; Baragli, A.; Colzi, A.; Griffon, N.; Corsini, G.U.; Sokoloff, P.; Levenson, R.; et al. D2/D3 Dopamine Receptor Heterodimers Exhibit Unique Functional Properties. *J. Biol. Chem.* **2001**, *276*, 30308–30314. [CrossRef]
32. Hasbi, A.; Fan, T.; Alijaniaram, M.; Nguyen, T.; Perreault, M.L.; O'Dowd, B.F.; George, S.R. Calcium signaling cascade links do-pamine D1-D2 receptor heteromer to striatal BDNF production and neuronal growth. *Proc. Natl. Acad. Sci. USA* **2009**, *106*, 21377–21382. [CrossRef] [PubMed]
33. Borroto-Escuela, D.O.; Van Craenenbroeck, K.; Romero-Fernandez, W.; Guidolin, D.; Woods, A.S.; Rivera, A.; Haegeman, G.; Agnati, L.F.; Tarakanov, A.O.; Fuxe, K. Dopamine D2 and D4 receptor heteromerization and its allosteric receptor–receptor inter-actions. *Biochem. Biophys. Res. Commun.* **2011**, *404*, 928–934. [CrossRef] [PubMed]
34. Ginés, S.; Hillion, J.; Torvinen, M.; Le Crom, S.; Casadó, V.; Canela, E.I.; Rondin, S.; Lew, J.Y.; Watson, S.; Zoli, M.; et al. Dopamine D1 and adenosine A1 receptors form functionally interacting heteromeric complexes. *Proc. Natl. Acad. Sci. USA* **2000**, *97*, 8606–8611. [CrossRef] [PubMed]
35. Hillion, J.; Canals, M.; Torvinen, M.; Casadó, V.; Scott, R.; Terasmaa, A.; Hansson, A.; Watson, S.; Olah, M.E.; Mallol, J.; et al. Coaggregation, Cointernalization, and Codesensitization of Adenosine A2A Receptors and Dopamine D2Receptors. *J. Biol. Chem.* **2002**, *277*, 18091–18097. [CrossRef] [PubMed]
36. Ferrada, C.; Moreno, E.; Casadó, V.; Bongers, G.; Cortés, A.; Mallol, J.; Canela, E.I.; Leurs, R.; Ferré, S.; Lluís, C.; et al. Marked changes in signal transduction upon heteromerization of dopamine D1 and histamine H3 receptors. *Br. J. Pharmacol.* **2009**, *157*, 64–75. [CrossRef]
37. Ferrada, C.; Ferré, S.; Casadó, V.; Cortés, A.; Justinova, Z.; Barnes, C.; Canela, E.I.; Goldberg, S.R.; Leurs, R.; Lluis, C.; et al. Inter-actions between histamine H3 and dopamine D2 receptors and the implications for striatal function. *Neuropharmacology* **2008**, *55*, 190–197. [CrossRef]
38. Borroto-Escuela, D.O.; Brito, I.; Romero-Fernandez, W.; Di Palma, M.; Oflijan, J.; Skieterska, K.; Duchou, J.; Van Craenenbroeck, K.; Suárez-Boomgaard, D.; Rivera, A.; et al. The G protein-coupled receptor heterodimer network (GPCR-HetNet) and its hub com-ponents. *Int. J. Mol. Sci.* **2014**, *15*, 8570–8590. [CrossRef]
39. Gonzalez, S.; Moreno-Delgado, D.; Moreno, E.; Pérez-Capote, K.; Franco, R.; Mallol, J.; Cortés, A.; Casadó, V.; Lluis, C.; Ortiz, J.; et al. Circadian-Related Heteromerization of Adrenergic and Dopamine D4 Receptors Modulates Melatonin Synthesis and Release in the Pineal Gland. *PLoS Biol.* **2012**, *10*, e1001347. [CrossRef] [PubMed]
40. Navarro, G.; Borroto-Escuela, D.O.D.O.; Fuxe, K.; Franco, R. Purinergic signaling in Parkinson's disease. Relevance for treatment. *Neuropharmacology* **2015**, *104*, 161–168. [CrossRef]
41. Fuxe, K.; Agnati, L.; Jacobsen, K.; Hillion, J.; Canals, M.; Torvinen, M.; Tinner-Staines, B.; Staines, W.; Rosin, D.; Terasmaa, A.; et al. Receptor heteromerization in adenosine A2A receptor signaling: Relevance for striatal function and Parkinson's disease. *Neurology* **2003**, *61*, S19–S23. [CrossRef] [PubMed]
42. Zeppelin, T.; Ladefoged, L.K.; Sinning, S.; Periole, X.; Schiøtt, B. A direct interaction of cholesterol with the dopamine transporter prevents its out-to-inward transition. *PLoS Comput. Biol.* **2018**, *14*, e1005907. [CrossRef]
43. Orłowski, A.; Grzybek, M.; Bunker, A.; Pasenkiewicz-Gierula, M.; Vattulainen, I.; Männistö, P.T.; Róg, T. Strong preferences of dopamine and l-dopa towards lipid head group: Importance of lipid composition and implication for neurotransmitter metabolism. *J. Neurochem.* **2012**, *122*, 681–690. [CrossRef]
44. Zhuge, W.; Wen, F.; Ni, Z.; Zheng, Z.; Zhu, X.; Lin, J.; Wang, J.; Zhuge, Q.; Ding, S. Dopamine Burden Triggers Cholesterol Overload Following Disruption of Synaptogenesis in Minimal Hepatic Encephalopathy. *Neuroscience* **2019**, *410*, 1–15. [CrossRef]
45. Björkhem, I.; Lövgren-Sandblom, A.; Leoni, V.; Meaney, S.; Brodin, L.; Salveson, L.; Winge, K.; Pålhagen, S.; Svenningsson, P. Oxysterols and Parkinson's disease: Evidence that levels of 24S-hydroxycholesterol in cerebrospinal fluid correlates with the duration of the disease. *Neurosci. Lett.* **2013**, *555*, 102–105. [CrossRef] [PubMed]
46. Cheng, D.; Kim, W.S.; Garner, B. Regulation of α-synuclein expression by liver X receptor ligands in vitro. *NeuroReport* **2008**, *19*, 1685–1689. [CrossRef] [PubMed]
47. Schommer, J.; Marwarha, G.; Schommer, T.; Flick, T.; Lund, J.; Ghribi, O. 27-Hydroxycholesterol increases α-synuclein protein levels through proteasomal inhibition in human dopaminergic neurons. *BMC Neurosci.* **2018**, *19*, 17. [CrossRef]

48. Marwarha, G.; Rhen, T.; Schommer, T.; Ghribi, O. The oxysterol 27-hydroxycholesterol regulates α-synuclein and tyrosine hy-droxylase expression levels in human neuroblastoma cells through modulation of liver X receptors and estrogen receptors–relevance to Parkinson's disease. *J. Neurochem.* **2011**, *119*, 1119–1136. [CrossRef]
49. Nakamura, K.; Mori, F.; Tanji, K.; Miki, Y.; Yamada, M.; Kakita, A.; Takahashi, H.; Utsumi, J.; Sasaki, H.; Wakabayashi, K. Iso-pentenyl diphosphate isomerase, a cholesterol synthesizing enzyme, is localized in Lewy bodies. *Neuropathology* **2015**, *35*, 432–440. [CrossRef]
50. Scott, D.; Roy, S. α-Synuclein inhibits intersynaptic vesicle mobility and maintains recycling-pool homeostasis. *J. Neurosci.* **2012**, *32*, 10129–10135. [CrossRef]
51. Krüger, R.; Vieira-Saecker, A.M.; Kuhn, W.; Berg, D.; Müller, T.; Kühnl, N.; Fuchs, G.A.; Storch, A.; Hungs, M.; Woitallam, D.; et al. Increased susceptibility to sporadic Parkinson's disease by a certain combined alpha-synuclein/apolipoprotein E genotype. *Ann. Neurol.* **1999**, *45*, 611–617. [CrossRef]
52. Fantini, J.; Carlus, D.; Yahi, N. The fusogenic tilted peptide (67–78) of α-synuclein is a cholesterol binding domain. *Biochim. Biophys. Acta (BBA) Biomembr.* **2011**, *1808*, 2343–2351. [CrossRef]
53. Hsiao, J.-H.T.; Halliday, G.M.; Kim, W.S. α-Synuclein Regulates Neuronal Cholesterol Efflux. *Molecules* **2017**, *22*, 1769. [CrossRef] [PubMed]
54. Sui, Y.-T.; Bullock, K.M.; Erickson, M.A.; Zhang, J.; Banks, W. Alpha synuclein is transported into and out of the brain by the blood–brain barrier. *Peptides* **2014**, *62*, 197–202. [CrossRef] [PubMed]
55. Barceló-Coblijn, G.; Golovko, M.Y.; Weinhofer, I.; Berger, J.; Murphy, E.J. Brain neutral lipids mass is increased in α-synuclein gene-ablated mice. *J. Neurochem.* **2006**, *101*, 132–141. [CrossRef] [PubMed]
56. Van Maarschalkerweerd, A.; Vetri, V.; Vestergaard, B. Cholesterol facilitates interactions between α-synuclein oligomers and charge-neutral membranes. *FEBS Lett.* **2015**, *589*, 2661–2667. [CrossRef]
57. Emamzadeh, F.N.; Aojula, H.; McHugh, P.C.; Allsop, D. Effects of different isoforms of apoE on aggregation of the α-synuclein protein implicated in Parkinson's disease. *Neurosci Lett.* **2016**, *618*, 146–151. [CrossRef] [PubMed]
58. Heverin, M.; Bogdanovic, N.; Lütjohann, D.; Bayer, T.; Pikuleva, I.; Bretillon, L.; Diczfalusy, U.; Winblad, B.; Björkhem, I. Changes in the levels of cerebral and extracerebral sterols in the brain of patients with Alzheimer's disease. *J. Lipid Res.* **2004**, *45*, 186–193. [CrossRef]
59. Lütjohann, D.; Von Bergmann, K. 24S-Hydroxycholesterol: A Marker of Brain Cholesterol Metabolism. *Pharmacopsychiatry* **2003**, *36*, 102–106. [CrossRef]
60. Sokratian, A.; Ziaee, J.; Kelly, K.; Chang, A.; Bryant, N.; Wang, S.; Xu, E.; Li, J.Y.; Wang, S.-H.; Ervin, J.; et al. Heterogeneity in α-synuclein fibril activity correlates to disease phenotypes in Lewy body dementia. *Acta Neuropathol.* **2021**, *141*, 547–564. [CrossRef]
61. Sierra, S.; Ramos, M.C.; Molina, P.; Esteo, C.; Vázquez, J.A.; Burgos, J.S. Statins as Neuroprotectants: A Comparative In Vitro Study of Lipophilicity, Blood-Brain-Barrier Penetration, Lowering of Brain Cholesterol, and Decrease of Neuron Cell Death. *J. Alzheimer's Dis.* **2011**, *23*, 307–318. [CrossRef]
62. Yan, J.; Xu, Y.; Zhu, C.; Zhang, L.; Wu, A.; Yang, Y.; Xiong, Z.; Deng, C.; Huang, X.-F.; Yenari, M.A.; et al. Simvastatin Prevents Dopaminergic Neurodegeneration in Experimental Parkinsonian Models: The Association with Anti-Inflammatory Responses. *PLoS ONE* **2011**, *6*, e20945. [CrossRef] [PubMed]
63. Yan, J.; Sun, J.; Huang, L.; Fu, Q.; Du, G. Simvastatin prevents neuroinflammation by inhibiting N-methyl-D-aspartic acid receptor 1 in 6-hydroxydopamine-treated PC12 cells. *J. Neurosci. Res.* **2014**, *92*, 634–640. [CrossRef]
64. Fassbender, K.; Simons, M.; Bergmann, C.; Stroick, M.; Lutjohann, D.; Keller, P.; Runz, H.; Kuhl, S.; Bertsch, T.; von Bergmann, K.; et al. Simvastatin strongly reduces levels of Alzheimer's disease beta-amyloid peptides Abeta 42 and Abeta 40 in vitro and in vivo. *Proc. Natl. Acad. Sci. USA* **2001**, *98*, 5856–5861. [CrossRef]
65. Kojro, E.; Gimpl, G.; Lammich, S.; Marz, W.; Fahrenholz, F. Low cholesterol stimulates the nonamyloidogenic pathway by its effect on the -secretase ADAM 10. *Proc. Natl. Acad. Sci. USA* **2001**, *98*, 5815–5820. [CrossRef] [PubMed]
66. Wolozin, B.; Kellman, W.; Ruosseau, P.; Celesia, G.G.; Siegel, G. Decreased Prevalence of Alzheimer Disease Associated With 3-Hydroxy-3-Methyglutaryl Coenzyme A Reductase Inhibitors. *Arch. Neurol.* **2000**, *57*, 1439–1443. [CrossRef]
67. Rockwood, K.; Kirkland, S.; Hogan, D.B.; Macknight, C.; Merry, H.; Verreault, R.; Wolfson, C.; McDowell, I. Use of Lipid-Lowering Agents, Indication Bias, and the Risk of Dementia in Community-Dwelling Elderly People. *Arch. Neurol.* **2002**, *59*, 223–227. [CrossRef] [PubMed]
68. Rea, T.D.; Breitner, J.C.; Psaty, B.M.; Fitzpatrick, A.L.; Lopez, O.L.; Newman, A.B.; Hazzard, W.R.; Zandi, P.P.; Burke, G.L.; Lyketsos, C.G.; et al. Statin use and the risk of incident dementia: The Cardiovascular Health Study. *Arch. Neurol.* **2005**, *62*, 1047–1051. [CrossRef]
69. Lin, F.C.; Chuang, Y.S.; Hsieh, H.M.; Lee, T.C.; Chiu, K.F.; Liu, C.K.; Wu, M.T. Early Statin Use and the Progression of Alzheimer Disease: A Total Population-Based Case-Control Study. *Medicine* **2015**, *94*, e2143. [CrossRef] [PubMed]
70. Sheng, Z.; Jia, X.; Kang, M. Statin use and risk of Parkinson's disease: A meta-analysis. *Behav. Brain Res.* **2016**, *309*, 29–34. [CrossRef]
71. Haag, M.D.M.; Hofman, A.; Koudstaal, P.J.; Stricker, B.H.C.; Breteler, M.M.B. Statins are associated with a reduced risk of Alzheimer disease regardless of lipophilicity. The Rotterdam Study. *J. Neurol. Neurosurg. Psychiatry* **2008**, *80*, 13–17. [CrossRef] [PubMed]

72. Huang, X.; Alonso, A.; Guo, X.; Umbach, D.M.; Lichtenstein, M.L.; Ballantyne, C.M.; Mailman, R.B.; Mosley, T.H.; Chen, H. Statins, plasma cholesterol, and risk of Parkinson's disease: A prospective study. *Mov. Disord.* **2015**, *30*, 552–559. [CrossRef] [PubMed]
73. Liu, G.; Sterling, N.W.; Kong, L.; Lewis, M.M.; Mailman, R.B.; Chen, H.; Leslie, D.; Huang, X. Statins may facilitate Parkinson's disease: Insight gained from a large, national claims database. *Mov. Disord.* **2017**, *32*, 913–917. [CrossRef] [PubMed]
74. Rozani, V.; Giladi, N.; El-Ad, B.; Gurevich, T.; Tsamir, J.; Hemo, B.; Peretz, C. Statin adherence and the risk of Parkinson's disease: A population-based cohort study. *PLoS ONE* **2017**, *12*, e0175054. [CrossRef]
75. Yan, J.; Qiao, L.; Tian, J.; Liu, A.; Wu, J.; Huang, J.; Shen, M.; Lai, X. Effect of statins on Parkinson's disease: A systematic review and meta-analysis. *Medicine* **2019**, *98*, e14852. [CrossRef] [PubMed]
76. Bai, S.; Song, Y.; Huang, X.; Peng, L.; Jia, J.; Liu, Y.; Lu, H. Statin Use and the Risk of Parkinson's Disease: An Updated Meta-Analysis. *PLoS ONE* **2016**, *11*, e0152564. [CrossRef]
77. Feldman, H.; Doody, R.S.; Kivipelto, M.; Sparks, D.L.; Waters, D.D.; Jones, R.W.; Schwam, E.; Schindler, R.; Hey-Hadavi, J.; Demicco, D.A.; et al. Randomized controlled trial of atorvastatin in mild to moderate Alzheimer disease: LEADe. *Neurology* **2010**, *74*, 956–964. [CrossRef]
78. Sparks, D.L.; Sabbagh, M.N.; Connor, D.J.; Lopez, J.; Launer, L.J.; Browne, P.; Wasser, D.; Johnson-Traver, S.; Lochhead, J.; Ziol-wolski, C. Atorvastatin for the treatment of mild to moderate Alzheimer disease: Preliminary results. *Arch. Neurol.* **2005**, *62*, 753–757. [CrossRef]
79. Friedhoff, L.T.; Cullen, E.I.; Geoghagen, N.S.; Buxbaum, J.D. Treatment with controlled-release lovastatin decreases serum con-centrations of human beta-amyloid (A beta) peptide. *Int. J. Neuropsychopharmacol.* **2001**, *4*, 127–130. [CrossRef]
80. Appleton, J.P.; Scutt, P.; Sprigg, N.; Bath, P.M. Hypercholesterolaemia and vascular dementia. *Clin. Sci.* **2017**, *131*, 1561–1578. [CrossRef]
81. Du, S.-Q.; Wang, X.-R.; Xiao, L.-Y.; Tu, J.-F.; Zhu, W.; He, T.; Liu, C.-Z. Molecular Mechanisms of Vascular Dementia: What Can Be Learned from Animal Models of Chronic Cerebral Hypoperfusion? *Mol. Neurobiol.* **2016**, *54*, 3670–3682. [CrossRef] [PubMed]
82. Maurer, S.V.; Williams, C.L. The Cholinergic System Modulates Memory and Hippocampal Plasticity via Its Interactions with Non-Neuronal Cells. *Front. Immunol.* **2017**, *8*, 1489. [CrossRef] [PubMed]
83. Sun, Y.; Zhao, Z.; Li, Q.; Wang, C.; Ge, X.; Wang, X.; Wang, G.; Qin, Y. Dl-3-n-butylphthalide regulates cholinergic dysfunction in chronic cerebral hypoperfusion rats. *J. Int. Med. Res.* **2020**, *48*, 300060520936177. [CrossRef] [PubMed]
84. Picciotto, M.R.; Higley, M.J.; Mineur, Y.S. Acetylcholine as a Neuromodulator: Cholinergic Signaling Shapes Nervous System Function and Behavior. *Neuron* **2012**, *76*, 116–129. [CrossRef]
85. Wess, J. Novel insights into muscarinic acetylcholine receptor function using gene targeting technology. *Trends Pharmacol. Sci.* **2003**, *24*, 414–420. [CrossRef]
86. Picciotto, M.R.; Caldarone, B.J.; King, S.L.; Zachariou, V. Nicotinic Receptors in the Brain Links between Molecular Biology and Behavior. *Neuropsychopharmacolohy* **2000**, *22*, 451–465. [CrossRef]
87. Everitt, B.J.; Robbins, T.W. Central Cholinergic Systems and Cognition. *Annu. Rev. Psychol.* **1997**, *48*, 649–684. [CrossRef] [PubMed]
88. Sato, A.; Sato, Y.; Uchida, S. Activation of the intracerebral cholinergic nerve fibers originating in the basal forebrain increases regional cerebral blood flow in the rat's cortex and hippocampus. *Neurosci. Lett.* **2004**, *361*, 90–93. [CrossRef]
89. Sato, A.; Sato, Y.; Uchida, S. Regulation of regional cerebral blood flow by cholinergic fibers originating in the basal forebrain. *Int. J. Dev. Neurosci.* **2001**, *19*, 327–337. [CrossRef]
90. Pavlov, V.A.; Tracey, K.J. Controlling inflammation: The cholinergic anti-inflammatory pathway. *Biochem. Soc. Trans.* **2006**, *34*, 1037–1040. [CrossRef]
91. Perry, E.K.; Gibson, P.H.; Blessed, G.; Perry, R.H.; Tomlinson, B.E. Neurotransmitter enzyme abnormalities in senile dementia. Choline acetyltransferase and glutamic acid decarboxylase activities in necropsy brain tissue. *J. Neurol. Sci.* **1977**, *34*, 247–265. [CrossRef]
92. Sharp, S.I.; Francis, P.T.; Elliott, M.S.; Kalaria, R.N.; Bajic, N.; Hortobágyi, T.; Ballard, C.G. Choline Acetyltransferase Activity in Vascular Dementia and Stroke. *Dement. Geriatr. Cogn. Disord.* **2009**, *28*, 233–238. [CrossRef] [PubMed]
93. Tohgi, H.; Abe, T.; Kimura, M.; Saheki, M.; Takahashi, S. Cerebrospinal fluid acetylcholine and choline in vascular dementia of Binswanger and multiple small infarct types as compared with Alzheimer-type dementia. *J. Neural. Transm.* **1996**, *103*, 1211–1220. [CrossRef] [PubMed]
94. Jia, J.P.; Jia, J.M.; Zhou, W.D.; Xu, M.; Chu, C.B.; Yan, X.; Sun, Y.X. Differential acetylcholine and choline concentrations in the cerebrospinal fluid of patients with Alzheimer's disease and vascular dementia. *Chin. Med. J.* **2004**, *117*, 1161–1164.
95. Sakurada, T.; Alufuzoff, I.; Winblad, B.; Nordberg, A. Substance P-like immunoreactivity, choline acetyltransferase activity and cholinergic muscarinic receptors in Alzheimer's disease and multi-infarct dementia. *Brain Res.* **1990**, *521*, 329–332. [CrossRef]
96. Waller, S.B.; Ball, M.J.; Reynolds, M.A.; London, E.D. Muscarinic Binding and Choline Acetyltransferase in Postmortem Brains of Demented Patients. *Can. J. Neurol. Sci. J. Can. Sci. Neurol.* **1986**, *13*, 528–532. [CrossRef]
97. Martin-Ruiz, C.; Court, J.; Lee, M.; Piggott, M.; Johnson, M.; Ballard, C.; Kalaria, R.; Perry, R.; Perry, E. Nicotinic receptors in de-mentia of Alzheimer, Lewy body and vascular types. *Acta Neurol. Scand. Suppl.* **2000**, *176*, 34–41. [CrossRef]
98. Damodaran, T.; Müller, C.P.; Hassan, Z. Chronic cerebral hypoperfusion-induced memory impairment and hippocampal long-term potentiation deficits are improved by cholinergic stimulation in rats. *Pharmacol. Rep.* **2019**, *71*, 443–448. [CrossRef]
99. Sodero, A.O.; Barrantes, F.J. Pleiotropic effects of statins on brain cells. *Biochim. Biophys. Acta (BBA) Biomembr.* **2020**, *1862*, 183340. [CrossRef]

100. El-Dessouki, A.M.; Galal, M.A.; Awad, A.S.; Zaki, H.F. Neuroprotective Effects of Simvastatin and Cilostazol in l-Methionine-Induced Vascular Dementia in Rats. *Mol. Neurobiol.* **2016**, *54*, 5074–5084. [CrossRef]
101. Muldoon, M.F.; Barger, S.D.; Ryan, C.M.; Flory, J.D.; Lehoczky, J.P.; Matthews, K.A.; Manuck, S.B. Effects of lovastatin on cognitive function and psychological well-being. *Am. J. Med.* **2000**, *108*, 538–546. [CrossRef]
102. Collins, R.; Reith, C.; Emberson, J.; Armitage, J.; Baigent, C.; Blackwell, L.; Blumenthal, R.; Danesh, J.; Smith, G.D.; DeMets, D.; et al. Interpretation of the evidence for the efficacy and safety of statin therapy. *Lancet* **2016**, *388*, 2532–2561. [CrossRef]
103. Sinha, K.; Sun, C.; Kamari, R.; Bettermann, K. Current status and future prospects of pathophysiology-based neuroprotective drugs for the treatment of vascular dementia. *Drug Discov. Today* **2020**, *25*, 793–799. [CrossRef] [PubMed]
104. Davoudian, P.A.; Wilkinson, S.T. *Clinical Overview of NMDA-R Antagonists and Clinical Practice*; Elsevier BV: Amsterdam, The Netherlands, 2020; Volume 89, pp. 103–129.
105. Meldrum, B.S. Glutamate as a Neurotransmitter in the Brain: Review of Physiology and Pathology. *J. Nutr.* **2000**, *130*, 1007S–1015S. [CrossRef] [PubMed]
106. Gutierrez-Vargas, J.A.; Muñoz-Manco, J.I.; Garcia-Segura, L.M.; Cardona-Gómez, G.P. GluN2B N-methyl-D-aspartic acid receptor subunit mediates atorvastatin-Induced neuroprotection after focal cerebral ischemia. *J. Neurosci. Res.* **2014**, *92*, 1529–1548. [CrossRef]
107. Kristiansen, L.V.; Huerta, I.; Beneyto, M.; Meador-Woodruff, J.H. NMDA receptors and schizophrenia. *Curr. Opin. Pharmacol.* **2007**, *7*, 48–55. [CrossRef] [PubMed]
108. Salussolia, C.L.; Prodromou, M.L.; Borker, P.; Wollmuth, L.P. Arrangement of Subunits in Functional NMDA Receptors. *J. Neurosci.* **2011**, *31*, 11295–11304. [CrossRef]
109. Groc, L.; Bard, L.; Choquet, D. Surface trafficking of N-methyl-d-aspartate receptors: Physiological and pathological perspectives. *Neuroscience* **2009**, *158*, 4–18. [CrossRef]
110. Loftis, J.M.; Janowsky, A. The N-methyl-d-aspartate receptor subunit NR2B: Localization, functional properties, regulation, and clinical implications. *Pharmacol. Ther.* **2003**, *97*, 55–85. [CrossRef]
111. Furukawa, H.; Singh, S.K.; Mancusso, R.; Gouaux, E. Subunit arrangement and function in NMDA receptors. *Nat. Cell Biol.* **2005**, *438*, 185–192. [CrossRef]
112. Kalia, L.V.; Kalia, S.K.; Salter, M.W. NMDA receptors in clinical neurology: Excitatory times ahead. *Lancet Neurol.* **2008**, *7*, 742–755. [CrossRef]
113. Dobrek, Ł.; Thor, P. Glutamate NMDA Receptors in Pathophysiology and Pharmacotherapy of Selected Nervous System Diseases. *PHMD* **2011**, *65*, 338–346.
114. Lau, C.G.; Zukin, R.S. NMDA receptor trafficking in synaptic plasticity and neuropsychiatric disorders. *Nat. Rev. Neurosci.* **2007**, *8*, 413–426. [CrossRef]
115. Dong, X.-X.; Wang, Y.; Qin, Z.-H. Molecular mechanisms of excitotoxicity and their relevance to pathogenesis of neurodegenerative diseases. *Acta Pharmacol. Sin.* **2009**, *30*, 379–387. [CrossRef]
116. Reynolds, I.J.; Hastings, T.G. Glutamate induces the production of reactive oxygen species in cultured forebrain neurons following NMDA receptor activation. *J. Neurosci.* **1995**, *15*, 3318–3327. [CrossRef] [PubMed]
117. Donnan, G.A.; Fisher, M.; Malcolm Macleod, S.M.D. Emergency and Comprehensive Care for Stroke Needed. *Lancet* **2008**, *373*, 1612–1623. [CrossRef]
118. Lo, E.H.; Moskowitz, M.A.; Jacobs, T.P. Exciting, Radical, Suicidal: How Brain Cells Die after Stroke. *Stroke* **2005**, *36*, 189–192. [CrossRef]
119. Lai, T.W.; Zhang, S.; Wang, Y.T. Excitotoxicity and stroke: Identifying novel targets for neuroprotection. *Prog. Neurobiol.* **2014**, *115*, 157–188. [CrossRef]
120. Hoskison, M.; Yanagawa, Y.; Obata, K.; Shuttleworth, C. Calcium-dependent NMDA-induced dendritic injury and MAP2 loss in acute hippocampal slices. *Neuroscience* **2007**, *145*, 66–79. [CrossRef]
121. Jurado, F.W.; Cardona-go, G.P. P120 Catenin/a N-Catenin Are Molecular Targets in the Neuroprotection and Neuronal Plasticity Mediated by Atorvastatin after Focal Cerebral Ischemia. *J. Neurosci. Res.* **2010**, *88*, 3621–3634.
122. Valerio, A.; Bertolotti, P.; Delbarba, A.; Perego, C.; Dossena, M.; Ragni, M.; Spano, P.; Carruba, M.O.; De Simoni, M.G.; Nisoli, E. Glycogen synthase kinase-3 inhibition reduces ischemic cerebral damage, restores impaired mitochondrial biogenesis and prevents ROS production. *J. Neurochem.* **2011**, *116*, 1148–1159. [CrossRef] [PubMed]
123. Tramacere, I.; Boncoraglio, G.B.; Banzi, R.; Del Giovane, C.; Kwag, K.H.; Squizzato, A.; Moja, L. Comparison of statins for secondary prevention in patients with ischemic stroke or transient ischemic attack: A systematic review and network meta-analysis. *BMC Med.* **2019**, *17*, 1–12. [CrossRef] [PubMed]
124. Yebyo, H.G.; Aschmann, H.E.; Kaufmann, M.; Puhan, M.A. Comparative effectiveness and safety of statins as a class and of specific statins for primary prevention of cardiovascular disease: A systematic review, meta-analysis, and network meta-analysis of randomized trials with 94,283 participants. *Am. Hear. J.* **2019**, *210*, 18–28. [CrossRef]
125. Wang, C.-Y.; Liu, P.-Y.; Liao, J.K. Pleiotropic effects of statin therapy: Molecular mechanisms and clinical results. *Trends Mol. Med.* **2008**, *14*, 37–44. [CrossRef] [PubMed]
126. Gutiérrez-Vargas, J.A.; Cespedes-Rubio, A.; Cardona-Gómez, G.P. Perspective of synaptic protection after post-infarction treatment with statins. *J. Transl. Med.* **2015**, *13*, 1–9. [CrossRef] [PubMed]

127. Tuttolomondo, A.; Di Raimondo, D.; Pecoraro, R.; Maida, C.; Arnao, V.; Corte, V.D.; Simonetta, I.; Corpora, F.; Di Bona, D.; Maugeri, R.; et al. Early High-Dosage Atorvastatin Treatment Improved Serum Immune-Inflammatory Markers and Functional Outcome in Acute Ischemic Strokes Classified as Large Artery Atherosclerotic Stroke: A Randomized Trial. *Medicine* **2016**, *95*, e3186. [CrossRef] [PubMed]
128. Campos-Martorell, M.; Salvador, N.; Monge, M.; Canals, F.; García-Bonilla, L.; Hernández-Guillamon, M.; Ayuso, M.I.; Chacon, P.; Rosell, A.; Alcázar, A.; et al. Brain proteomics identifies potential simvastatin targets in acute phase of stroke in a rat embolic model. *J. Neurochem.* **2014**, *130*, 301–312. [CrossRef]
129. Ploughman, M.; Windle, V.; MacLellan, C.L.; White, N.; Doré, J.J.; Corbett, D. Brain-Derived Neurotrophic Factor Contributes to Recovery of Skilled Reaching after Focal Ischemia in Rats. *Stroke* **2009**, *40*, 1490–1495. [CrossRef]
130. Hannon, J.; Hoyer, D. Molecularbiology of 5-HT receptors. *Behav. Brain Res.* **2008**, *195*, 198–213. [CrossRef]
131. Abela, A.R.; Browne, C.J.; Sargin, D.; Prevot, T.D.; Ji, X.D.; Li, Z.; Lambe, E.K.; Fletcher, P.J. Median raphe serotonin neurons promote anxiety-like behavior via inputs to the dorsal hippocampus. *Neuropharmacology* **2020**, *168*, 107985. [CrossRef]
132. Rang, H.P.; Dale, M.M.; Ritter, J.M.; Flower, R.J.; Henderson, G. *Rang & Dale's pharmacology*, 7th ed.; Elsevier Churchill Livingstone: Edinburgh, UK, 2012; pp. 199–200.
133. Huang, K.W.; Ochandarena, N.E.; Philson, A.C.; Hyun, M.; Birnbaum, J.E.; Cicconet, M.; Sabatini, B.L. Molecular and anatomicalorganization of the dorsalraphenucleus. *Elife* **2019**, *8*, e46464. [CrossRef] [PubMed]
134. Borroto-Escuela, D.O.; Ambrogini, P.; Chruścicka, B.; Lindskog, M.; Crespo-Ramirez, M.; Hernández-Mondragón, J.C.; Perez de la Mora, M.; Schellekens, H.; Fuxe, K. The Role of Central Serotonin Neurons and 5-HT Heteroreceptor Complexes in the Pathophysiology of Depression: A HistoricalPerspective and Future Prospects. *Int. J. Mol. Sci.* **2021**, *22*, 1927. [CrossRef]
135. He, J.; Hommen, F.; Lauer, N.; Balmert, S.; Scholz, H. Serotonin transporter dependent modulation of food-seeking behavior. *PLoS ONE* **2020**, *15*, e0227554. [CrossRef] [PubMed]
136. Paulus, E.V.; Mintz, E.M. Circadianrhythms of clockgeneexpression in the cerebellum of serotonin-deficient Pet-1 knockout mice. *Brain Res.* **2016**, *1630*, 10–17. [CrossRef] [PubMed]
137. Pourhamzeh, M.; Moravej, F.G.; Arabi, M.; Shahriari, E.; Mehrabi, S.; Ward, R.; Ahadi, R.; Joghataei, M.T. The Roles of Serotonin in Neuropsychiatric Disorders. *Cell. Mol. Neurobiol.* **2021**, 1–22. [CrossRef]
138. Müller, H.K.; Wiborg, O.; Haase, J. Subcellular Redistribution of the Serotonin Transporter by Secretory Carrier Membrane Protein 2. *J. Biol. Chem.* **2006**, *281*, 28901–28909. [CrossRef] [PubMed]
139. White, K.J.; Walline, C.C.; Barker, E.L. Serotonin transporters: Implications for antidepressantdrug development. *AAPS J.* **2005**, *7*, e421–433. [CrossRef]
140. Deveau, C.M.; Rodriguez, E.; Schroering, A.; Yamamoto, B.K. Serotonin transporter regulation by cholesterol-independent lipid signaling. *Biochem. Pharmacol.* **2021**, *183*, 114349. [CrossRef] [PubMed]
141. Johnson-Anuna, L.N.; Eckert, G.P.; Keller, J.H.; Igbavboa, U.; Franke, C.; Fechner, T.; Schubert-Zsilavecz, M.; Karas, M.; Müller, W.E.; Wood, W.G. Chronic administration of statins altersmultiplegene expression patterns in mouse cerebral cortex. *J. Pharmacol. Exp. Ther.* **2005**, *312*, 786–793. [CrossRef]
142. Molero, Y.; Cipriani, A.; Larsson, H.; Lichtenstein, P.; D'Onofrio, B.M.; Fazel, S. Associations between statin use and suicidality, depression, anxiety, and seizures: A Swedish total-population cohort study. *Lancet Psychiatry* **2020**, *7*, 982–990. [CrossRef]
143. Köhler-Forsberg, O.; Otte, C.; Gold, S.M.; Østergaard, S.D. Statins in the treatment of depression: Hype or hope? *Pharmacol. Ther.* **2020**, *215*, 107625. [CrossRef] [PubMed]
144. Jialal, I.; Stein, D.; Balis, D.; Grundy, S.M.; Adams-Huet, B.; Devaraj, S. Effect of hydroxymethylglutarylcoenzyme a reductase inhibitor therapy on high sensitive C reactive protein levels. *Circulation* **2001**, *103*, 1933–1935. [CrossRef]
145. Shishehbor, M.H.; Aviles, R.J.; Brennan, M.L.; Fu, X.; Goormastic, M.; Pearce, G.L.; Gokce, N.; Keaney, J.F.; Penn, M.S.; Sprecher, D.L.; et al. Association of nitrotyrosinelevels with cardiovasculardisease and modulation by statintherapy. *JAMA* **2003**, *289*, 1675–1680. [CrossRef]
146. Ferro, D.; Parrotto, S.; Basili, S.; Alessandri, C.; Violi, F. Simvastatininhibits the monocyteexpression of proinflammatorycytokines in patients with hypercholesterolemia. *J. Am. Coll. Cardiol.* **2000**, *36*, 427–431. [CrossRef]
147. Weitz-Schmidt, G.; Welzenbach, K.; Brinkmann, V.; Kamata, T.; Kallen, J.; Bruns, C.; Cottens, S.; Takada, Y.; Hommel, U. Statins selectively inhibit leukocyte function antigen-1 by binding to a novel regulatory integrinsite. *Nat. Med.* **2001**, *6*, 687–692. [CrossRef] [PubMed]
148. Bu, D.X.; Tarrio, M.; Grabie, N.; Zhang, Y.; Yamazaki, H.; Stavrakis, G.; Maganto-Garcia, E.; Pepper-Cunningham, Z.; Jarolim, P.; Aikawa, M.; et al. Statin-induced Krüppel-like factor 2 expression in human and mouse T cells reduces inflammatory and pathogenic responses. *J. Clin. Investig.* **2010**, *120*, 1961–1970. [CrossRef]
149. van Agtmaal, M.J.M.; Houben, A.J.H.M.; Pouwer, F.; Stehouwer, C.D.A.; Schram, M.T. Association of Microvascular Dysfunction With Late-Life Depression: A Systematic Review and Meta-analysis. *JAMA Psychiatry* **2017**, *74*, 729–739. [CrossRef]

molecules

Review

Arterial Blood Pressure Variability and Other Vascular Factors Contribution to the Cognitive Decline in Parkinson's Disease

Anna Pierzchlińska [1,*], Magdalena Kwaśniak-Butowska [2,3], Jarosław Sławek [2,3], Marek Droździk [4,*] and Monika Białecka [1]

1 Department of Pharmacokinetics and Therapeutic Drug Monitoring, Pomeranian Medical University, Aleja Powstańców Wlkp 72, 70-111 Szczecin, Poland; monika-bialecka@post.pl
2 Division of Neurological and Psychiatric Nursing, Medical University of Gdansk, Aleja Jana Pawła II 50, 80-462 Gdansk, Poland; magdalena.butowska@gumed.edu.pl (M.K.-B.); jaroslaw.slawek@gumed.edu.pl (J.S.)
3 Department of Neurology, St Adalbert Hospital, Aleja Jana Pawła II 50, 80-462 Gdansk, Poland
4 Department of Experimental and Clinical Pharmacology, Pomeranian Medical University, Aleja Powstańców Wlkp 72, 70-111 Szczecin, Poland
* Correspondence: anna.pierzchlinska@pum.edu.pl (A.P.); drozdzik@pum.edu.pl (M.D.)

Abstract: Dementia is one of the most disabling non-motor symptoms in Parkinson's disease (PD). Unlike in Alzheimer's disease, the vascular pathology in PD is less documented. Due to the uncertain role of commonly investigated metabolic or vascular factors, e.g., hypertension or diabetes, other factors corresponding to PD dementia have been proposed. Associated dysautonomia and dopaminergic treatment seem to have an impact on diurnal blood pressure (BP) variability, which may presumably contribute to white matter hyperintensities (WMH) development and cognitive decline. We aim to review possible vascular and metabolic factors: Renin-angiotensin-aldosterone system, vascular endothelial growth factor (VEGF), hyperhomocysteinemia (HHcy), as well as the dopaminergic treatment, in the etiopathogenesis of PD dementia. Additionally, we focus on the role of polymorphisms within the genes for catechol-*O*-methyltransferase (*COMT*), apolipoprotein E (*APOE*), vascular endothelial growth factor (*VEGF*), and for renin-angiotensin-aldosterone system components, and their contribution to cognitive decline in PD. Determining vascular risk factors and their contribution to the cognitive impairment in PD may result in screening, as well as preventive measures.

Keywords: white matter hyperintensities; dysautonomia; genetic polymorphisms; dementia; levodopa; renin-angiotensin system; orthostatic hypotension

Citation: Pierzchlińska, A.; Kwaśniak-Butowska, M.; Sławek, J.; Droździk, M.; Białecka, M. Arterial Blood Pressure Variability and Other Vascular Factors Contribution to the Cognitive Decline in Parkinson's Disease. *Molecules* **2021**, *26*, 1523. https://doi.org/10.3390/molecules26061523

Academic Editors: Alicja Nowaczyk and Grzegorz Grześk

Received: 14 February 2021
Accepted: 9 March 2021
Published: 10 March 2021

1. Introduction

Parkinson's disease (PD) is a neurodegenerative disorder with a wide spectrum of motor (bradykinesia, tremor, rigidity, loss of postural stability) and non-motor (cognitive decline, depression, dysautonomia, psychosis) symptoms. Parkinson's disease dementia mostly affects the executive and visuospatial functions, as well as attention. However, the impairment in memory and language functions are less pronounced than in Alzheimer's disease (AD) [1]. Dementia in PD is six times more common than in age-matched general population [2]. As a result of an 8-year prospective study, the cumulative prevalence of dementia was assessed to be 78% [3]. According to a 5-year prospective study in more than 400 patients with PD, the risk factors for dementia included older age, longer disease duration, later age-at-onset and higher daily levodopa (L-dopa) dosage [4]. In contrast to Alzheimer's disease, vascular contribution to PD dementia is not so obvious. The available data demonstrate the multifactorial origin of PD dementia: The combination of pathological findings of Alzheimer-like and cortical Lewy-bodies, but also a possible role of vascular burden due to hyperhomocysteinemia and dysautonomia with abnormal blood pressure (BP) variability [5,6]. In this review paper, the authors present the current state of information about the role of BP variability and other vascular risk factors, as well as selected genetic polymorphisms, in the pathogenesis of PD dementia.

2. Blood Pressure Variability

In healthy individuals a compensatory mechanism, involving the sympathetic and parasympathetic systems, provides an adequate response of BP and cerebral perfusion to environmental (e.g., seasons, altitude), physical (e.g., posture), and emotional factors. The size and patterns of these BP variations constitute BP variability, which occurs within seconds and minutes (very short-term), along 24 h (short-term), between days (mid-term), months or even years (long-term; visit-to-visit BP variability) [7].

Numerous studies have shown a dysfunctional response of autonomic nervous system controlling blood pressure in PD [8,9]. Dysautonomia in PD is manifested, among others, in orthostatic hypotension (OH), supine hypertension or loss of circadian rhythm of BP, which may be the results of both autonomic nervous system dysfunction and pharmacological management, including dopaminergic medications.

Orthostatic hypotension is defined as a systolic pressure fall of at least 20 mmHg and/or diastolic pressure fall of 10 mmHg upon standing or passive tilting. Supine hypertension in PD is often associated with OH and causes an increase in BP when lying down—to at least 150 mmHg in systolic and/or 90 mmHg in diastolic BP. This phenomenon often remains unrecognized, thus an ambulatory 24-h BP monitoring provides a valuable insight into the BP alterations and enables non-pharmacological and pharmacological management. Supine hypertension can be additionally worsened by the drugs prescribed against OH. On the other hand, the treatment of hypertension may worsen OH, thus it should include non-pharmacological measures as a priority [8]. Four clinical trials have addressed OH in conditions with dysautonomia, including PD, and have posted results by the time of this review (clinicaltrials.gov: NCT00738062, NCT00782340, NCT01176240, NCT00633880). In all of them droxidopa—a precursor of norepinephrine—was compared with placebo. The results showed some discrepancies, as only two of the trials established significant clinical changes favoring droxidopa in terms of increasing upright systolic BP, ameliorating symptoms associated with OH and improving daily life activities (i.e., standing, walking) (NCT00782340, NCT00633880) [10].

Evaluating the circadian blood pressure profile in healthy subjects demonstrated a physiological decrease of arterial BP at night, while sleeping (dipping) [11]. This phenomenon is influenced by several factors, and we briefly describe only some of them. First of all, photoreceptor cells in retina detect the environmental darkness, subsequently, the information is conveyed via the suprachiasmatic nucleus—the central oscillator—to the pineal gland, which reacts by producing melatonin. Melatonin decreases BP by its impact on vasodilation, nitric oxide, and norepinephrine levels. Accordingly, the pivotal role in the circadian BP pattern is exerted by the sympathetic nervous system with norepinephrine and epinephrine having the lowest levels in the evening and the highest in the morning. Sleep itself affects BP, decreasing its values especially during the deep sleep stages [12]. Similarly, physical activity may change the circadian rhythm—people who work at night, are likely to have blunted nocturnal drop in systolic BP. Dipping depends also on the BP liability upon dietary sodium intake and endothelial function [13]. The loss of night BP reduction (non-dipping) has been recognized as a risk factor of cardiovascular pathologies, e.g., left ventricle hypertrophy [14]. Nocturnal hypertension is usually diagnosed when BP is higher than 120/70 mmHg [8]; whereas the term "non-dipping" relates to a relative difference between daytime and nighttime BP (i.e., <10% of difference). It is often associated with other cardiovascular autonomic abnormalities, such as OH and supine hypertension [15]. The 24-h BP monitoring showed that over 70% of PD patients did not have a proper circadian BP profile compared to 48% in the control group [16]. The analysis performed by Berganzo et al. revealed that the most frequent phenotype among the PD patients was non-dipper, while the number of the risers (mean arterial BP higher in the night than during the day) was the same as subjects having the physiological diurnal pattern [16]. Orthostatic hypotension was more prevalent in non-dippers and risers; those phenotypes administrated a higher dose of dopaminergic treatment; however, none of the associations reached statistical significance.

Neurocirculatory abnormalities in PD have been linked to cognitive impairment. In patients with early stage of the disease, who were not receiving dopaminergic medication, dementia was significantly more often in the subjects with OH or supine hypertension [17]. Strikingly, none of the patients suffering from both OH and supine hypertension was cognitively intact. The disruption of the nocturnal BP fall was related to worse visuospatial memory registration; however, mild cognitive impairment (MCI) or dementia were similarly frequent in dipper and non-dipper groups. Anang et al. carried out a prospective research with a comprehensive assessment of 80 PD patients who were cognitively intact at baseline [18]. After 4.4 years' follow-up, higher BP at the entry and OH were predisposing factors for cognitive decline. Some of the cross-sectional studies reviewed by Udow et al. did not provide a correlation linking OH in PD with cognitive impairment assessed with Mini–Mental State Examination (MMSE) [19]. On the other hand, in analyses using more detailed neuropsychological tests OH was associated with worse performance. In one of the recent studies the riser pattern in PD was significantly correlated with dementia, whereas the dipper status was much less common in demented (3.7%) than non-demented (23.6%) subjects [20]. The authors found no association between dementia and non-dipper or extreme dipper (nocturnal BP lower >20% compared to daytime) phenotypes. Both OH and supine hypertension were significantly more prevalent in the dementia group. Thus, cardiovascular autonomic dysfunction can be considered as a plausible predictor of PD dementia.

3. The Role of Levodopa in Neurocirculatory Abnormalities and Cognitive Decline in Parkinson's Disease

The dopaminergic medications used in the treatment of PD produce positive effects on PD motor manifestations, but at the same time may promote the development of side effects, e.g., dyskinesia may enhance autonomic disturbances [21]. Positron emission tomography (PET) and functional magnetic resonance imaging (fMRI) in experimental models and in PD patients have shown changes in dopaminergic synapses during long-term administration of L-dopa. The chronic use of L-dopa resulted in endothelial cell proliferation, promoted angiogenesis in the striatum and other structures of the basal ganglia in animals with L-dopa–induced dyskinesia [22]. Animal models have also evidenced that chronic L-dopa treatment induced expression of vascular endothelial growth factor (VEGF) in the basal ganglia in a dose-dependent manner [23]. VEGF exerts angiogenic activity and is essential for vasculogenesis. It can also enhance blood–brain barrier permeability, which in turn increases the bioavailability of L-dopa to the central nervous system (CNS). In the aforementioned model, VEGF was expressed predominantly in astrocytes and astrocytic processes around blood vessels. Administration of a VEGF signaling inhibitor blocked the appearance of markers of blood–brain barrier permeability (albumin extravasation) as well as of angiogenic response—nestin (a marker of immature endothelial cells) and VEGF expression. Furthermore, it was found that VEGF inhibition significantly attenuated the expression of dyskinesia in animal models with L-dopa-induced dyskinesia. Human tissue from the autopsies of chronically L-dopa-treated PD patients established increased nestin staining and *VEGF* mRNA expression in the striatum [23,24]. Pulsatile stimulation of dopamine receptors, which may be a result of abnormal L-dopa pharmacokinetics in the absence of efficient, endogenous regulatory mechanisms, is regarded as the main mechanism of peak-of-dose choreic dyskinesia (the result of D-receptor hypersensitivity or excessive dopamine release). Chronic L-dopa administration, apart from inducing angiogenesis and changes in blood–brain barrier permeability, stimulates vasodilation through D1 receptor agonist action, thus increasing regional blood flow [24].

According to a 5-year prospective study higher L-dopa dose was established as one of dementia risk factors in PD—the mean L-dopa dosage equivalent (LDE) was 514 mg per day, whereas non-demented patients received 316 mg of LDE per day [4]. Moreover, L-dopa-induced dyskinesia were correlated with the progression of cognitive decline, especially executive functions [25]. Daily changes in BP, dipper or non-dipper phenotype, OH and supine hypertension may modulate CNS blood flow, and thus affect L-dopa distribution, which may result in cognitive performance deterioration, and other side effects. Up to now, no studies have addressed the role of BP variability, especially nocturnal BP reduction, in the development of L-dopa complications, e.g., peak-of-dose dyskinesia due to impaired drug distribution.

Dopaminergic treatment was suggested to exacerbate dysautonomia in PD; L-dopa may worsen or cause OH [26], however, Goldstein et al. indicated that OH occurs independently from L-dopa treatment [27]. Although L-dopa is well known for its BP decreasing function [9,28], the available literature does not give a clear answer to the question whether it decreases supine hypertension [28,29]. There are some discrepancies on the role of dopamine agonists as well. Non-ergot derivatives of dopamine agonists possibly influence cardiovascular functions less, compared to ergot-derivatives [30]. Nevertheless, the side effects of non-ergot derivatives depend on the affinity to dopaminergic and α-adrenergic receptors [31]. Although non-ergot dopamine agonists were generally correlated with OH occurrence, rotigotine was showed to improve the abnormal 24-h BP pattern in PD patients [32]. On the other hand, rotigotine may increase the risk of the atrioventricular block. Pramipexole in turn, due to its high affinity towards α2-adrenergic receptors, may decrease the adrenergic tone and myocardial contractility, facilitating heart failure occurrence. Pramipexole may unmask a subclinical heart failure or exacerbate preexisting cardiovascular comorbidities [31]. Another non-ergot dopamine agonist—apomorphine—was suggested to prolong QT interval; however, no causality has been established [31,33]. Undoubtedly, the aforementioned cardiovascular side effects influence BP and may lead to the impairments within the cerebrovascular functions, such as episodes of hypo- and hyperperfusion.

The relationship between dopaminergic treatment and the BP variability needs to be further assessed. It seems important because disturbances in the diurnal BP pattern, especially nocturnal hypertension, are associated with an increased risk of cerebrovascular complications. Nevertheless, despite many side effects, levodopa is still the most often prescribed antiparkinsonian medication due to its effectiveness against motor symptoms. Non-ergot derivatives are in turn beneficial in treating non-motor symptoms, e.g., depression, sleep disorders, and nocturnal akinesia [31]. In most cases positive effects of dopaminergic medication (L-dopa and dopamine agonists) surpass potential side effects in the cardiovascular system, however, the risk must be always individually estimated.

4. White Matter Hyperintensities

Shimada et al. documented that an absent or insufficient nocturnal BP fall in elderly hypertensives was associated with a silent cerebrovascular damage seen in MRI as white matter hyperintensities (WMH) [34]. In recent years, WMH appearance has become the radiological marker of CNS ischemia. White matter hyperintensities are more frequently observed in subjects over 60 years of age with cardiovascular disease, diabetes, hyperhomocysteinemia, and other vascular risk factors [35,36]. Chronic ischemia being a consequence of BP variability was established as one of the possible factors leading to the development of WMH. In addition to a non-dipper phenotype, an excessive nocturnal BP fall of more than 20% compared to daytime BP values was found to be an important risk factor of WMH. The extreme dipper phenotype also was proven to be a risk factor for clinically silent brain ischemia episodes, particularly those associated with more extensive white matter damage, and can be related to nocturnal cerebral hypoperfusion [37,38]. Studies analyzing neurocirculatory abnormalities in PD demonstrated a correlation between WMH and OH [17,39]. Cerebral hypoxia along with hypoperfusion were proposed as mechanisms linking OH and WMH [40]. Indeed, hippocampal atrophy was correlated with WMH in the study performed by Sławek et al. [41]. Furthermore, WMH in PD was also associated with other cardiovascular dysautonomic features, as supine hypertension [17] or nocturnal hypertension [42]. Up to date, the only study examining nighttime BP fall and WMH in PD showed no correlation between non-dipping status and WMH [42].

According to the meta-analysis performed by Debette and Markus, WMH predicted faster decline in global cognitive performance and executive function [43]. In PD associated dysautonomia and dopaminergic medication-induced hypotension may be responsible for WMH formation and cognitive decline. In a prospective study in PD patients a significant relationship between increased WMH volume and cognitive burden was demonstrated. Moreover, the risk for the development of MCI in the course of PD was higher in the subjects with greater WMH [44]. Subsequent studies supported the finding, demonstrating a significant correlation between WMH and MCI or dementia in PD [45,46]

Cardiovascular dysautonomia in PD, along with dopaminergic therapy, leading to episodes of cerebral hypo- and hyperperfusion, may be one of the most important pathophysiological mechanisms leading to WMH and, presumably, dementia.

The studies on the impact of BP variability on cognition and WMH in PD are summarized in Table 1.

Table 1. Studies on the impact of blood pressure (BP) variability and white matter hyperintensities (WMH) on cognitive performance in Parkinson's disease (PD).

		Blood Pressure Variability	
Authors (year), Type of the Study	**Subjects**	**Factor**	**Outcome**
Oka et al. (2020) [47], retrospective study	PD = 75 (de novo) DLB = 24	Circadian blood pressure variability. Supine hypertension.	Better performance assessed with MMSE positively associated with the percentage of nocturnal BP fall in PD. No correlation with SH. Nocturnal BP fall (%) positively associated with better performance in Frontal Assessment Battery. SH negatively correlated with Frontal Assessment Battery.
Sforza et al. (2018) [48], retrospective study	PD = 28	Orthostatic hypotension.	In upright position, PD-OH(+) performed worse at the Stroop's test word reading time and number of errors at the interference section compared to PD-OH(−).
Tanaka et al. (2018) [20], retrospective study	PD-NCI = 110 PDD = 27	Circadian blood pressure variability. Orthostatic hypotension.	The riser pattern associated with dementia. Coexistence of the riser pattern and OH more associated with dementia than the riser pattern alone.
Centi et al. (2017) [49], retrospective study	PD-OH(+) = 18 PD-OH(−) = 19 controls = 18	Orthostatic hypotension.	Upright posture correlated with the deficits in sustained attention and response inhibition, reduced semantic fluency and verbal memory in the PD-OH(+). OH correlated with the deficits in executive function, memory and visuospatial function.
Anang et al. (2014) [18], prospective study	PD = 80 (dementia free at baseline)	Orthostatic hypotension.	OH strongly associated with dementia risk.
Pilleri et al. (2013) [50], retrospective study	PD = 48	Orthostatic hypotension.	PD-OH(+) performed significantly worse in sustained attention, visuospatial and verbal memory, compared with PD-OH(−).
Kim et al. (2012) [17], retrospective study	PD-NCI = 25 PD-MCI = 48 PDD = 14	Circadian blood pressure variability, supine hypertension and orthostatic hypotension.	The OH group had more severe impairment in verbal immediate/delayed memory. Dementia significantly more prevalent in patients having OH, SH or OH + SH. Non-dipping not associated with cognitive impairment.
Allcock et al. (2006) [51], retrospective study	PD-OH(+) = 87 PD-OH(−) = 88	Orthostatic hypotension.	OH(+) subjects worse in sustained attention and visual episodic memory. OH not associated with the MMSE score, the prevalence of dementia, or the simple and choice reaction times, working memory or long term memory.
		White Matter Hyperintensities	
Authors (Year), Type of the Study	**Subjects**	**Factor**	**Outcome**
Nicoletti et al. (2021) [52], prospective study	PD-NCI = 84 PD-MCI = 55	WMH	WMH was a predictor of PDD development.
Huang et al. (2020) [53], retrospective study	Early PD: PD-NCI = 81 PD-MCI = 94	WMH	PD-MCI associated with the periventricular WMH but not with total WMH. Periventricular WMH associated with worse executive function and visuospatial function.
Ramirez et al. (2020) [54], retrospective study	PD = 139	WMH	WMH negatively associated with global cognition.

Table 1. *Cont.*

Dadar et al. (2020) [55], prospective study	PD = 50 controls = 45	WMH	No correlation between WMH and total Dementia Rating Scale. Greater WMH burden in patients diagnosed with dementia at 36 months.
Linortner et al. (2020) [56], retrospective study	PD = 85 controls = 18	WMH	Dementia and executive impairment significantly more prevalent in PD patients with WMH than without WMH. WMH associated with worse performance in Symbol Digit Modalities and Stroop tests.
Lee et al. (2020) [57], retrospective study	PD = 136 (de novo)	WMH	Performance in language function, frontal/executive and visual memory associated with the severity of WMH.
Chahine et al. (2019) [58], prospective study	PD = 141 controls = 63	WMH	Annual rate of change in global cognition correlated with WMH. Higher temporal WMH associated with greater decline over time in verbal memory.
Hanning et al. (2019) [59], prospective study	Drug-naïve: PD-NCI = 79 PD-MCI = 29 controls = 107	WMH (volume and CHIPS score)	No association between global or localised WMH and cognitive decline, both cross-sectional and longitudinal.
Pozorski et al. (2019) [60], prospective study	PD = 29 controls = 42	WMH	Greater regional and global WMH at baseline more strongly associated with lower executive function in PD than in controls. Increased regional WMH more strongly associated with impaired memory performance in PD relative to controls. Longitudinally, no associations between WMH and cognitive change.
Stojkovic et al. (2018) [61], retrospective study	PD-NCI = 49 PD-MCI = 61 PDD = 23	WMH	PDD patients had significantly greater whole brain WMH than PD-NCI subjects.
Dadar et al. (2018) [62], prospective study	PD = 365 (de novo) controls = 174	WMH	PD subjects with greater WMH had significantly more severe cognitive decline than PD subjects with low WMH load or controls with high WMH load.
Ham et al. (2016) [63], retrospective study	PD = 171 (non-demented)	WMH	Total WMH and deep WMH associated with worse performance in semantic fluency.
Mak et al. (2015) [64], retrospective study	PD-NCI = 65 PD-MCI = 25	WMH	Greater total and periventricular WMH in PD-MCI than in PD-NCI. Spatial distribution of WMH associated with global cognition, performance on the Frontal Assessment Battery and Fruit Fluency.
Sunwoo et al. (2014) [45], prospective study	PD-NCI = 46 PD-MCI = 65	WMH (volume and CHIPS score)	The progression from PD-MCI to PDD correlated with WMH volume and CHIPS score. In PD-MCI patients WMH volume and CHIPS score associated with longitudinal decline in general cognition, semantic fluency and Stroop test scores.
Kandiah et al. (2013) [44], prospective study	PD-NCI = 67 PD-MCI = 24	WMH	PD-MCI patients had significantly greater volume of periventricular and deep subcortical WMH than PD-NCI. Regional WMH significantly greater among PD-MCI in the frontal, parietal and occipital regions.
Sławek et al. (2013) [41], retrospective study	PD-NCI = 135 PDD = 57 controls = 184	WMH	WMH significantly greater in PDD than PD-NCI group.
Kim et al. (2012) [17], retrospective study	PD-NCI = 25 PD-MCI = 48 PDD = 14	WMH (CHIPS score)	The severity of WMH in the periventricular and subcortical white matter higher in PDD than in PD-NCI or PD-MCI. No difference in WMH between PD-NCI and PD-MCI.
Shin et al. (2012) [65], retrospective study	PD-NCI = 44 PD-MCI = 87 PDD = 40	WMH (CHIPS score)	The CHIPS score significantly higher in PDD than in PD-NCI or PD-MCI. WMH negatively associated with performance in MMSE. The CHIPS score correlated with the performance in contrasting programme and forward digit span tests.
Lee et al. (2010) [66], retrospective study	PD-NCI = 11 PD-MCI = 25 PDD = 35	WMH	Greater total and periventricular WMH in the PDD group compared to PD-MCI and PD-NCI groups. No difference in WMH between PD-MCI and PD-NCI groups.
Dalaker et al. (2009) [67], retrospective study	Drug-naïve: PD-NCI = 133 PD-MCI = 30 controls = 102	WMH	No differences between the groups in total volume or spatial distribution of WMH. No correlation between WMH and cognitive functions.
Beyer et al. (2006) [68], retrospective study	PD-NCI = 19 PDD = 16 controls = 20	WMH	PDD group had significantly more WMH in deep white matter and periventricular areas than the PD-NCI group.

Table 1. *Cont.*

Interaction between WMH and BP Variability			
Authors (year), type of the study	**Subjects**	**Factor**	**Outcome**
Dadar et al. (2020) [69], prospective study	PD = 365 (de novo) controls = 174	WMH Orthostatic hypotension.	A correlation between WMH burden and worse Montreal Cognitive Assessment (MoCA) score in PD over time. WMH linked with diastolic OH. Direct effect of diastolic OH on the rate of cognitive decline via WMH burden.
Oh et al. (2013) [39], retrospective study	PD = 117	WMH Orthostatic hypotension, supine hypertension.	Orthostatic hypotension and supine hypertension correlated with WMH score.
Oh et al. (2013) [42], retrospective study	Drug-naïve: PD = 129	WMH Circadian blood pressure variability.	Nocturnal hypertension associated with WMH in the basal ganglia. No influence of the non-dipping pattern on WMH. Nighttime systolic BP closely correlated with WMH.
Kim et al. (2012) [17], retrospective study	PD-NCI = 25 PD-MCI = 48 PDD = 14	WMH (CHIPS score) Circadian blood pressure variability, supine hypertension and orthostatic hypotension.	WMH significantly more severe in patients having OH, SH or OH + SH. No difference in WMH between the dippers and non-dippers.

BP—blood pressure; DLB—dementia with Lewy Bodies; CHIPS—Cholinergic Pathways Hyperintensities Scale, measures the extent of WMH in the periventricular and subcortical white matter; MCI—mild cognitive impairment; MMSE—Mini-Mental State Examination; NCI—no cognitive impairment; OH(+)—with orthostatic hypotension; OH(−)—without orthostatic hypotension; PDD—PD dementia; WMH—white matter hyperintensities.

5. Metabolic and Vascular Risk Factors

The etiology of cognitive impairment in PD presumably involves other than dopamine-dependent mechanisms, from which factors affecting the cerebrovascular status seem highly probable (Figure 1) [61]. Hypertension, diabetes mellitus and hypercholesterolemia lead to structural changes in the vessels [52], hypoperfusion, endothelial disorders, and altered blood–brain barrier permeability [70]. This results in cerebrovascular pathologies, seen as WMH—a marker of cognitive deterioration [52].

Vascular risk factors and their significance in PD and PD dementia have been investigated in several analyses, one of which was a cohort study on Finnish population assessing the impact of diabetes on PD occurrence. The hazard ratio of PD among patients with type 2 diabetes at baseline was estimated as 1.83 (95% CI 1.21–2.76) [71]. However, in the Nurses' Health Study and the Health Professionals Follow-up Study the relationship between PD and self-reported diabetes was not confirmed [72]. In the same analysis self-reported history of hypertension or high cholesterol levels were not established as PD risk factors either. In the meta-analysis performed by Cereda et al. diabetes was correlated with PD, although the diagnosis of idiopathic PD without imaging techniques in some studies seemed to be uncertain, since diabetes might lead to microvascular complications with parkinsonism as clinical outcome [73]. The impact of diabetes on PD dementia in a meta-analysis by Xu et al. was not confirmed, in contrast to hypertension (OR 1.57, 95% CI 1.11–2.22) [74]. The relationship between hypertension and cognitive performance was additionally found in Doiron et al. research [70]. In this prospective study, the history of hypertension was followed by lower Z-scores on immediate and delayed free recall, recognition, and verbal fluency tests. However, the numbers of years with hyperlipidemia did not correlate with a change in any of the Z-scores at the 24-month follow-up. In a prospective research, hypertension was correlated with an increased risk of the MCI development in PD patients, whereas MCI and WMH predicted the conversion to PDD [52]. No impact of hypertension on the progression from MCI to PDD was established. Thus, it is likely that hypertension contributes to increasing WMH, which in turn modulates the risk of dementia. On the other hand, vascular factors (e.g., smoking status, body mass index, hypertension, and diabetes)—calculated together into Framingham General Cardiovascular Disease Risk Score—increased the risk of both MCI and dementia in PD [61]. Homocysteine (Hcy) is an established risk factor for vascular damage. Additionally, it has been correlated with neurodegeneration related to oxidative stress, calcium accumulation and apoptosis [75]. An elevated concentration of homocysteine (hyperhomocysteinemia: HHcy;

value over 15 μmol/L of blood) was more frequently observed in PD dementia than in PD patients without dementia [41]. Hcy elevated levels might result from L-dopa methylation by catechol-*O*-methyltransferase (COMT), but the authors assessed the correlation between Hcy levels and L-dopa dose as weak (coefficient of determination R2 = 0.12). However, an increase in Hcy level was established for the treatment with duodenal levodopa gel (duodopa), due to its formulation which negatively affects the absorption of B6 vitamin and folate, necessary for reducing Hcy levels [76,77]. The correlation between Hcy and cognitive status in PD was demonstrated in a meta-analysis performed by Xie et al., with suggestion that the detrimental effect of HHcy could be mitigated with folate and/or B12 vitamin supplementation [78].

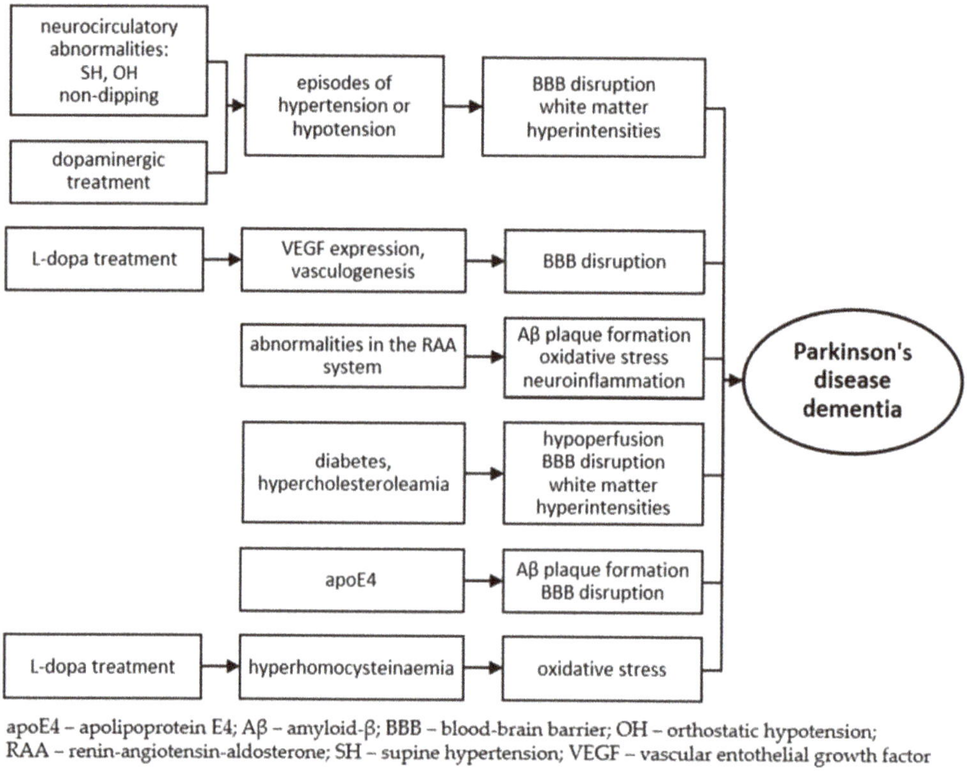

Figure 1. Possible vascular-related mechanisms leading to dementia in Parkinson's disease.

The plasma and tissue renin–angiotensin–aldosterone (RAA) system has recently emerged as another risk factor for PD and PD dementia. It plays a key role in controlling BP as well as water and electrolytes homeostasis. The conversion of angiotensinogen to angiotensin II (AngII) is catalyzed by renin, and then angiotensin converting enzyme (ACE). The resultant AngII binds to type 1 or 2 angiotensin receptors (AT1R, AT2R), expressed among others in peripheral vessels, heart, kidneys and CNS. Initially, the effects of the RAA system in CNS were considered to be mediated only through circumventricular organs, since active products of this system do not cross the blood–brain barrier [79]. However, at this moment it is known that the brain has an independent local RAA system, and the existence of the intracellular RAA system has been confirmed. As demonstrated in the experimental model, angiotensinogen in CNS is produced by astrocytes with a limited contribution from neurons, and central AngII levels may be even higher than the peripheral concentration [80]. The role of the RAA system in the nigro-striatal pathway seems to be of particular interest. Dopamine deficiency leads to compensatory RAA system hyperreactivity and an increased expression of AT1R and AT2R [81]. In neurons, interaction of AngII with its receptor AT1 leads to activation of neuronal NADPH oxidase and production of reactive oxygen species (ROS). This triggers oxidative stress and inflammatory processes that are additionally enhanced by ROS from other sources i.e., mitochondria or activated microglia. Free radicals from the latter are released extracellularly, and consequently, may lead to progressive damage to dopaminergic neurons [79].

Experimental and clinical evidence demonstrates beneficial effects of AT1 receptor blocking or converting enzyme inhibition on RAA system function, and dopamine concentration in striatum, as well as a reduction in inflammatory processes [79,82]. The RAA system is closely linked to VEGF synthesis, and like AngII, VEGF stimulates angiogenesis, affects permeability of blood vessels and blood brain barrier function. Janelidze et al. established the correlation between cerebrospinal fluid (CSF) biomarkers of angiogenesis and PD with and without dementia [40]. Levels of VEGF, placental growth factor (PlGF), and one of VEGF receptors (VEGFR-2) were significantly higher in both demented and non-demented PD patients comparing to the control group. However, no difference was observed between PD and PD dementia groups. In another study, the CSF level of VEGF was considerably higher in PD dementia (grouped together with patients with Lewy bodies dementia) than in the control subjects [83]. VEGF was suggested as a potent trigger of vascular leakage and blood–brain barrier dysfunction, which is in line with elevated endothelial cell nuclei and vessels in the substantia nigra pars compacta of PD patients found in post-mortem studies [23,84]. Moreover, it was noted that patients with diastolic OH had increased levels of VEGF and PlGF in comparison with subjects without OH. Insufficient autoregulation of cerebral blood flow in PD patients results in hypoxia-induced VEGF signaling and, consequently, in an angiogenic response [40].

Some proteins from the VEGF family demonstrate neuroprotective activity (VEGF-B), as revealed in diencephalon cell cultures exposed to rotenone (widely used as an experimental model of PD). The neuroprotective effect of VEGF on 6-hydroxydopamine (6-OHDA) treated dopaminergic neurons was reported to be mediated by both direct and indirect vascular and neuronal mechanisms. The neuroprotective effect of VEGF in PD models was dose-dependent, i.e., the low dose protected dopaminergic neurons, whereas the high dose induced severe brain edema [85]. Excessive activation of the tissue and/or plasma RAA system resulting from dopamine deficiency may lead to the fostering of processes damaging dopamine neurons. This in turn may increase the risk of L-dopa-induced side effects (e.g., dyskinesia) due to both increased neurodegeneration and changes in L-dopa distribution within CNS (pulsatile dopamine receptor stimulation).

Muñoz et al. demonstrated that administration of candesartan, AT1 receptor blocker, significantly reduced dyskinesia in the 6-OHDA induced, experimental model of PD [86]. In animals with dyskinesia, higher concentrations of VEGF and IL-1β within striatum and substantia nigra were found. Furthermore, animals treated with candesartan along with L-dopa were characterized by lower levels of VEGF, IL-1β, and less severe dyskinesia compared to animals receiving only L-dopa. L-dopa monotherapy reduces the activity of the RAA system. It is likely that the effects of L-dopa on angiogenesis in the course of chronic treatment cannot be eliminated, but can be mitigated by AT1R blockade. Moreover, the reduction of L-dopa-induced dyskinesia did not diminish L-dopa effectiveness against motor symptoms. Taking into consideration the aforesaid facts that long-term L-dopa treatment is a risk factor for developing PD dementia and that L-dopa-induced dyskinesia correlate with cognitive decline, it is possible that blocking AT1R may decrease the risk of cognitive decline.

A recent prospective study assessed the impact of several angiotensin II-stimulating (thiazides, dihydropyridine calcium channel blockers, AT1R blockers) and angiotensin II-inhibiting (ACE inhibitors, β-blockers, nondihydropyridine calcium channel blockers) antihypertensive drugs on the risk of dementia in older people (70–78 years at baseline) [87]. Subjects administrating AngII-stimulating antihypertensives had significantly lower risk of developing dementia compared to AngII-inhibiting drugs, independently of systolic BP or the baseline history of stroke, diabetes or CV diseases. As for the individual types of antihypertensives, the only significant decrease of dementia risk was associated with dihydropyridine calcium channel blockers. The beneficial role of upregulating AngII may result from the neuroprotection connected with AT2R. On the other hand, as ACE was showed to degrade amyloid-β (Aβ) in experimental models, the use of ACE inhibitors may promote Aβ plaque formation [87,88]. Regardless of the pivotal role of Aβ in AD, its deposition in PD was associated with cognitive decline [89]. However, in the aforementioned prospective study, the incidence rate of dementia in the group using ACE inhibitors did not differ from other types of antihypertensive drugs [87]. Moreover, Zhuang et al. showed in their meta-analysis that ACE inhibitors, as well as AT1R blockade, lowered the risk of AD, and AT1R blockade additionally decreased the risk of cognitive impairment associated with age [90]. Thus, the possible involvement of ACE in cognitive impairment and the effects exerted by ACE inhibitors seem to be far from being elucidated.

6. Genetic Factors

Although several causative genes for PD have been found, they scarcely account for some of the familial cases, whereas for the idiopathic form of PD and PD dementia, only susceptibility genes have been established, though not without inconsistency. Among the analyzed susceptibility genes are these coding for catechol-*O*-methyltransferase (*COMT*), apolipoprotein E (*APOE*), vascular endothelial growth factor (*VEGF*) and for renin–angiotensin–aldosterone system.

6.1. COMT

Catechol-O-methyltransferase (COMT) catalyzes the transfer of a methyl group from S-adenosyl-methionine to a hydroxyl group on a catecholamine (e.g., dopamine, norepinephrine, or catechol estrogen), thus regulating dopamine level in the prefrontal cortex, and is also a crucial enzyme involved in L-dopa metabolism [91,92]. Furthermore, the methylation of L-dopa is followed by the production of S-adenosylhomocysteine, hydrolyzed to homocysteine, which in turn may be responsible for HHcy in L-dopa medicated PD patients. However, homocysteine levels can be reduced by concurrent administration of COMT inhibitors in PD patients [93]. A common polymorphism in *COMT* gene—a G→A substitution (rs4680) results in an amino acid codon alteration (Val158Met in the membrane-bound form of COMT), and according to Chen et al., significantly lower enzymatic activity in homozygous *COMT*-Met in comparison with homozygous *COMT*-Val in post-mortem human prefrontal cortex tissues [91]. The dopaminergic imaging study demonstrated that Met homozygotes were characterized by an increased level of caudate striatal dopamine transporter (DAT), and a slightly protective effect on dementia was found for homozygous *COMT*-Met carriers [94]. Additionally, in a prospective analysis, Val homozygotes were at greater risk of developing PD-MCI than the other *COMT* genotypes, although the correlation with PD dementia was not observed [95]. Interestingly, Williams-Gray et al. [96] demonstrated in their longitudinal CamPaIGN study a varying impact of *COMT* alleles in relation to the disease duration. In "early" disease (<1.6 years), there was a significant decrease in the Tower of London (TOL; test of planning) scores with an increasing number of Met alleles, whereas no effect was observed in the "later" disease group (>1.6 years). Moreover, after 5.2-year follow-up, Met homozygotes were more likely to improve the TOL test score, in contrast to Val homozygotes or heterozygotes. The observed difference is possibly a consequence of an inverted U-shaped relationship between dopamine levels and prefrontal function, assessed mainly by working memory [96].

The *COMT* polymorphism seems to affect Hcy total level as well. Tunbridge et al. established that Val carriers had 1 μmol/L higher Hcy plasma values compared with Met homozygotes [92]. Additionally, the effect correlated with a polymorphism in methylenetetrahydrofolate reductase (*MTHFR* 677C > T; rs1801133) gene, which is commonly analysed with regard to Hcy/folate metabolism, resulting in the highest Hcy level among PD patients with both *MTHFR* 677TT and *COMT*-Val genotypes [92,97]. This indicates a necessity of COMT inhibitors administration, especially in patients at the greatest genetic risk for developing HHcy. However, in another study, significantly higher Hcy plasma levels were observed only in PD patients with *MTHFR* 677TT and low activity-determining *COMT* genotypes (based on the genotyping of four *COMT* single nucleotide polymorphisms—SNPs: rs4680, rs6269, rs4633 and rs4818) at the same time. The authors showed a correlation between Hcy levels and PD dementia, although none of the analyzed polymorphisms had an impact on cognitive impairment [97].

6.2. *APOE*

Apolipoprotein E (apoE) is associated with cerebrovascular and neurodegenerative diseases, such as late onset AD and PD [98,99]. The *APOE* gene polymorphism is identified in the form of three major alleles *APOE2*, *APOE3*, and *APOE4*, which determine three protein isoforms (E2, E3, and E4, resp.) and six possible genotypes (*e2/e2*, *e2/e3*, *e2/e4*, *e3/e3*, *e3/e4*, and *e4/e4*). Several studies showed that the *e2* allele is associated with a higher risk of PD [100,101], whereas in others, the *e4* allele was a risk factor. However, the data is inconsistent [102,103]. It was suggested that *APOE4* expression exerts detrimental effects on the cerebrovascular system, including blood–brain barrier impairments [104]. Indeed, Bell et al. showed that mice expressing human *APOE4* had altered blood–brain barrier permeability and reduced cerebral blood flow compared with animals expressing *APOE2* or *APOE3* [105]. In addition, apoE mediates the clearance of Aβ across blood–brain barrier, through binding to its liver receptor (low-density lipoprotein receptor-related protein-1—LRP1), and that *APOE4* allele contributes to cerebral accumulation of Aβ [105].

In a study performed by Janelidze et al., blood–brain barrier permeability characterized by the use of the cerebrospinal fluid/plasma albumin ratio (Qalb) differed significantly in groups with dementia (AD, dementia with Lewy bodies or PD dementia, vascular dementia or frontotemporal dementia) compared to healthy controls, although no impact of *APOE4* allele on Qalb was found [83]. Nevertheless, Qalb seemed to correlate with CSF biomarkers of angiogenesis or endothelial damage, i.e., intracellular adhesion molecule 1 (ICAM-1), vascular cell adhesion molecule 1 (VCAM-1) and VEGF, in all diagnostic groups. Those results support the role of the blood–brain barrier leakage in dementia, including PD dementia.

Despite some discrepancy in the studies assessing the role of *APOE4* in cognitive status of PD patients, possibly due to different diagnostic criteria for dementia [106], two meta-analyses [101,107] showed an over-representation of *APOE4* carriers in PD dementia groups compared to cognitively normal PD patients. Additionally, the most recent meta-analysis revealed that *APOE4* was a risk factor for PD dementia development regardless of the population origin [107].

6.3. *VEGF*

Variability in *VEGF* expression, induced by specific *VEGFA* variants, is involved in angiogenesis-related disorders. At least 30 SNPs in this gene have been described, and some SNPs can alter VEGF serum levels. Three common SNPs, namely −2578C/A in the promoter region (rs699947), −634C/G in the 5-untranslated region (rs2010963) and +936C/T in the 3-untranslated region (rs3025039) are related to VEGF protein production [108,109], although no association between VEGF serum level and PD has been established so far [110]. Some *VEGF* SNPs have been examined as susceptibility factors to AD. Del Bo et al. found a correlation between AD and −2578A/A and −1198C/T genotypes [111]. Although the VEGF serum level did not differ between AD patients and controls, increased values were correlated with *VEGF* polymorphisms, which had previously been described as associated with AD. Furthermore, a link between the severity of cognitive impairment and VEGF level was determined in Alvarez et al. study—the protein values were higher in AD than in MCI patients and in the controls [112]. The number of wild-type *VEGF* −2578C alleles was positively associated with total grey matter volume, total white matter volume and total arterial blood volume in young adults [113]. Considering that brain atrophy, thus smaller brain volume, correlates with cognitive decline in in PD [114], this can suggest a protective role of the *C* allele.

In the studies on *VEGF* genetic polymorphisms in PD patients, rs3025039 was the only *VEGF* polymorphism determined to correlate with PD development [110,111,115]. *VEGF* gene expression interacted with the genetic susceptibility factor for PD dementia. i.e., *APOE4*, on global cognition in AD, but not on AD neuropathology suggesting independence of the interaction from AD neuropathology [116]. However, no research has analyzed the impact of *VEGF* polymorphisms on cognitive performance or dementia in PD.

6.4. RAA System Genes

The neuroprotective effects of ACE inhibitors or AT1R antagonists observed in animal PD models suggest that abnormalities in the RAA system may promote the PD development [117]. Over the past several years, numerous polymorphic loci in genes encoding various components of the RAA system were defined, e.g., an insertion/deletion polymorphism in angiotensin converting enzyme gene (*ACE*) [118] or SNPs in angiotensin II receptor type 1 (*AGTR1*) [119], angiotensin II receptor type 2 (*AGTR2*) [120] or in angiotensinogen (*AGT*) [121] genes.

The insertion/deletion polymorphism in the angiotensin-converting enzyme gene (*ACE* I/D) was the first in the RAA system to be examined as a potential susceptibility factor in PD [122]. Though no association was found by Mellick et al. in an Australian population [122], or Pascale et al. in an Italian one [123], a study in a Chinese population showed an increased frequency of *DD* genotype in PD compared to the control group [124]. This discrepancy may result from differences in *ACE* I/D polymorphism frequency among the respective populations, since the prevalence of the *D* allele is estimated to be 50–58% in Caucasians and 35–39% in a Chinese population [124].

On the other hand, in a Swedish study the *II* homozygotes had a two-fold higher risk of dementia (including AD and vascular dementia) than the other *ACE* I/D carriers [125]. However, the polymorphism was not associated with dementia in the follow-up. Similarly, the *CC* genotype of *AGTR1* rs5186 was associated with dementia only at baseline [126]. Three other SNPs in *AGTR1* (rs2638363, rs1492103, rs2675511) were signs of worse episodic memory performance in a 4 years' follow-up and additionally correlated with a hippocampal atrophy in older adults [127].

Purandure et al. reported a link between *ACE* I/D polymorphism and WMH in patients of Caucasian origin with AD or vascular dementia [128]. White matter hyperintensities were more severe in patients carrying the *DD* than *ID* ($p = 0.01$) or *II* genotype ($p = 0.009$) and the correlation remained significant after a correction for cardiovascular risk factors, thus suggesting other mechanisms contributing to WMH development. It is worth mentioning that carriers of both *APOE4* genotype and *ACE I* allele were at higher risk of developing late-onset AD [129].

Other *ACE* polymorphisms (rs4362), along with the SNP in the angiotensinogen gene (*AGT* rs699) and the SNP in angiotensin II receptor type 1 gene (*AGTR1* rs5182) were evaluated in older Australians [130]. A male-only relationship between *AGT* rs699 and *ACE* rs4362 polymorphisms and WMH was found, independently of hypertension. Moreover, the authors reported a synergistic effect of *AGT* rs699 and *AGTR1* rs5182 on WMH. Although it was established that *ACE* I/D polymorphism accounts for 47% of the variation in ACE serum level [131], other genetic polymorphisms, including synonymous ones, can affect gene expression and protein synthesis. Therefore, they may exert an impact on WMH and cognitive functions.

The available literature does not provide a comprehensive assessment of variability in genes encoding the RAA system components and their associations with BP variability in the course of PD or cognitive decline in PD (Table 2).

Table 2. Genetic factors influencing vascular functions and cognitive decline in PD.

Gene	Name of the Protein	Function of the Protein	Role in Cognitive Decline	References
COMT	catechol-*O*-methyltransferase	metabolism of catecholamines and L-dopa, involved in Hcy synthesis	polymorphism associated with Hcy overproduction	[92]
APOE	apolipoprotein E	component of several lipoproteins	*APOE4* variant linked to Aβ accumulation and BBB disruption	[105]
VEGF	vascular endothelial growth factor	angiogenic activity, essential in vasculogenesis.	microvascular pathologies, BBB disruption	[23]
MTHFR	methylenetetrahydrofolate reductase	Hcy and folate metabolism	polymorphism correlated with HHcy	[132]
ACE	angiotensin converting enzyme	catalyzes AII synthesis; its inhibitors lower BP	Aβ degradation; polymorphism associated with WMH	[87,130]
AGT	angiotensinogen	precursor of all components within the RAA system	polymorphism associated with WMH	[130]
AGTR1	angiotensin receptor type 1	AII receptor	oxidative stress and neuroinflammation; polymorphisms associated with hippocampal atrophy	[79,127]
AGTR2	angiotensin receptor type 2	AII receptor	possible neuroprotection	[87]
HMGCR	HMG-CoA reductase	rate-controlling enzyme in the cholesterol synthesis pathway	polymorphism decreases cholesterol production	[133]

AII—angiotensin II; Aβ—amyloid-β; BBB—blood–brain barrier; Hcy—homocysteine; HHcy—hyperhomocysteinemia; HMG-CoA—3-hydroxy-3-methylglutaryl-CoA; RAA—renin-angiotensin-aldosterone; WMH—white matter hyperintensities.

7. Conclusions

There is a growing demand to determine factors predisposing to the development of PD dementia. The impact of abnormal circadian BP variability observed in PD patients seems to contribute to WMH, which in turn may be a radiological marker for cognitive decline. Many of the presented factors, correlating with WMH hyperintensities and/or cognitive decline in PD, may and should be treated as far as possible (Figure 2). Hypertension, OH, supine hypertension and the absence of nocturnal BP fall can be diagnosed by an ambulatory 24-h BP monitoring and then managed by both nonpharmacological and pharmacological measures. Similarly, the impact of hyperhomocysteinemia—a metabolic risk factor for dementia in PD—may be possibly alleviated by more frequent blood concentration assessments and folate and/or B12 vitamin supplementation. As for the genetic risk factors, they may serve as markers of cognitive decline in PD or indicate a future direction for specific treatment, e.g., AGT1 receptor blockers and inhibitors of the RAA system. In summary, knowledge on vascular risk factors and their contribution to the cognitive impairment in PD may result in prophylaxis and better screening methods. However, this matter needs to be addressed in future studies, including clinical trials.

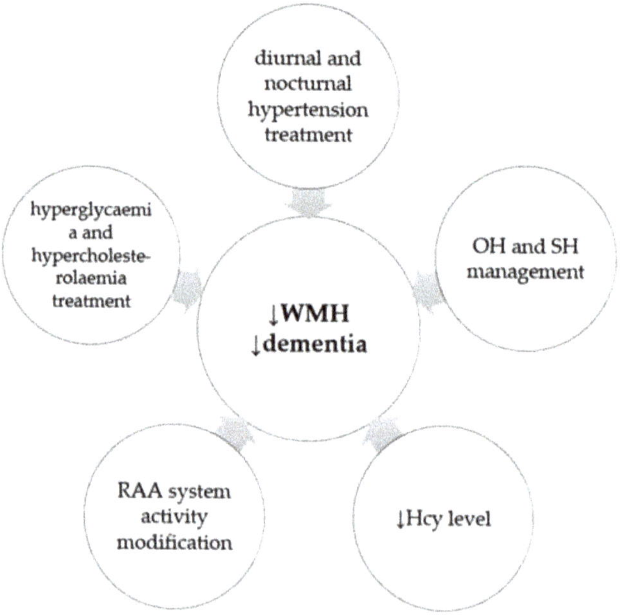

Figure 2. Possible measures decreasing the risk of developing WMH, and/or dementia, in Parkinson's disease.

Author Contributions: Conceptualization, M.B. and J.S.; investigation, A.P. and M.K.-B.; writing—original draft preparation, A.P.; writing—review and editing, J.S., M.D. and M.B.; supervision, M.B. All authors have read and agreed to the published version of the manuscript.

Funding: This research received no external funding.

Institutional Review Board Statement: Not applicable.

Informed Consent Statement: Not applicable.

Data Availability Statement: Not applicable.

Acknowledgments: Not applicable.

Conflicts of Interest: The authors declare no conflict of interest.

References

1. Poewe, W.; Gauthier, S.; Aarsland, D.; Leverenz, J.B.; Barone, P.; Weintraub, D.; Tolosa, E.; Dubois, B. Diagnosis and management of Parkinson's disease dementia. *Int. J. Clin. Pract.* **2008**, *62*, 1581–1587. [CrossRef]
2. Emre, M. Dementia associated with Parkinson's disease. *Lancet Neurol.* **2003**, *2*, 229–237. [CrossRef]
3. Aarsland, D.; Andersen, K.; Larsen, J.P.; Lolk, A.; Kragh-Sørensen, P. Prevalence and characteristics of dementia in Parkinson disease: An 8-year prospective study. *Arch. Neurol.* **2003**, *60*, 387–392. [CrossRef] [PubMed]
4. Zhu, K.; van Hilten, J.J.; Marinus, J. Predictors of dementia in Parkinson's disease; findings from a 5-year prospective study using the SCOPA-COG. *Parkinsonism Relat. Disord.* **2014**, *20*, 980–985. [CrossRef]
5. Horvath, J.; Herrmann, F.R.; Burkhard, P.R.; Bouras, C.; Kövari, E. Neuropathology of dementia in a large cohort of patients with Parkinson's disease. *Parkinsonism Relat. Disord.* **2013**, *19*, 864–868. [CrossRef] [PubMed]
6. Hanganu, A.; Bedetti, C.; Jubault, T.; Gagnon, J.F.; Mejia-Constain, B.; Degroot, C.; Lafontaine, A.L.; Chouinard, S.; Monchi, O. Mild cognitive impairment in patients with Parkinson's disease is associated with increased cortical degeneration. *Mov. Disord.* **2013**, *28*, 1360–1369. [CrossRef]
7. Parati, G.; Stergiou, G.S.; Dolan, E.; Bilo, G. Blood pressure variability: Clinical relevance and application. *J. Clin. Hypertens.* **2018**, *20*, 1133–1137. [CrossRef]
8. Pathak, A.; Senard, J.M. Blood pressure disorders during Parkinson's disease: Epidemiology, pathophysiology and management. *Expert Rev. Neurother.* **2006**, *6*, 1173–1180. [CrossRef]

9. Jain, S.; Goldstein, D.S. Cardiovascular dysautonomia in Parkinson disease: From pathophysiology to pathogenesis. *Neurobiol. Dis.* **2012**, *46*, 572–580. [CrossRef] [PubMed]
10. Biaggioni, I.; Arthur Hewitt, L.; Rowse, G.J.; Kaufmann, H. Integrated analysis of droxidopa trials for neurogenic orthostatic hypotension. *BMC Neurol.* **2017**, *17*, 90. [CrossRef]
11. Milazzo, V.; Di Stefano, C.; Vallelonga, F.; Sobrero, G.; Zibetti, M.; Romagnolo, A.; Merola, A.; Milan, A.; Espay, A.J.; Lopiano, L.; et al. Reverse blood pressure dipping as marker of dysautonomia in Parkinson disease. *Parkinsonism Relat. Disord.* **2018**, *56*, 82–87. [CrossRef] [PubMed]
12. Fabbian, F.; Smolensky, M.H.; Tiseo, R.; Pala, M.; Manfredini, R.; Portaluppi, F. Dipper and non-dipper blood pressure 24-hour patterns: Circadian rhythm-dependent physiologic and pathophysiologic mechanisms. *Chronobiol. Int.* **2013**, *30*, 17–30. [CrossRef]
13. Agarwal, R. Regulation of circadian blood pressure: From mice to astronauts. *Curr. Opin. Nephrol. Hypertens.* **2010**, *19*, 51–58. [CrossRef] [PubMed]
14. Kuwajima, I.; Suzuki, Y.; Shimosawa, T.; Kanemaru, A.; Hoshino, S.; Kuramoto, K. Diminished nocturnal decline in blood pressure in elderly hypertensive patients with left ventricular hypertrophy. *Am. Heart. J.* **1992**, *123*, 1307–1311. [CrossRef]
15. Fanciulli, A.; Strano, S.; Ndayisaba, J.P.; Goebel, G.; Gioffrè, L.; Rizzo, M.; Colosimo, C.; Caltagirone, C.; Poewe, W.; Wenning, G.K.; et al. Detecting nocturnal hypertension in Parkinson's disease and multiple system atrophy: Proposal of a decision-support algorithm. *J. Neurol.* **2014**, *261*, 1291–1299. [CrossRef]
16. Berganzo, K.; Díez-Arrola, B.; Tijero, B.; Somme, J.; Lezcano, E.; Llorens, V.; Ugarriza, I.; Ciordia, R.; Gómez-Esteban, J.C.; Zarranz, J.J. Nocturnal hypertension and dysautonomia in patients with Parkinson's disease: Are they related? *J. Neurol.* **2013**, *260*, 1752–1756. [CrossRef]
17. Kim, J.S.; Oh, Y.S.; Lee, K.S.; Kim, Y.I.; Yang, D.W.; Goldstein, D.S. Association of cognitive dysfunction with neurocirculatory abnormalities in early Parkinson disease. *Neurology* **2012**, *79*, 1323–1331. [CrossRef]
18. Anang, J.B.; Gagnon, J.F.; Bertrand, J.A.; Romenets, S.R.; Latreille, V.; Panisset, M.; Montplaisir, J.; Postuma, R.B. Predictors of dementia in Parkinson disease: A prospective cohort study. *Neurology* **2014**, *83*, 1253–1260. [CrossRef]
19. Udow, S.J.; Robertson, A.D.; MacIntosh, B.J.; Espay, A.J.; Rowe, J.B.; Lang, A.E.; Masellis, M. 'Under pressure': Is there a link between orthostatic hypotension and cognitive impairment in α-synucleinopathies? *J. Neurol. Neurosurg. Psychiatry* **2016**, *87*, 1311–1321. [CrossRef]
20. Tanaka, R.; Shimo, Y.; Yamashiro, K.; Ogawa, T.; Nishioka, K.; Oyama, G.; Umemura, A.; Hattori, N. Association between abnormal nocturnal blood pressure profile and dementia in Parkinson's disease. *Parkinsonism Relat. Disord.* **2018**, *46*, 24–29. [CrossRef]
21. Calabresi, P.; Di Filippo, M.; Ghiglieri, V.; Tambasco, N.; Picconi, B. Levodopa-induced dyskinesias in patients with Parkinson's disease: Filling the bench-to-bedside gap. *Lancet Neurol.* **2010**, *9*, 1106–1117. [CrossRef]
22. Westin, J.E.; Lindgren, H.S.; Gardi, J.; Nyengaard, J.R.; Brundin, P.; Mohapel, P.; Cenci, M.A. Endothelial Proliferation and Increased Blood-Brain Barrier Permeability in the Basal Ganglia in a Rat Model of 3,4-Dihydroxyphenyl-L-Alanine-Induced Dyskinesia. *J. Neurosci.* **2006**, *26*, 9448–9461. [CrossRef] [PubMed]
23. Ohlin, K.E.; Francardo, V.; Lindgren, H.S.; Sillivan, S.E.; O'Sullivan, S.S.; Luksik, A.S.; Vassoler, F.M.; Lees, A.J.; Konradi, C.; Cenci, M.A. Vascular endothelial growth factor is upregulated by L-dopa in the parkinsonian brain: Implications for the development of dyskinesia. *Brain* **2011**, *134*, 2339–2357. [CrossRef] [PubMed]
24. Ko, J.H.; Lerner, R.P.; Eidelberg, D. Effects of levodopa on regional cerebral metabolism and blood flow. *Mov. Disord.* **2015**, *30*, 54–63. [CrossRef] [PubMed]
25. Yoo, H.S.; Chung, S.J.; Lee, Y.H.; Lee, H.S.; Ye, B.S.; Sohn, Y.H.; Lee, P.H. Levodopa induced dyskinesia is closely linked to progression of frontal dysfunction in PD. *Neurology* **2019**, *92*, e1468–e1478. [CrossRef] [PubMed]
26. Espay, A.J.; LeWitt, P.A.; Hauser, R.A.; Merola, A.; Masellis, M.; Lang, A.E. Neurogenic orthostatic hypotension and supine hypertension in Parkinson's disease and related synucleinopathies: Prioritisation of treatment targets. *Lancet Neurol.* **2016**, *15*, 954–966. [CrossRef]
27. Goldstein, D.S.; Eldadah, B.A.; Holmes, C.; Pechnik, S.; Moak, J.; Saleem, A.; Sharabi, Y. Neurocirculatory abnormalities in Parkinson disease with orthostatic hypotension: Independence from levodopa treatment. *Hypertension* **2005**, *46*, 1333–1339. [CrossRef]
28. Wolf, J.P.; Bouhaddi, M.; Louisy, F.; Mikehiev, A.; Mourot, L.; Cappelle, S.; Vuillier, F.; Andre, P.; Rumbach, L.; Regnard, J. Side-effects of L-dopa on venous tone in Parkinson's disease: A leg-weighing assessment. *Clin. Sci.* **2006**, *110*, 369–377. [CrossRef]
29. Fanciulli, A.; Göbel, G.; Ndayisaba, J.P.; Granata, R.; Duerr, S.; Strano, S.; Colosimo, C.; Poewe, W.; Pontieri, F.E.; Wenning, G.K. Supine hypertension in Parkinson's disease and multiple system atrophy. *Clin. Auton. Res.* **2016**, *26*, 97–105. [CrossRef]
30. Montastruc, F.; Moulis, F.; Araujo, M.; Chebane, L.; Rascol, O.; Montastruc, J.L. Ergot and non-ergot dopamine agonists and heart failure in patients with Parkinson's disease. *Eur. J. Clin. Pharmacol.* **2017**, *73*, 99–103. [CrossRef] [PubMed]
31. Torti, M.; Bravi, D.; Vacca, L.; Stocchi, F. Are All Dopamine Agonists Essentially the Same? *Drugs* **2019**, *79*, 693–703. [CrossRef]
32. Oka, H.; Nakahara, A.; Umehara, T. Rotigotine Improves Abnormal Circadian Rhythm of Blood Pressure in Parkinson's Disease. *Eur. Neurol.* **2018**, *79*, 281–286. [CrossRef] [PubMed]
33. Watanabe, Y.; Nakamura, Y.; Cao, X.; Ohara, H.; Yamazaki, Y.; Murayama, N.; Sugiyama, Y.; Izumi-Nakaseko, H.; Ando, K.; Yamazaki, H.; et al. Intravenous Administration of Apomorphine Does NOT Induce Long QT Syndrome: Experimental Evidence from In Vivo Canine Models. *Basic Clin. Pharmacol. Toxicol.* **2015**, *116*, 468–475. [CrossRef] [PubMed]

34. Shimada, K.; Kawamoto, A.; Matsubayashi, K.; Nishinaga, M.; Kimura, S.; Ozawa, T. Diurnal blood pressure variations and silent cerebrovascular damage in elderly patients with hypertension. *J. Hypertens.* **1992**, *10*, 875–878.
35. Bohnen, N.I.; Albin, R.L. White matter lesions in Parkinson disease. *Nat. Rev. Neurol.* **2011**, *7*, 229–236. [CrossRef] [PubMed]
36. Bohnen, N.I.; Müller, M.L.; Zarzhevsky, N.; Koeppe, R.A.; Bogan, C.W.; Kilbourn, M.R.; Frey, K.A.; Albin, R.L. Leucoaraiosis, nigrostriatal denervation and motor symptoms in Parkinson's disease. *Brain* **2011**, *134*, 2358–2365. [CrossRef]
37. Siennicki-Lantz, A.; Reinprecht, F.; Axelsson, J.; Elmståhl, S. Cerebral perfusion in the elderly with nocturnal blood pressure fall. *Eur. J. Neurol.* **2007**, *14*, 715–720. [CrossRef]
38. Axelsson, J.; Reinprecht, F.; Siennicki-Lantz, A.; Elmståhl, S. Lower cognitive performance in 81-year-old men with greater nocturnal blood pressure dipping. *Int. J. Gen. Med.* **2009**, *1*, 69–75. [CrossRef]
39. Oh, Y.S.; Kim, J.S.; Lee, K.S. Orthostatic and supine blood pressures are associated with white matter hyperintensities in Parkinson disease. *J. Mov. Disord.* **2013**, *6*, 23–27. [CrossRef]
40. Janelidze, S.; Lindqvist, D.; Francardo, V.; Hall, S.; Zetterberg, H.; Blennow, K.; Adler, C.H.; Beach, T.G.; Serrano, G.E.; van Westen, D.; et al. Increased CSF biomarkers of angiogenesis in Parkinson disease. *Neurology* **2015**, *85*, 1834–1842. [CrossRef] [PubMed]
41. Sławek, J.; Roszmann, A.; Robowski, P.; Dubaniewicz, M.; Sitek, E.J.; Honczarenko, K.; Gorzkowska, A.; Budrewicz, S.; Mak, M.; Gołąb-Janowska, M.; et al. The impact of MRI white matter hyperintensities on dementia in Parkinson's disease in relation to the homocysteine level and other vascular risk factors. *Neurodegener. Dis.* **2013**, *12*, 1–12. [CrossRef] [PubMed]
42. Oh, Y.S.; Kim, J.S.; Yang, D.W.; Koo, J.S.; Kim, Y.I.; Jung, H.O.; Lee, K.S. Nighttime blood pressure and white matter hyperintensities in patients with Parkinson disease. *Chronobiol. Int.* **2013**, *30*, 811–817. [CrossRef] [PubMed]
43. Debette, S.; Markus, H.S. The clinical importance of white matter hyperintensities on brain magnetic resonance imaging: Systematic review and meta-analysis. *BMJ* **2010**, *341*, c3666. [CrossRef]
44. Kandiah, N.; Mak, E.; Ng, A.; Huang, S.; Au, W.L.; Sitoh, Y.Y.; Tan, L.C. Cerebral white matter hyperintensity in Parkinson's disease: A major risk factor for mild cognitive impairment. *Parkinsonism Relat. Disord.* **2013**, *19*, 680–683. [CrossRef]
45. Sunwoo, M.K.; Jeon, S.; Ham, J.H.; Hong, J.Y.; Lee, J.E.; Lee, J.M.; Sohn, Y.H.; Lee, P.H. The burden of white matter hyperintensities is a predictor of progressive mild cognitive impairment in patients with Parkinson's disease. *Eur. J. Neurol.* **2014**, *21*, 922-e50. [CrossRef] [PubMed]
46. Compta, Y.; Buongiorno, M.; Bargalló, N.; Valldeoriola, F.; Muñoz, E.; Tolosa, E.; Ríos, J.; Cámara, A.; Fernández, M.; Martí, M.J. White matter hyperintensities, cerebrospinal amyloid-β and dementia in Parkinson's disease. *J. Neurol. Sci.* **2016**, *367*, 284–290. [CrossRef] [PubMed]
47. Oka, H.; Umehara, T.; Nakahara, A.; Matsuno, H. Comparisons of cardiovascular dysautonomia and cognitive impairment between de novo Parkinson's disease and de novo dementia with Lewy bodies. *BMC Neurol.* **2020**, *20*, 350. [CrossRef]
48. Sforza, M.; Assogna, F.; Rinaldi, D.; Sette, G.; Tagliente, S.; Pontieri, F. Orthostatic hypotension acutely impairs executive functions in Parkinson's disease. *Neurol. Sci.* **2018**, *39*, 1459–1462. [CrossRef]
49. Centi, J.; Freeman, R.; Gibbons, C.H.; Neargarder, S.; Canova, A.O.; Cronin-Golomb, A. Effects of orthostatic hypotension on cognition in Parkinson disease. *Neurology* **2017**, *88*, 17–24. [CrossRef] [PubMed]
50. Pilleri, M.; Facchini, S.; Gasparoli, E.; Biundo, R.; Bernardi, L.; Marchetti, M.; Formento, P.; Antonini, A. Cognitive and MRI correlates of orthostatic hypotension in Parkinson's disease. *J. Neurol.* **2013**, *260*, 253–259. [CrossRef]
51. Allcock, L.M.; Kenny, R.A.; Mosimann, U.P.; Tordoff, S.; Wesnes, K.A.; Hildreth, A.J.; Burn, D.J. Orthostatic hypotension in Parkinson's disease: Association with cognitive decline? *Int. J. Geriatr. Psychiatry* **2006**, *21*, 778–783. [CrossRef]
52. Nicoletti, A.; Luca, A.; Baschi, R.; Cicero, C.E.; Mostile, G.; Davì, M.; La Bianca, G.; Restivo, V.; Zappia, M.; Monastero, R. Vascular risk factors, white matter lesions and cognitive impairment in Parkinson's disease: The PACOS longitudinal study. *J. Neurol.* **2021**, *268*, 549–558. [CrossRef] [PubMed]
53. Huang, X.; Wen, M.C.; Ng, S.Y.; Hartono, S.; Chia, N.S.; Choi, X.; Tay, K.Y.; Au, W.L.; Chan, L.L.; Tan, E.K.; et al. Periventricular white matter hyperintensity burden and cognitive impairment in early Parkinson's disease. *Eur. J. Neurol.* **2020**, *27*, 959–966. [CrossRef]
54. Ramirez, J.; Dilliott, A.A.; Binns, M.A.; Breen, D.P.; Evans, E.C.; Beaton, D.; McLaughlin, P.M.; Kwan, D.; Holmes, M.F.; Ozzoude, M.; et al. Parkinson's Disease, NOTCH3 Genetic Variants, and White Matter Hyperintensities. *Mov. Disord.* **2020**, *35*, 2090–2095. [CrossRef] [PubMed]
55. Dadar, M.; Gee, M.; Shuaib, A.; Duchesne, S.; Camicioli, R. Cognitive and motor correlates of grey and white matter pathology in Parkinson's disease. *Neuroimage Clin.* **2020**, *27*, 102353. [CrossRef]
56. Linortner, P.; McDaniel, C.; Shahid, M.; Levine, T.F.; Tian, L.; Cholerton, B.; Poston, K.L. White Matter Hyperintensities Related to Parkinson's Disease Executive Function. *Mov. Disord. Clin. Pract.* **2020**, *7*, 629–638. [CrossRef] [PubMed]
57. Lee, Y.H.; Lee, W.J.; Chung, S.J.; Yoo, H.S.; Jung, J.H.; Baik, K.; Sohn, Y.H.; Seong, J.K.; Lee, P.H. Microstructural Connectivity is More Related to Cognition than Conventional MRI in Parkinson's Disease. *J. Parkinsons Dis.* **2020**. [CrossRef]
58. Chahine, L.M.; Dos Santos, C.; Fullard, M.; Scordia, C.; Weintraub, D.; Erus, G.; Rosenthal, L.; Davatzikos, C.; McMillan, C.T. Modifiable vascular risk factors, white matter disease and cognition in early Parkinson's disease. *Eur. J. Neurol.* **2019**, *26*, 246-e18. [CrossRef] [PubMed]
59. Hanning, U.; Teuber, A.; Lang, E.; Trenkwalder, C.; Mollenhauer, B.; Minnerup, H. White matter hyperintensities are not associated with cognitive decline in early Parkinson's disease—The DeNoPa cohort. *Parkinsonism Relat. Disord.* **2019**, *69*, 61–67. [CrossRef]

60. Pozorski, V.; Oh, J.M.; Okonkwo, O.; Krislov, S.; Barzgari, A.; Theisen, F.; Sojkova, J.; Bendlin, B.B.; Johnson, S.C.; Gallagher, C.L. Cross-sectional and longitudinal associations between total and regional white matter hyperintensity volume and cognitive and motor function in Parkinson's disease. *Neuroimage Clin.* **2019**, *23*, 101870. [CrossRef] [PubMed]
61. Stojkovic, T.; Stefanova, E.; Soldatovic, I.; Markovic, V.; Stankovic, I.; Petrovic, I.; Agosta, F.; Galantucci, S.; Filippi, M.; Kostic, V. Exploring the relationship between motor impairment, vascular burden and cognition in Parkinson's disease. *J. Neurol.* **2018**, *265*, 1320–1327. [CrossRef] [PubMed]
62. Dadar, M.; Zeighami, Y.; Yau, Y.; Fereshtehnejad, S.M.; Maranzano, J.; Postuma, R.B.; Dagher, A.; Collins, D.L. White matter hyperintensities are linked to future cognitive decline in de novo Parkinson's disease patients. *Neuroimage Clin.* **2018**, *20*, 892–900. [CrossRef] [PubMed]
63. Ham, J.H.; Lee, J.J.; Sunwoo, M.K.; Hong, J.Y.; Sohn, Y.H.; Lee, P.H. Effect of olfactory impairment and white matter hyperintensities on cognition in Parkinson's disease. *Parkinsonism Relat. Disord.* **2016**, *24*, 95–99. [CrossRef] [PubMed]
64. Mak, E.; Dwyer, M.G.; Ramasamy, D.P.; Au, W.L.; Tan, L.C.; Zivadinov, R.; Kandiah, N. White Matter Hyperintensities and Mild Cognitive Impairment in Parkinson's Disease. *J. Neuroimaging* **2015**, *25*, 754–760. [CrossRef]
65. Shin, J.; Choi, S.; Lee, J.E.; Lee, H.S.; Sohn, Y.H.; Lee, P.H. Subcortical white matter hyperintensities within the cholinergic pathways of Parkinson's disease patients according to cognitive status. *J. Neurol. Neurosurg. Psychiatry* **2012**, *83*, 315–321. [CrossRef] [PubMed]
66. Lee, S.J.; Kim, J.S.; Yoo, J.Y.; Song, I.U.; Kim, B.S.; Jung, S.L.; Yang, D.W.; Kim, Y.I.; Jeong, D.S.; Lee, K.S. Influence of white matter hyperintensities on the cognition of patients with Parkinson disease. *Alzheimer Dis. Assoc. Disord.* **2010**, *24*, 227–233. [CrossRef]
67. Dalaker, T.O.; Larsen, J.P.; Dwyer, M.G.; Aarsland, D.; Beyer, M.K.; Alves, G.; Bronnick, K.; Tysnes, O.B.; Zivadinov, R. White matter hyperintensities do not impact cognitive function in patients with newly diagnosed Parkinson's disease. *Neuroimage* **2009**, *47*, 2083–2089. [CrossRef] [PubMed]
68. Beyer, M.K.; Aarsland, D.; Greve, O.J.; Larsen, J.P. Visual rating of white matter hyperintensities in Parkinson's disease. *Mov. Disord.* **2006**, *21*, 223–229. [CrossRef]
69. Dadar, M.; Fereshtehnejad, S.M.; Zeighami, Y.; Dagher, A.; Postuma, R.B.; Collins, D.L. White Matter Hyperintensities Mediate Impact of Dysautonomia on Cognition in Parkinson's Disease. *Mov. Disord. Clin. Pract.* **2020**, *7*, 639–647. [CrossRef]
70. Doiron, M.; Langlois, M.; Dupré, N.; Simard, M. The influence of vascular risk factors on cognitive function in early Parkinson's disease. *Int. J. Geriatr. Psychiatry* **2018**, *33*, 288–297. [CrossRef]
71. Hu, G.; Jousilahti, P.; Bidel, S.; Antikainen, R.; Tuomilehto, J. Type 2 diabetes and the risk of Parkinson's disease. *Diabetes Care* **2007**, *30*, 842–847. [CrossRef] [PubMed]
72. Simon, K.C.; Chen, H.; Schwarzschild, M.; Ascherio, A. Hypertension, hypercholesterolemia, diabetes, and risk of Parkinson disease. *Neurology* **2007**, *69*, 1688–1695. [CrossRef]
73. Cereda, E.; Barichella, M.; Pedrolli, C.; Klersy, C.; Cassani, E.; Caccialanza, R.; Pezzoli, G. Diabetes and risk of Parkinson's disease: A systematic review and meta-analysis. *Diabetes Care* **2011**, *34*, 2614–2623. [CrossRef]
74. Xu, Y.; Yang, J.; Shang, H. Meta-analysis of risk factors for Parkinson's disease dementia. *Transl. Neurodegener.* **2016**, *5*, 11. [CrossRef] [PubMed]
75. Sławek, J.; Białecka, M. Homocysteine and Dementia. In *Diet and Nutrition in Dementia and Cognitive Decline*; Martin, C.R., Preedy, V.R., Eds.; Academic Press: Cambridge, MA, USA, 2015; Chapter 57; pp. 611–621. [CrossRef]
76. Nyholm, D. Duodopa® treatment for advanced Parkinson's disease: A review of efficacy and safety. *Parkinsonism Relat. Disord.* **2012**, *18*, 916–929. [CrossRef] [PubMed]
77. Klostermann, F.; Jugel, C.; Müller, T.; Marzinzik, F. Malnutritional neuropathy under intestinal levodopa infusion. *J. Neural. Transm.* **2012**, *119*, 369–372. [CrossRef] [PubMed]
78. Xie, Y.; Feng, H.; Peng, S.; Xiao, J.; Zhang, J. Association of plasma homocysteine, vitamin B12 and folate levels with cognitive function in Parkinson's disease: A meta-analysis. *Neurosci. Lett.* **2017**, *636*, 190–195. [CrossRef]
79. Labandeira-Garcia, J.L.; Rodriguez-Pallares, J.; Dominguez-Meijide, A.; Valenzuela, R.; Villar-Cheda, B.; Rodríguez-Perez, A.I. Dopamine-Angiotensin interactions in the basal ganglia and their relevance for Parkinson's disease. *Mov. Disord.* **2013**, *28*, 1337–1342. [CrossRef] [PubMed]
80. Milsted, A.; Barna, B.P.; Ransohoff, R.M.; Brosnihan, K.B.; Ferrario, C.M. Astrocyte cultures derived from human brain tissue express angiotensinogen mRNA. *Proc. Natl. Acad. Sci. USA* **1990**, *87*, 5720–5723. [CrossRef] [PubMed]
81. Labandeira-García, J.L.; Garrido-Gil, P.; Rodriguez-Pallares, J.; Valenzuela, R.; Borrajo, A.; Rodríguez-Perez, A.I. Brain renin-angiotensin system and dopaminergic cell vulnerability. *Front. Neuroanat.* **2014**, *8*, 67. [CrossRef]
82. Villar-Cheda, B.; Valenzuela, R.; Rodriguez-Perez, A.I.; Guerra, M.J.; Labandeira-Garcia, J.L. Aging-related changes in the nigral angiotensin system enhances proinflammatory and pro-oxidative markers and 6-OHDA-induced dopaminergic degeneration. *Neurobiol. Aging* **2012**, *33*, 204.e1–204.e11. [CrossRef]
83. Janelidze, S.; Hertze, J.; Nägga, K.; Nilsson, K.; Nilsson, C.; Swedish BioFINDER Study Group; Wennström, M.; van Westen, D.; Blennow, K.; Zetterberg, H.; et al. Increased blood-brain barrier permeability is associated with dementia and diabetes but not amyloid pathology or APOE genotype. *Neurobiol. Aging* **2017**, *51*, 104–112. [CrossRef]
84. Faucheux, B.A.; Bonnet, A.M.; Agid, Y.; Hirsch, E.C. Blood vessels change in the mesencephalon of patients with Parkinson's disease. *Lancet* **1999**, *353*, 981–982. [CrossRef]

85. Yasuhara, T.; Shingo, T.; Muraoka, K.; wen Ji, Y.; Kameda, M.; Takeuchi, A.; Yano, A.; Nishio, S.; Matsui, T.; Miyoshi, Y.; et al. The differences between high and low-dose administration of VEGF to dopaminergic neurons of in vitro and in vivo Parkinson's disease model. *Brain Res.* **2005**, *1038*, 1–10. [CrossRef]
86. Muñoz, A.; Garrido-Gil, P.; Dominguez-Meijide, A.; Labandeira-Garcia, J.L. Angiotensin type 1 receptor blockage reduces l-dopa-induced dyskinesia in the 6-OHDA model of Parkinson's disease. Involvement of vascular endothelial growth factor and interleukin-1β. *Exp. Neurol.* **2014**, *261*, 720–732. [CrossRef] [PubMed]
87. Van Dalen, J.W.; Marcum, Z.A.; Gray, S.L.; Barthold, D.; Moll van Charante, E.P.; van Gool, W.A.; Crane, P.K.; Larson, E.B.; Richard, E. Association of Angiotensin II-Stimulating Antihypertensive Use and Dementia Risk: Post Hoc Analysis of the PreDIVA Trial. *Neurology* **2021**, *96*, e67–e80. [CrossRef]
88. Kehoe, P.G. The Coming of Age of the Angiotensin Hypothesis in Alzheimer's Disease: Progress Toward Disease Prevention and Treatment? *J. Alzheimers Dis.* **2018**, *62*, 1443–1466. [CrossRef]
89. Lim, E.W.; Aarsland, D.; Ffytche, D.; Taddei, R.N.; van Wamelen, D.J.; Wan, Y.M.; Tan, E.K.; Ray Chaudhuri, K.; Kings Parcog groupMDS Nonmotor Study Group. Amyloid-β and Parkinson's disease. *J. Neurol.* **2019**, *266*, 2605–2619. [CrossRef] [PubMed]
90. Zhuang, S.; Wang, H.F.; Wang, X.; Li, J.; Xing, C.M. The association of renin-angiotensin system blockade use with the risks of cognitive impairment of aging and Alzheimer's disease: A meta-analysis. *J. Clin. Neurosci.* **2016**, *33*, 32–38. [CrossRef] [PubMed]
91. Chen, J.; Lipska, B.K.; Halim, N.; Ma, Q.D.; Matsumoto, M.; Melhem, S.; Kolachana, B.S.; Hyde, T.M.; Herman, M.M.; Apud, J.; et al. Functional analysis of genetic variation in catechol-O-methyltransferase (COMT): Effects on mRNA, protein, and enzyme activity in postmortem human brain. *Am. J. Hum. Genet.* **2004**, *75*, 807–821. [CrossRef] [PubMed]
92. Tunbridge, E.M.; Harrison, P.J.; Warden, D.R.; Johnston, C.; Refsum, H.; Smith, A.D. Polymorphisms in the catechol-O-methyltransferase (COMT) gene influence plasma total homocysteine levels. *Am. J. Med. Genet. B Neuropsychiatr. Genet.* **2008**, *147B*, 996–999. [CrossRef]
93. Lamberti, P.; Zoccolella, S.; Iliceto, G.; Armenise, E.; Fraddosio, A.; de Mari, M.; Livrea, P. Effects of levodopa and COMT inhibitors on plasma homocysteine in Parkinson's disease patients. *Mov. Disord.* **2005**, *20*, 69–72. [CrossRef]
94. Huertas, I.; Jesús, S.; García-Gómez, F.J.; Lojo, J.A.; Bernal-Bernal, I.; Bonilla-Toribio, M.; Martín-Rodriguez, J.F.; García-Solís, D.; Gómez-Garre, P.; Mir, P. Genetic factors influencing frontostriatal dysfunction and the development of dementia in Parkinson's disease. *PLoS ONE* **2017**, *12*, e0175560. [CrossRef]
95. Bäckström, D.; Eriksson Domellöf, M.; Granåsen, G.; Linder, J.; Mayans, S.; Elgh, E.; Zetterberg, H.; Blennow, K.; Forsgren, L. Polymorphisms in dopamine-associated genes and cognitive decline in Parkinson's disease. *Acta Neurol. Scand.* **2018**, *137*, 91–98. [CrossRef]
96. Williams-Gray, C.H.; Evans, J.R.; Goris, A.; Foltynie, T.; Ban, M.; Robbins, T.W.; Brayne, C.; Kolachana, B.S.; Weinberger, D.R.; Sawcer, S.J.; et al. The distinct cognitive syndromes of Parkinson's disease: 5 year follow-up of the CamPaIGN cohort. *Brain* **2009**, *132*, 2958–2969. [CrossRef]
97. Białecka, M.; Kurzawski, M.; Roszmann, A.; Robowski, P.; Sitek, E.J.; Honczarenko, K.; Gorzkowska, A.; Budrewicz, S.; Mak, M.; Jarosz, M.; et al. Association of COMT, MTHFR, and SLC19A1(RFC-1) polymorphisms with homocysteine blood levels and cognitive impairment in Parkinson's disease. *Pharmacogenet. Genom.* **2012**, *22*, 716–724. [CrossRef]
98. Mata, I.F.; Leverenz, J.B.; Weintraub, D.; Trojanowski, J.Q.; Hurtig, H.I.; Van Deerlin, V.M.; Ritz, B.; Rausch, R.; Rhodes, S.L.; Factor, S.A.; et al. APOE, MAPT, and SNCA genes and cognitive performance in Parkinson disease. *JAMA Neurol.* **2014**, *71*, 1405–1412. [CrossRef]
99. Zlokovic, B.V. Cerebrovascular effects of apolipoprotein E: Implications for Alzheimer disease. *JAMA Neurol.* **2013**, *70*, 440–444. [CrossRef] [PubMed]
100. Huang, X.; Chen, P.C.; Poole, C. APOE-[epsilon]2 allele associated with higher prevalence of sporadic Parkinson disease. *Neurology* **2004**, *62*, 2198–2202. [CrossRef] [PubMed]
101. Williams-Gray, C.H.; Goris, A.; Saiki, M.; Foltynie, T.; Compston, D.A.; Sawcer, S.J.; Barker, R.A. Apolipoprotein E genotype as a risk factor for susceptibility to and dementia in Parkinson's disease. *J. Neurol.* **2009**, *256*, 493–498. [CrossRef] [PubMed]
102. Li, Y.J.; Hauser, M.A.; Scott, W.K.; Martin, E.R.; Booze, M.W.; Qin, X.J.; Walter, J.W.; Nance, M.A.; Hubble, J.P.; Koller, W.C.; et al. Apolipoprotein E controls the risk and age at onset of Parkinson disease. *Neurology* **2004**, *62*, 2005–2009. [CrossRef]
103. Pankratz, N.; Byder, L.; Halter, C.; Rudolph, A.; Shults, C.W.; Conneally, P.M.; Foroud, T.; Nichols, W.C. Presence of an APOE4 allele results in significantly earlier onset of Parkinson's disease and a higher risk with dementia. *Mov. Disord.* **2006**, *21*, 45–49. [CrossRef]
104. Alata, W.; Ye, Y.; St-Amour, I.; Vandal, M.; Calon, F. Human apolipoprotein E ε4 expression impairs cerebral vascularization and blood-brain barrier function in mice. *J. Cereb. Blood Flow Metab.* **2015**, *35*, 86–94. [CrossRef] [PubMed]
105. Bell, R.D.; Winkler, E.A.; Singh, I.; Sagare, A.P.; Deane, R.; Wu, Z.; Holtzman, D.M.; Betsholtz, C.; Armulik, A.; Sallstrom, J.; et al. Apolipoprotein E controls cerebrovascular integrity via cyclophilin A. *Nature* **2012**, *485*, 512–516. [CrossRef] [PubMed]
106. Pierzchlińska, A.; Białecka, M.; Kurzawski, M.; Sławek, J. The impact of Apolipoprotein E alleles on cognitive performance in patients with Parkinson's disease. *Neurol. Neurochir. Pol.* **2018**, *52*, 477–482. [CrossRef]
107. Pang, S.; Li, J.; Zhang, Y.; Chen, J. Meta-Analysis of the Relationship between the APOE Gene and the Onset of Parkinson's Disease Dementia. *Parkinsons Dis.* **2018**, *2018*, 9497147. [CrossRef] [PubMed]

108. Koukourakis, M.I.; Papazoglou, D.; Giatromanolaki, A.; Bougioukas, G.; Maltezos, E.; Sivridis, E. VEGF gene sequence variation defines VEGF gene expression status and angiogenic activity in non-small cell lung cancer. *Lung Cancer* **2004**, *46*, 293–298. [CrossRef]
109. Renner, W.; Kotschan, S.; Hoffmann, C.; Obermayer-Pietsch, B.; Pilger, E. A common 936 C/T mutation in the gene for vascular endothelial growth factor is associated with vascular endothelial growth factor plasma levels. *J. Vasc. Res.* **2000**, *37*, 443–448. [CrossRef] [PubMed]
110. Mihci, E.; Ozkaynak, S.S.; Sallakci, N.; Kizilay, F.; Yavuzer, U. VEGF polymorphisms and serum VEGF levels in Parkinson's disease. *Neurosci. Lett.* **2011**, *494*, 1–5. [CrossRef]
111. Del Bo, R.; Scarlato, M.; Ghezzi, S.; Martinelli Boneschi, F.; Fenoglio, C.; Galbiati, S.; Virgilio, R.; Galimberti, D.; Galimberti, G.; Crimi, M.; et al. Vascular endothelial growth factor gene variability is associated with increased risk for AD. *Ann. Neurol.* **2005**, *57*, 373–380. [CrossRef] [PubMed]
112. Alvarez, X.A.; Alvarez, I.; Aleixandre, M.; Linares, C.; Muresanu, D.; Winter, S.; Moessler, H. Severity-Related Increase and Cognitive Correlates of Serum VEGF Levels in Alzheimer's Disease ApoE4 Carriers. *J. Alzheimers Dis.* **2018**, *63*, 1003–1013. [CrossRef]
113. Takeuchi, H.; Tomita, H.; Taki, Y.; Kikuchi, Y.; Ono, C.; Yu, Z.; Sekiguchi, A.; Nouchi, R.; Kotozaki, Y.; Nakagawa, S.; et al. The VEGF gene polymorphism impacts brain volume and arterial blood volume. *Hum. Brain Mapp.* **2017**, *38*, 3516–3526. [CrossRef]
114. Donzuso, G.; Monastero, R.; Cicero, C.E.; Luca, A.; Mostile, G.; Giuliano, L.; Baschi, R.; Caccamo, M.; Gagliardo, C.; Palmucci, S.; et al. Neuroanatomical changes in early Parkinson's disease with mild cognitive impairment: A VBM study; the Parkinson's Disease Cognitive Impairment Study (PaCoS). *Neurol. Sci.* **2021**. [CrossRef] [PubMed]
115. Wu, Y.; Zhang, Y.; Han, X.; Li, X.; Xue, L.; Xie, A. Association of VEGF gene polymorphisms with sporadic Parkinson's disease in Chinese Han population. *Neurol. Sci.* **2016**, *37*, 1923–1929. [CrossRef]
116. Moore, A.M.; Mahoney, E.; Dumitrescu, L.; De Jager, P.L.; Koran, M.; Petyuk, V.A.; Robinson, R.A.; Ruderfer, D.M.; Cox, N.J.; Schneider, J.A.; et al. APOE ε4-specific associations of VEGF gene family expression with cognitive aging and Alzheimer's disease. *Neurobiol. Aging* **2020**, *87*, 18–25. [CrossRef] [PubMed]
117. Perez-Lloret, S.; Otero-Losada, M.; Toblli, J.E.; Capani, F. Renin-angiotensin system as a potential target for new therapeutic approaches in Parkinson's disease. *Expert Opin. Investig. Drugs* **2017**, *26*, 1163–1173. [CrossRef]
118. Rigat, B.; Hubert, C.; Corvol, P.; Soubrier, R. PCR detection of the insertion/deletion polymorphism of the human angiotensin converting enzyme gene (DCP1) (dipeptidyl carboxypeptidase 1). *Nucleic Acids Res.* **1992**, *20*, 1433. [CrossRef] [PubMed]
119. Bonnardeaux, A.; Davies, E.; Jeunemaitre, X.; Féry, I.; Charru, A.; Clauser, E.; Tiret, L.; Cambien, F.; Corvol, P.; Soubrier, F. Angiotensin II type 1 receptor gene polymorphisms in human essential hypertension. *Hypertension* **1994**, *24*, 63–69. [CrossRef]
120. Schmieder, R.E.; Erdmann, J.; Delles, C.; Jacobi, J.; Fleck, E.; Hilgers, K.; Regitz-Zagrosek, V. Effect of the angiotensin II type 2-receptor gene (+1675 G/A) on left ventricular structure in humans. *J. Am. Coll. Cardiol.* **2001**, *37*, 175–182. [CrossRef]
121. Caulfield, M.; Lavender, P.; Farrall, M.; Munroe, P.; Lawson, M.; Turner, P.; Clark, A.J. Linkage of the angiotensinogen gene to essential hypertension. *N. Engl. J. Med.* **1994**, *330*, 1629–1633. [CrossRef]
122. Mellick, G.D.; Buchanan, D.D.; McCann, S.J.; Davis, D.R.; Le Couteur, D.G.; Chan, D.; Johnson, A.G. The ACE deletion polymorphism is not associated with Parkinson's disease. *Eur. Neurol.* **1999**, *41*, 103–106. [CrossRef]
123. Pascale, E.; Purcaro, C.; Passarelli, E.; Guglielmi, R.; Vestri, A.R.; Passarelli, F.; Meco, G. Genetic polymorphism of Angiotensin-Converting Enzyme is not associated with the development of Parkinson's disease and of L-dopa-induced adverse effects. *J. Neurol. Sci.* **2009**, *276*, 18–21. [CrossRef]
124. Lin, J.J.; Yueh, K.C.; Chang, D.C.; Lin, S.Z. Association between genetic polymorphism of angiotensin-converting enzyme gene and Parkinson's disease. *J. Neurol. Sci.* **2002**, *199*, 25–29. [CrossRef]
125. Gustafson, D.R.; Melchior, L.; Eriksson, E.; Sundh, V.; Blennow, K.; Skoog, I. The ACE Insertion Deletion polymorphism relates to dementia by metabolic phenotype, APOEepsilon4, and age of dementia onset. *Neurobiol. Aging* **2010**, *31*, 910–916. [CrossRef]
126. Zettergren, A.; Kern, S.; Gustafson, D.; Gudmundsson, P.; Sigström, R.; Östling, S.; Eriksson, E.; Zetterberg, H.; Blennow, K.; Skoog, I. The ACE Gene Is Associated with Late-Life Major Depression and Age at Dementia Onset in a Population-Based Cohort. *Am. J. Geriatr. Psychiatry* **2017**, *25*, 170–177. [CrossRef] [PubMed]
127. Zannas, A.S.; McQuoid, D.R.; Payne, M.E.; MacFall, J.R.; Ashley-Koch, A.; Steffens, D.C.; Potter, G.G.; Taylor, W.D. Association of gene variants of the renin-angiotensin system with accelerated hippocampal volume loss and cognitive decline in old age. *Am. J. Psychiatry* **2014**, *171*, 1214–1221. [CrossRef] [PubMed]
128. Purandare, N.; Oude Voshaar, R.C.; Davidson, Y.; Gibbons, L.; Hardicre, J.; Byrne, J.; McCollum, C.; Jackson, A.; Burns, A.; Mann, D.M. Deletion/insertion polymorphism of the angiotensin-converting enzyme gene and white matter hyperintensities in dementia: A pilot study. *J. Am. Geriatr. Soc.* **2006**, *54*, 1395–1400. [CrossRef] [PubMed]
129. Wang, B.; Jin, F.; Yang, Z.; Lu, Z.; Kan, R.; Li, S.; Zheng, C.; Wang, L. The insertion polymorphism in angiotensin-converting enzyme gene associated with the APOE epsilon 4 allele increases the risk of late-onset Alzheimer disease. *J. Mol. Neurosci.* **2006**, *30*, 267–271. [CrossRef]
130. Assareh, A.A.; Mather, K.A.; Crawford, J.D.; Wen, W.; Anstey, K.J.; Easteal, S.; Tan, X.; Mack, H.A.; Kwok, J.B.; Schofield, P.R.; et al. Renin-angiotensin system genetic polymorphisms and brain white matter lesions in older Australians. *Am. J. Hypertens.* **2014**, *27*, 1191–1198. [CrossRef] [PubMed]

131. Rigat, B.; Hubert, C.; Alhenc-Gelas, F.; Cambien, F.; Corvol, P.; Soubrier, F. An insertion/deletion polymorphism in the angiotensin I-converting enzyme gene accounting for half the variance of serum enzyme levels. *J. Clin. Investig.* **1990**, *86*, 1343–1346. [CrossRef]
132. Rai, V. Methylenetetrahydrofolate Reductase (MTHFR) C677T Polymorphism and Alzheimer Disease Risk: A Meta-Analysis. *Mol. Neurobiol.* **2017**, *54*, 1173–1186. [CrossRef] [PubMed]
133. Wright, S.M.; Jensen, S.L.; Cockriel, K.L.; Davis, B.; Tschanz, J.T.; Munger, R.G.; Corcoran, C.D.; Kauwe, J. Association study of rs3846662 with Alzheimer's disease in a population-based cohort: The Cache County Study. *Neurobiol. Aging* **2019**, *84*, 242.e1–242.e6. [CrossRef] [PubMed]

MDPI
St. Alban-Anlage 66
4052 Basel
Switzerland
Tel. +41 61 683 77 34
Fax +41 61 302 89 18
www.mdpi.com

Molecules Editorial Office
E-mail: molecules@mdpi.com
www.mdpi.com/journal/molecules

MDPI

www.ingramcontent.com/pod-product-compliance
Lightning Source LLC
LaVergne TN
LVHW070708100526
838202LV00013B/1050
* 9 7 8 3 0 3 6 5 4 2 7 7 5 *